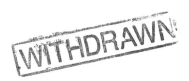
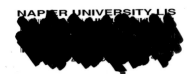

Management of Cleft Lip and Palate

Management of Cleft Lip and Palate

Edited by

A.C.H. WATSON
Honorary Consultant Plastic Surgeon,
Royal Hospital for Sick Children, Ediburgh

D.A. SELL
Head of Speech and Language Therapy Department,
Great Ormond Street Hospital, London, Visiting Professor, Division of
Psychology and Speech and Language Therapy, De Montfort University,
Leicester and Honorary Senior Lecturer, Institute of Child Health,
University College, London

AND

P. GRUNWELL
Professor of Clinical Linguistics, De Montfort University, Leicester

W

WHURR PUBLISHERS

LONDON AND PHILADELPHIA

© 2001 Whurr Publishers
First published 2001 by
Whurr Publishers Ltd
19b Compton Terrace, London N1 2UN, England and
325 Chestnut Street, Philadelphia PA 19106, USA

British Library Cataloguing in Publication Data
A catalogue record for this book is available from the
British Library.

ISBN: 1 86156 158 X

Printed and bound in the UK by Athenaeum Press Ltd,
Gateshead, Tyne & Wear

Contents

Contributors

Patricia Bannister, RN, SCM, HV, AdDipN, MSc Adv Dip Counselling
Department of Orthodontics, Turner Dental Hospital, Manchester

Eileen Bradbury, PhD
Health Psychologist, Turner Dental School, Manchester

Lynn S. Chitty, PhD, MRCOG
Senior Lecturer and Consultant in Genetics and Fetal Medicine, Department of Clinical Genetics, Institute of Child Health, London

Gareth Davies
Chief Executive, Cleft Lip and Palate Association

David R. Griffin, FRCOG
Consultant Obstetrician and Gynaecologist, Watford General Hospital, Watford

Brigitte Griffiths, FDS, BDS, PhD
Consultant Prosthodontist, Eastman Dental Hospital and Honorary Consultant in Restorative Dentistry, Great Ormond Street Hospital, London

Pamela Grunwell, PhD, MA, BA(Hon), HonFCSLT, FRSA
Professor of Clinical Linguistics and formerly Head of Department of Human Communication, De Montfort University, Leicester

Alex Habel, MB, ChB, FRCP
Consultant Paediatrician, Great Ormond Street Hospital, London

Anne Harding, PhD, MRCSLT
Senior Specialist Speech and Language Therapist, Addenbrookes Hospital, Cambridge and North Herts NHS Trust, Stevenage; Senior Research Fellow, Department of Human Communication, De Montfort University, Leicester

Ian S. Hathorn, BDS, FDSRCS, DOrth
Consultant Orthodontist, Bristol Dental Hospital, Bristol

Melissa Lees, MBBS, DCH, MRCP, MSc, MD, FRACP
Specialist Registrar in Clinical Genetics, Great Ormond Street Hospital NHS Trust.

Glenn E. Lello, BDS, FDSRCS, FRCS, MBChB, PhD
Consultant Maxillofacial Surgeon, St John's Hospital, Livingston, West Lothian

Penny Lennox, BM BCL, BA, FRCS
Specialist Registrar in ENT, Royal National Throat, Nose and Ear Hospital, London

Micheal Mars, BDS, FDS, DOrth, PhD
Consultant Orthodontist, Great Ormond Street Hospital, London

Vanessa Martin, BA Hons, RGN, RSCN, DPSN
Clinical Nurse Specialist, Nottingham City Hospital, Nottingham

Nigel S.G. Mercer, MB ChB, ChM, FRCS
Consultant Plastic Surgeon, Frenchay Healthcare Trust, Bristol

Ron W. Pigott, MB, FRCSI
Honorary Consultant Plastic Surgeon, South Western Regional Health Authority

Jane Russell, PhD, FRCSLT
Senior Specialist Speech and Language Therapist, Birmingham Children's Hospital NHS Trust

Debbie A. Sell, PhD, FRCSLT
Head of Speech and Language Therapy Department, Great Ormond Street Hospital, London; Honorary Senior Lecturer, Institute of Child Health, University of London; Visiting Professor, Department of Human Communication, De Montfort University, Leicester

Gunvor Semb, DDS, PhD
    Senior Lecturer in Craniofacial Anomalies, Turner Dental School, Manchester

William C. Shaw, PhD, MScD, BDS, FSD, DOrth, RCSEng
    Professor of Orthodontics and Dentofacial Development, Turner Dental School, Manchester

Brian C. Sommerlad, MB, BS, FRCS
    Consultant Plastic Surgeon, Broomfield Hospital, Essex and Great Ormond Street Hospital, London

Antony C.H. Watson, MB, ChB, FRCSEd
    Honorary Consultant Plastic Surgeon, Royal Hospital for Sick Children, Edinburgh

Preface

This book is a successor to *Advances in the Management of Cleft Palate*, edited by Margaret Edwards and Tony Watson and published in 1980, but it is different enough for its new publishers and editors to feel that its name should be changed. The previous book itself succeeded Muriel Morley's classic *Cleft Palate and Speech*, which had run to seven editions. In the late 1970s it was recognized that it was no longer possible for a single author to review the advances in management of such a complex deformity and this is just as true today.

The aim of the present book is the same as before: to provide an up-to-date review of all aspects of the management of clefts. We have dropped 'Advances' from the title because we include much more core information alongside recent research. We have increased the number of chapters from 19 to 25 and our contributors represent a wider range of professions associated with the care of cleft lip and palate. There are new chapters on genetics by Melissa Lees, on antenatal sonographic diagnosis by Lynn Chitty and David Griffin, and on psychological aspects by Eileen Bradbury. The role of the paediatrician is covered by Alex Habel and that of the parent support group by Gareth Davies, Chairman of the Cleft Lip and Palate Association in the UK. Indeed this book provides largely a British perspective on this condition.

Although there have been significant advances in the last 20 years in several aspects of the management of clefts, overall improvement in the scientific basis for treatment has been disappointing. There is a great variety of management protocols and there has been a striking lack of randomized controlled trials comparing their effectiveness. William Shaw and Gunvor Semb address this issue in the final chapter of the book.

The way in which patients with cleft lip and palate are managed in the UK is about to change dramatically following the government's acceptance of the CSAG report published in 1998. Care, which has been fragmented, will be concentrated in fewer centres, ensuring greater experience for each team, opportunities for better record keeping, audit and involvement in clinical trials and, one hopes for the patient, better outcomes. Several of this book's contributors were involved in the preparation of the report and its ethos is reflected in the text.

In the last 20 years there has been an increasing emphasis on the importance of the multidisciplinary team in the care of clefts and we have reflected this in the range of contributors. We hope that we have provided a valuable introduction to the condition for members of all specialties involved in the care of young people with these deformities and that individual members of the cleft team will gain a greater insight into the work of their colleagues. The book is not designed to give detailed descriptions of operative and other techniques but the references will lead the interested reader to this information.

It remains for us to thank all our contributors and our patient publishers. Furthermore, this book would not have been written without the enormous amount of help given by Anne Watson, Terry Willetts and Andrew, Jack and Freddie Pegram, who struggled uncomplainingly with manuscripts, faxes, e-mails, references and editorial whims. We would also like to record our gratitude to David Cowan and Barbara Cadge for their invaluable advice. We are grateful to our families and colleagues who allowed us time and put up with our absences. We give them all our heartfelt thanks.

Tony Watson
Debbie Sell
Pam Grunwell

PART I
THE NATURE OF CLEFT LIP AND PALATE

CHAPTER 1

Embryology, Aetiology and Incidence

A.C.H. WATSON

Introduction

A knowledge of the main steps in the normal development of the face is an essential aid to understanding the abnormalities that make up the deformities of cleft lip and palate. Rational treatment is based on this knowledge and research into the causes of these malformations gives hope for their prevention.

The changes in appearance of the embryo face have been established for over a century (His, 1874), but it is only in the last 25 years that investigations have shown how many of these changes come about and how normal development may fail (Ferguson, 1991, 1993).

Initial development of the head and face

It is between the fifth and ninth weeks of pregnancy that the most important alterations are taking place in the developing face. At the end of the fourth week the embryo, which is only about 3.5 mm long, has nothing resembling a face, while by the end of the eighth week it is 30 mm long and the face is fully formed (Figure 1.1). The palate is not be completed for another two weeks.

The cells that are to form the face can be identified at a much earlier stage. During the third week of embryonic life the *neural plate* appears at the head end of the embryo; this develops a midline groove with *neural folds* on each side which subsequently fuse to form a tube. *Neural crest cells* form from the *ectoderm* or outer layer of cells of the neural folds, migrate into the underlying tissue as *mesenchyme* and continue their migration into the developing structure of the head and neck, where they give rise to the neural, skeletal and connective tissues, including the dermis and

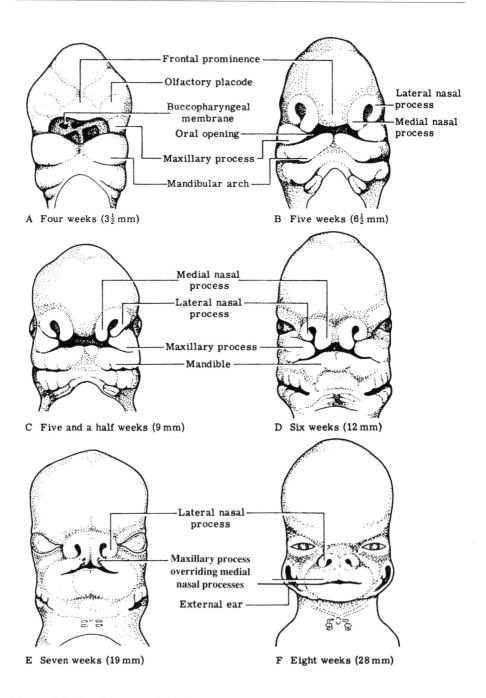

Figure 1.1. Development of the face. (Modified after Patten: *Human Embryology,* 3rd edition, by permission of McGraw-Hill Book Company.)

melanocytes. In particular, they provide the mesenchyme for the frontonasal, mandibular and maxillary processes (Figure 1.2). Although they do not produce the muscle cells or *myoblasts*, which are derived from *cranial mesoderm*, they do form the connective tissue support of the muscles which determines their form. Therefore, abnormalities of the facial muscles are usually due to interference with the migration or differentiation of neural crest cells. Ectoderm originating from the neural ridge (which overlies the neural folds) gives rise to the epithelium of the facial skin, nasal cavities and palate.

By the end of the third week the foregut of the embryo, which is lined by *entoderm*, ends blindly and is separated from a surface depression called the *stomatodeum* (lined by ectoderm) by the *buccopharyngeal membrane* (Figure 1.3). The breakdown of this membrane during the fourth week allows the two to communicate. Subsequent forward development of the tissues around the stomatodeum, due to the inflow of neural crest mesenchyme, results in the site of the buccopharyngeal membrane (i.e. the junction between ectoderm and entoderm) eventually lying in the region of the tonsils.

At four weeks a *frontal prominence* is present in the midline, forming the upper or cephalic boundary of the stomatodeum. On each side of this is a flattened area known as the *nasal* or *olfactory placode*, arising from ectoderm, which will eventually form the organs of smell high in the roof of

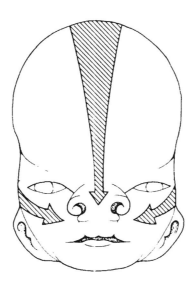

Figure 1.2. The migration of mesenchyme into the face. (After Stark in Converse (ed.) *Reconstructive Plastic Surgery* 2nd edition, 1977, by permission of WB Saunders Co.)

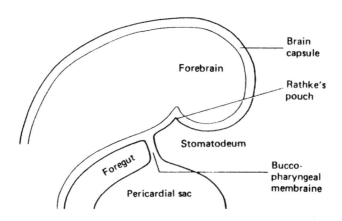

Figure 1.3. Diagrammatic representation of a sagittal section of the cranial end of a 3.5 week human embryo. (From Ferguson in Shaw, *Orthodontics and Occlusal Management,* 1993, by permission of Butterworth Heinemann.)

the nose (Figure 1.1A). During the fifth and sixth weeks the epithelium of the placode invaginates and horseshoe-shaped elevations develop around them, growing rapidly so that the placodes become recessed at the bottom of *nasal* or *olfactory pits*. The medial and lateral halves of these elevations are known respectively as *medial* and *lateral nasal processes* (Figure 1.1B, C, D). The area between the two nasal pits, including both medial nasal processes, is called the *frontonasal process*.

The medial nasal processes grow more rapidly than the lateral, and approach one another in the midline. Meanwhile the lower or caudal margin of the stomatodeum develops paired thickenings, the *mandibular arches*, which are the first of the *branchial arches*. They enlarge and coalesce in the midline. From the upper margin of the mandibular arches arise the *maxillary processes* which grow forwards towards the midline from the superolateral margins of the developing oral cavity, below the lateral nasal processes. Above them, the nasal pits continue to invaginate until they reach the roof of the oronasal cavity, where the two layers of epithelium form the *bucconasal membrane*. This ruptures and the resulting openings between nasal and oral cavities are called the *primary choanae*. Failure of breakdown leads to *choanal atresia*, where the nasal cavities end blindly.

The medial and lateral nasal processes and the maxillary process are all in continuity at their bases, but as they grow and project outwards slits develop between them. Eventually, as the mesenchyme continues to flow into the processes, their bases merge. More superficially, their tips come into contact across the slits, the epithelial cells separating them die and the processes fuse. Anything which interferes with the fusion of these processes may cause a cleft lip, the configuration and severity of which will depend on the nature and timing of the insult.

Further development of the lip and primary palate

The maxillary processes from each side continue to grow towards each other until they meet and fuse in front of the medial nasal processes. They will form the definitive upper lip. The frontonasal process does not contribute to the normal lip, but develops into the *primary palate*. This is the anterior part of the palate, the *premaxilla*, which lies in front of the incisive foramen and which includes the alveolus between the canine teeth on each side (Figure 1.4). The frontonasal process also forms the *primary nasal septum*, which is that part of the septum attached to the primary palate and lying between the invaginating nasal pits.

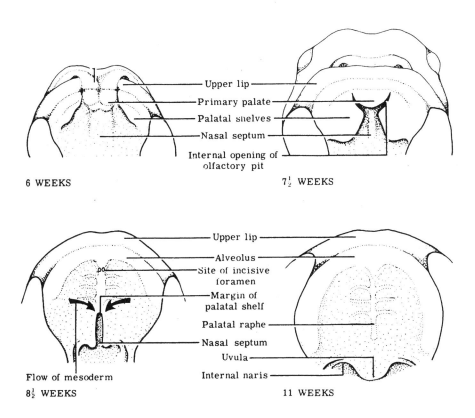

Figure 1.4. Development of the palate. (Adapted from Patten, *Human Embryology* 3rd edition, 1968, by permission of McGraw-Hill Book Company.)

If mesenchymal migration is inadequate or delayed the degree of clefting will depend on the extent of the deficiency. The mildest cleft will occur at the last place at which mesenchyme arrives – the vermilion – and if there is no mesodermal penetration at all, or if its arrival is greatly delayed, the cleft will involve lip, alveolus and palate as far back as the incisive foramen. In a bilateral cleft lip there is an abnormal element of lip tissue attached to the front of the premaxilla called the *prolabium*, which is derived from the frontonasal process and contains no muscle. The *philtrum* and *cupid's bow* of the normal lip develop much later and are caused by the pull of muscle fibres attached to the skin.

Development of the nose

After the breakdown of the bucconasal membrane the two anterior nares lie on each side of the primary nasal septum and communicate with the buccal cavity. Below and in front of them is the primary palate. Mesenchyme from the inner aspect of each maxillary process, the *tecto-septal process*, migrates upwards across the roof of the developing nasal cavity and meets its fellow from the opposite side, except in the region of the olfactory epithelium. The joined processes then grow downwards, merging with the posterior margins of the primary nasal septum to form the *secondary nasal septum*.

As the two medial nasal processes move closer together they merge and the furrow between them becomes filled in. From parts of this mass of mesoderm above the developing lip arise the columella (between the nostrils) and the nasal bridge. The lateral nasal processes give rise to the alae of the nose.

Development of the secondary palate

By the beginning of the seventh week the primitive lip and primary palate are formed and behind them there is a common cavity for nose and mouth. However, from the inner aspect of the maxillary process on each side, below the tecto-septal processes, are developing a pair of *palatal shelves* which are destined to fuse in the midline to complete the palate. Because this part of the palate forms after the anterior part it is known as the *secondary palate* (Figure 1.4).

At first the palatal shelves hang vertically down on each side of the developing tongue, but as the neck begins to extend during the eighth to ninth week the tongue moves downwards and the palatal shelves rapidly spring upwards above it to the horizontal position where they can grow towards each other (Figure 1.5). Recent research (Ferguson, 1988) has shown that shelf elevation is due to an intrinsic tension within the shelves that builds up until it can overcome the resistance of the tongue. This tension is partly generated by the production of hyaluronic acid in the extra-cellular matrix to a varying degree in different parts of the palate. The hyaluronic acid binds water and expands, causing a directional force. In addition, the mesenchymal cells themselves are contractile and contribute to the elevation. A third contributor to shelf elevation may be the commence-ment of head and jaw movements at about the same time; opening of the mouth will allow the tongue to descend and create room for the shelves above it.

At the correct time of shelf elevation the head is not growing in width, so that the growing horizontal shelves can meet easily. However, if shelf eleva-tion is delayed, it will occur at a time of rapid growth in the width of the

7 WEEKS

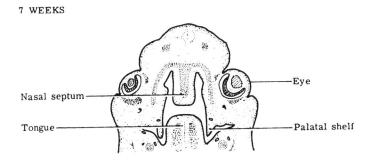

8½ WEEKS

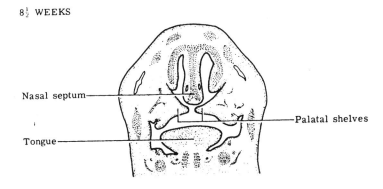

Figure 1.5. Downward movement of the tongue and elevation of palatal shelves during eighth to ninth week. (Adapted from Patten, *Human Embryology* 3rd edition, 1968, by permission of McGraw-Hill Book Company.)

head and the shelves may be unable to meet. As palatal elevation takes place in female embryos about seven days later than in males, this may explain the greater incidence of isolated cleft palate in females.

Once the palatal shelves have elevated, they normally make contact with each other and with the primary palate anteriorly and the free margins fuse together. The incisive foramen comes to lie at the junction of the primary and secondary palate in the midline. Fusion proceeds from front to back and, at the same time, the secondary nasal septum is growing downwards to fuse with the palatal shelves in the midline, completing the separation of the two nasal cavities.

The mechanism of fusion has been studied in some detail. Once the shelves have made contact their epithelia fuse to make an epithelial seam which then disrupts, partly by cell death and partly by migration of the cells, into the oral and nasal epithelium. Epithelial nests can sometimes be found at the sites of fusion, even in adult life. The disruption of the seam, and the subsequent differentiation of the epithelium, into squamous on the oral side and ciliated columnar on the nasal side, appears to be specified by the underlying mesenchymal cells. The mechanism is complex but involves changes in the extracellular matrix molecules and growth factors such as TGFα, TGFß and fibroblast growth factor. Specific epithelio-mesenchymal interactions lead to the development of bone in the hard palate and muscles in the soft palate, which form a sling across the midline. The mesoderm that forms these muscles has been shown to migrate from the pharyngeal walls and the palatal and pharyngeal muscles therefore have very close embryological links.

Innervation of the face

The sensory nerve supplying the face is the trigeminal nerve, which has three divisions. The ophthalmic division supplies tissue derived from the frontonasal process, and the maxillary and mandibular divisions supply the processes of the same name. The nerves follow the extensions of these processes, which explains the rather complicated sensory innervation of the nasal septum and palate. In a similar way, the motor innervation of the muscles of the soft palate and pharyngeal walls reflect their embryonic origins.

The causes of cleft lip and palate

Clefts of the lip and palate may be isolated deformities or may be part of a syndrome (see Lees, Chapter 6). Non-syndromic clefts are said to be *multifactorial* in origin; there may be a genetic predisposition with several genes being involved, and various environmental factors, acting at the relevant time of embryonic development, may contribute to cause a cleft, particularly in genetically predisposed patients. These include alcohol (Munger et al., 1996), maternal illness and smoking (Werler et al., 1990); several drugs have been implicated in animal studies but only phenytoin has been proved to be a cause in humans (see below). Folic acid may have a protective effect (MRC Vitamin Study, 1991).

Clefts of the lip, with or without cleft palate, form a different group from isolated clefts of the secondary palate, with a different incidence, genetic basis and sex distribution. However, the pathogenesis of all clefts is due to some form of interference with the normal development of the face and oral cavity, which can be classified in the following way.

Cleft lip, with or without cleft palate

Clefts are due to a failure of fusion of the medial nasal, lateral nasal and maxillary processes on one or both sides. Partial fusion will give rise to an incomplete cleft. A cleft of the secondary palate associated with a cleft of the lip and primary palate is thought to be due to the tongue tip being trapped in the cleft through the primary palate so that its descent and the associated elevation of the palatal shelves are significantly delayed. Failure of fusion may be caused by:

1. Hypoplasia of the facial processes: due either to a failure of migration of neural crest mesenchyme or interference with cellular proliferation within them. The lateral nasal processes are particularly susceptible as they have a growth spurt just before fusion is due to take place. The anti-epileptic drug phenytoin has been shown to cause cleft lip by interfering with this growth spurt (Strickler et al., 1985).
2. Variations in facial geometry. Increased facial width and variations in the orientation of the facial processes have been shown to cause clefts in mice and may be the reason for racial differences in the incidence of clefts.
3. Inability of the epithelium to take part in the process of fusion.
4. Excessive cell death in the mesenchymal seams coupled with mesenchymal deficiency may cause fused processes to rupture. If this is incomplete, a Simonart's band may result.

Isolated clefts of the secondary palate

These are due to a failure of the palatal shelves to fuse. Failure may be due to:
1. Hypoplasia of the palatal shelves caused either by a failure of mesenchymal migration or interference with cellular proliferation.

2. Failure of shelf elevation at the proper time, which may be due to defects in the complex intrinsic mechanism for shelf elevation or to external factors, in particular obstruction by the tongue. The tongue may be too big – macroglossia such as in Down's syndrome – or it may fail to descend. This can happen if the head cannot extend, due either to faulty growth of the cranial base or to constriction by a lack of amniotic fluid. Hypoplasia of the mandible, which may be caused by constriction or may be intrinsic, will also inhibit descent of the tongue. A combination of cleft palate with a small, retrodisplaced mandible is often associated with neonatal respiratory distress, and this is called the *Pierre Robin sequence* (see Lees, Chapter 6 and Habel, Chapter 9).

3. Excessive head width. Racial differences in the incidence of cleft palate correlate with head width. It is rare in blacks, more common in Caucasians and yet more frequent in Mongoloids. The greater frequency in females is probably related to the fact that palatal elevation occurs seven days later than in males, so that any delay in shelf elevation will leave the shelves with a gap that may be too wide to bridge.

4. Failure of fusion of the palatal shelves may occur even if their free margins meet. This may be due to interference with the mesenchymal–epithelial signalling mechanism, adhesiveness or migration of the epithelial cells, failure of differential gene expression or mechanical disruption.

5. Post-fusion rupture can result from excessive cell death in the epithelial seam, poor adhesion, attenuation of mesenchyme or excessive traction due to growth or movement.

The severity of a cleft depends on the severity of the insult to normal development. Minor interference will lead to an incomplete cleft, the mildest of all being the so-called *forme fruste* of the lip and the *submucous cleft* of the palate. All degrees of severity are possible between these and complete clefts and, because of the variety of causes, there can be wide variations in the amount of tissue deficiency and the configuration of the cleft, even in those that are superficially similar.

Distortions due to disturbed intrauterine growth

Although the cleft deformity is established in the first trimester of pregnancy, by the time the baby is born a number of other distortions have been superimposed on the primary deformity. Latham (1969, 1973) made detailed studies of the nature of the skeletal deformities, which are partly due to the disturbance of the normal attachments between structures that are actively growing. For example, the nasal septum appears to be a very important growth centre in embryonic and early fetal life. It is attached to the premaxilla by a well-defined ligament and its forward growth draws the premaxilla forward. Normally the forward movement of the premaxilla is restrained by its attachment to the maxillary processes, but when there is a cleft between the premaxilla and maxillary processes this constraint is lost. As a result, the premaxilla in a bilateral cleft lies too far forward, suspended from the tip of the septum, and the maxillary segments, deprived of the forward pull of the premaxilla, lie too far back. In the unilateral cleft the attachments on the non-cleft side restrain forward growth, so that the anterior nasal septum and premaxilla deviate towards the normal side. This in turn leads to the septum bulging into the cleft side of the nose more posteriorly. The maxillary process on the cleft side, lacking support from the premaxilla, may collapse in behind it.

Soft tissues can also play a part in producing secondary deformities *in utero*. The interruption of the normal rings of muscle in the cleft lip and soft palate can allow the two halves of a completely cleft maxilla to drift apart. The action of the tongue pushing up between the cleft palatal shelves can contribute to this deformity, and in addition may push the shelves into a more vertical position than normal.

An intriguing aspect of the cleft lip and palate deformity is the great variation in the extent and configuration of the deformity at birth. For all cases with a given type of cleft (e.g. a complete unilateral cleft), the intrauterine growth of normal structures around the cleft should exert the same influence on the eventual distortion, as the altered attachments and constraints are the same in all cases. The influence of disturbed muscular action may vary to some extent, but the most important factor is the difference between clefts established at the time they first appear. A relationship can be assumed between the extent of the primary mesodermal deficiency and the disturbance of growth potential in the tissues adjacent to the cleft. Unfortunately, at the present time the degree of this disturbance cannot be predicted and this enormously complicates studies of postnatal development. The problems are discussed in greater detail by Mars in Chapter 4.

Incidence of cleft lip and palate

Cleft lip and palate are among the most common of all congenital deformities, and the incidence appears to be slowly rising. The best data come from Denmark (Fogh-Andersen, 1943; Jensen et al., 1988), where the incidence rose from 1.45/1000 live births in 1942 to 1.89/1000 live births in 1981. This increasing incidence may in part be due to better reporting, but there is likely to be a true increase, perhaps because of an increase in environmental teratogens, lower neonatal mortality and increased marriage and childbearing among cleft patients, due to better care. Unfortunately, no other series has been published recording results over such a long period, and comparing incidences is fraught with problems due to variations in recording, whether stillbirths and abortions are included, failures in recording the type of cleft, the presence of syndromes or the sex of the patients. Nevertheless, information is available which shows that there are significant racial differences in incidence. Clefts of the lip and palate are most common in American Indians (3.7/1000 live births), then, in decreasing order of frequency, Japanese (2.7/1000), Maoris and Chinese (2.0/1000), Caucasians (1.7/1000) and blacks (0.4/1000) (cited in Vanderas, 1987).

In the Danish series, cleft lip, with or without cleft palate, CL(P), is more than twice as common in males as females, whereas isolated cleft palate, CP, is twice as common in females. The probable reason for this has been discussed. A unilateral cleft lip is twice as likely to be on the left as on the right, and the majority of these patients are left handed (Rintala, 1985). It is possible that there is a genetic link between CL(P) and asymmetric embryonic development.

In Denmark, isolated cleft palate made up 25% of the total, but in other series it varies – over 50% in Northern Ireland (Gregg et al., 1994) and the West of Scotland (Fitzpatrick et al., 1994), while in the Faroe Islands and Greenland it is 70–80% (Fogh-Andersen, 1980). In the UK, complete unilateral clefts of the lip and palate occur in about 15–20% of all clefts (Gregg et al., 1994; Bellis and Wolgemuth, 1998).

References

Bellis TH, Wolgemuth B (1999) The incidence of cleft lip and palate deformities in South East Scotland (1971–1990) British Journal of Orthodontics 26(2): 121–5.

Ferguson MJW (1988) Palatal development. Development 103: 41–60.

Ferguson MJW (1991) The orofacial region. In: Wigglesworth JS, Singer DB (eds) Textbook of Fetal and Perinatal Pathology. Oxford: Blackwell, pp. 843–880.

Ferguson MJW (1993) Craniofacial morphogensis and prenatal growth. In: Shaw WC (ed.) Orthodontics and Occlusal Management. London: Wright, pp. 1–25.

Fitzpatrick DR, Raine PAM, Boorman JG (1994) Facial clefts in the West of Scotland in the period 1980–1984: epidemiology and genetic diagnosis. Journal of Medical Genetics 31: 126–129.

Fogh-Andersen P (1943) Inheritance of Harelip and Cleft Palate. Copenhagen: Munksgaard.

Fogh-Andersen P (1980) Incidence and Aetiology. In: Edwards M, Watson ACH (eds) Advances in the Management of Cleft Palate. Edinburgh: Churchill Livingstone, pp. 43–48.

Gregg T, Boyd D, Richardson A (1994) The incidence of cleft lip and palate in Northern Ireland from 1980–1990. British Journal of Orthodontics 21: 387–392.

His W (1874) Unserer Koerperform und des Physiologische Problem inhrer Entstehung. Leipzig: Vogel.

Jensen BL, Kreiborg S, Dahl E, Fogh-Andersen P (1988) Cleft lip and palate in Denmark 1976–1981: Epidemiology, variability and early somatic development. Cleft Palate Journal 25: 258–269.

Latham RA (1969) The pathogenesis of the skeletal deformity associated with unilateral cleft lip and palate. Cleft Palate Journal 6: 404.

Latham RA (1973) Development and structure of the premaxillary deformity in bilateral cleft lip and palate. British Journal of Plastic Surgery 26: 1.

MRC Vitamin Study Research Group (1991) Prevention of neural tube defects: results of the Medical Research Council Vitamin Study. Lancet 338: 131–137.

Munger RG, Romiti PA, Daack-Hirsch S, Burns TL, Murray JC, Hanson J (1996) Maternal alcohol use in risk of orofacial cleft birth defects. Teratology 54: 27–33.

Rintala AE (1985) Relationship between side of the cleft and handedness of the patient. Cleft Palate Journal 22: 34–37.

Strickler SM, Dansky LV, Miller MA, Seni MH, Andermann E, Spielberg SP (1985) Genetic predisposition to phenytoin-induced birth defects. Lancet ii: 746–749.

Vanderas AP (1987) Incidence of cleft lip, cleft palate, and cleft lip and palate among races: a review. Cleft Palate Journal 24: 216–225.

Werler MM, Lammer EJ, Rosenberg L, Mitchell AA (1990) Maternal cigarette smoking during pregnancy in relation to oral clefts. American Journal of Epidemiology 132: 926–933.

CHAPTER 2

Classification

A.C.H. WATSON

There is an almost infinite variation in the presentation of clefts of the lip and palate, but it is necessary to classify them into groups in order to describe them, to study their causes, and to compare the results of their management. Simple classifications are valuable for everyday use; they are easy to understand and give broad groups with large numbers of patients in each of them, but they fail to distinguish between variations of severity within those groups. There has therefore been a tendency for systems of classification to be made more and more complicated in order to include every variation, with the result that they become more difficult to use as the groups they describe become smaller. For most purposes a compromise has to be reached between these two extremes.

Development of classification

Early attempts at classification of clefts (Davies and Ritchie, 1922; Veau, 1931) were simple but failed to include all types of clefts. A great step forward was made in 1942 when Fogh-Andersen published the results of his study of the incidence of cleft lip and palate in Denmark. He classified the clefts into:

(a) hare lip (including alveolus and as far back as the incisive foramen);
(b) hare lip and cleft palate;
(c) isolated clefts of the palate as far forward as the incisive foramen.

He showed that types (a) and (b) were quite distinct in their aetiology from type (c), and this classification, with its sound foundation on embryological and aetiological differences, is the basis for the variety of systems of nomenclature that are in use today.

The names introduced by Kernahan and Stark (1958) (Table 2.1) are probably those most commonly used at the present time. They called the lip, alveolar ridge and triangle of palate anterior to the incisive foramen the primary palate and the rest of the palate (derived from the palatal shelves of the embryo) the secondary palate.

Table 2.1. Kernahan and Stark's classification of clefts (1958)

Clefts of primary palate only
  Unilateral (right or left)
    Complete
    Incomplete
  Median
    Complete (premaxilla absent)
    Incomplete (premaxilla rudimentary)
  Bilateral
    Complete
    Incomplete

Clefts of secondary palate only
  Complete
  Incomplete
  Submucous

Clefts of primary and secondary palate
  Unilateral (right or left)
    Complete
    Incomplete
  Median
    Complete
    Incomplete
  Bilateral
    Complete
    Incomplete

Clefts of the primary palate may be complete or incomplete, and they may be unilateral, bilateral or median. Clefts of the secondary palate may be complete, incomplete or submucous.

Unfortunately, this simple and straightforward system has two significant disadvantages. The first is the possible confusion caused by calling the lip part of the primary palate. To call a cleft of the lip alone an incomplete cleft of the primary palate is obviously not ideal, but it is widely accepted. In an attempt to resolve this confusion, the American Cleft Palate Association (Harkins et al., 1960) recommended 'prepalate' and 'palate' for primary and secondary palates as an alternative, and the International Confederation for

Plastic and Reconstructive Surgery (1968) suggested 'anterior palate' for primary palate. This seems to have no advantage. Spina (1974) referred to pre-incisive foramen clefts, trans-incisive foramen clefts and post-incisive foramen clefts, terms that are precise but rather ponderous and have not been generally adopted.

The second disadvantage of Kernahan and Stark's classification is that, in its simplicity, it makes recording of fine detail difficult and cumbersome. For example, it has no subdivision between soft and hard palate, nor of lip and alveolus, and it does not offer an easy way of recording the degree of displacement of parts or of tissue deficiency. It was for this reason that the American Cleft Palate Association introduced their much more complex classification (Table 2.2). Berlin (1971) critically analysed the different classification systems in use at that time. He included McCabe's immensely detailed computer coding manual (McCabe, 1966), which must have been only one of many early efforts to record and store the information on computer. These systems were all daunting in their complexity.

Symbolic methods of recording clefts

In an attempt to simplify recording of data, Pfeifer (1964) proposed a symbolic method which was attractive in its simplicity (Figure 2.1a). Kernahan (1971) proposed a Striped Y classification (Figure 2.1b), and in the search for a way to identify more detail this was modified by Elsahy (1973) and again by Millard (1976) (Figure 2.1c). Millard used his modification throughout his book, and although it has lost some of the simplicity of Kernahan's original, it remains a fairly easily assimilated graphic representation of the cleft. It is concise and infinitely less intimidating than the lengthy tables needed to record the same details in words, and the numbering would allow simple storage and retrieval of information on computer.

Friedman et al. (1991) reviewed the development of symbolic representations of cleft lip and palate, which they felt had hitherto failed to address adequately the complex variations of those deformities that exist. They therefore introduced a new, even more complex, variation of the Striped Y, which required a separate descriptive coding sheet. This loses the benefit of a symbolic representation, which is easy to interpret. The Friedman et al. system seems to hold little advantage over the American Cleft Palate Association's immensely detailed classification if such detail is thought necessary. Although symbolic representation is less important in computerized databases of clefts, it can still be helpful to the person completing the form. Davison et al. (1998) have recently published a modification of Friedman's system which they state is simpler to use and gives as much detail (Figure 2.2). However, it remains very complex. Schwartz et al. (1993)

Table 2.2. American Cleft Palate Association's classification (1962)

Clefts of prepalate		
Cleft lip	Unilateral	Right, left
		Extent in thirds ($\frac{1}{3}$, $\frac{2}{3}$, $\frac{3}{3}$)
	Bilateral	Right, left
		Extent in thirds
Median	Extent in thirds	
Prolabium	Small, medium, large	
	Congenital scar	Right, left, median
		Extent in thirds
Cleft of alveolar	Unilateral	Right, left
process		Extent in thirds
	Median	Extent in thirds
		Submucous; right, left, median
Cleft of prepalate	Any combination of foregoing types	
	Prepalate protrusion	
	Prepalate rotation	
	Prepalate arrest (median cleft)	
Clefts of palate		
Cleft soft palate	Extent	Posteroanterior in thirds
		Width (maximum in mm)
	Palatal shortness	None, slight, moderate, marked
	Submucous cleft	Extent in thirds
Cleft hard palate	Extent	Posteroanterior in thirds
		Width (maximum in mm)
	Vomer attachment	Right, left, absent
	Submucous cleft	Extent in thirds
Cleft of soft and hard palate		
Clefts of prepalate and palate	Any combination of clefts described under clefts of prepalate and clefts of palate	

described a method of recording all the 63 variations of the original Striped Y on computer using only three digits, which they called the RPL system. In the United Kingdom, two groups have been working together to develop databases of clefts within their regions and have used variations of the Striped Y which, though differing in the amount of detail that they record, are simple to complete accurately and are mutually compatible. The Scottish Cleft Lip and Palate group (SCALP) has, since 1989, recorded details of all babies born with cleft lip and/or palate in Scotland. Their method of classifying clefts is shown in Figure 2.3. SCALP contributes its data to the Craniofacial Anomalies Register (CARE), a subcommittee of the Craniofacial

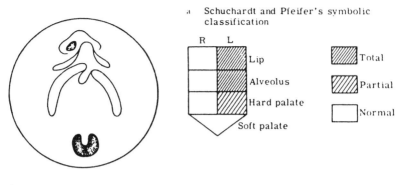

a   Schuchardt and Pfeifer's symbolic
    classification

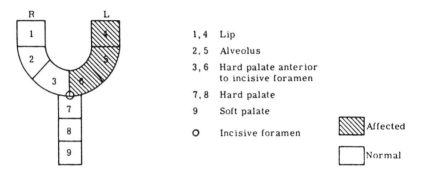

b   Kernahan's 'Striped Y' classification

1,4   Lip

2,5   Alveolus

3,6   Hard palate anterior
      to incisive foramen

7,8   Hard palate

9   Soft palate

O   Incisive foramen

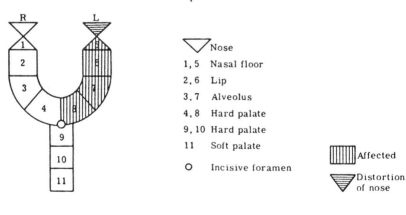

c   Millard's modification of the 'Striped Y'

1,5   Nasal floor

2,6   Lip

3,7   Alveolus

4,8   Hard palate

9,10 Hard palate

11   Soft palate

O   Incisive foramen

Figure 2.1. Symbolic methods of classifying cleft lip and palate. All can be reproduced
by a rubber stamp. Complete left-sided cleft of primary palate used as an example.

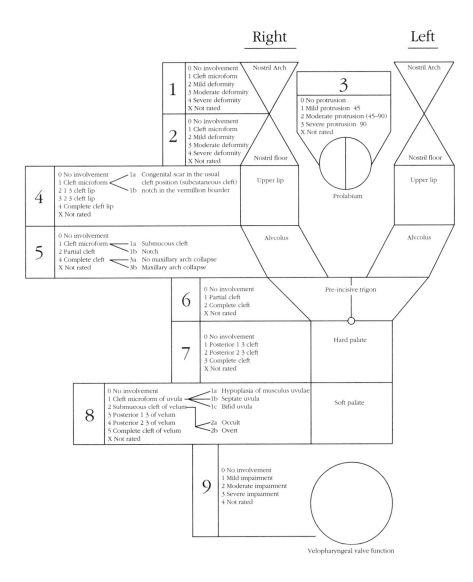

Figure 2.2. Davison et al.'s modification of Friedman's symbolic representation of cleft lip and palate anomalies. (Reproduced with permission of the British Journal of Plastic Surgery.)

CLEFT DIAGNOSIS:

<u>CODING:</u> for all categories   1 =Normal / No / Not present   9 = Not Known

		R	M	L
LOWER LIP	2 = Lip Pit	☐	☐	☐
ALAR DEFORMITY	2 = Present	☐		☐
NOSTRIL FLOOR CLEFT	2 = Present	☐		☐
SIMONARTS BAND (in otherwise complete cleft)	2 = Present	☐	☐	☐
LIP	2 = Microform : 3 = Partial : 4 = Complete	☐	☐	☐
ALVEOLUS/PRIMARY PALATE	2 = Notched : 3 = Partial : 4 = Complete bony cleft	☐	☐	☐
HARD PALATE VOMERINE ATTACHMENT	2 = Partial : 3 = None	☐		☐
HARD PALATE CLEFT EXTENT	2 = Notched : 3 = Partial : 4 = Complete bony cleft		☐	
SOFT PALATE CLEFT EXTENT	2 = Submucous : 3 = Partial : 4 = Complete cleft		☐	
BIFID UVULA	2 = Partial : 3 = Complete		☐	
CLEFT SHAPE (Isolated CP only)	2 = V - shaped : 3 = U - shaped		☐	
RESPIRATORY PROBLEMS	2 = Yes		☐	

Figure 2.3. SCALP symbolic classification of clefts. (Reproduced with permission of the Scottish Cleft Lip and Palate Group.)

Society of Great Britain, which is steadily getting closer to achieving its aim of recording every cleft in Britain. CARE's classification is shown in Figure 2.4. The data held on both these groups of patients should be comparable with any other group whose results are recorded using the Striped Y or one of its variants.

Conclusion

In deciding on a way of describing clefts it is important to distinguish between two quite separate requirements: there is the need in clinical practice to describe a particular cleft concisely and clearly to one's colleagues, and there is the different need to record the precise details of the deformity for research and audit purposes to allow later comparison of the progress of different groups of patients either within one unit or between different centres.

To fulfil the first requirement the Kernahan and Stark classification is satisfactory, although it may often be best to use terminology that is easily

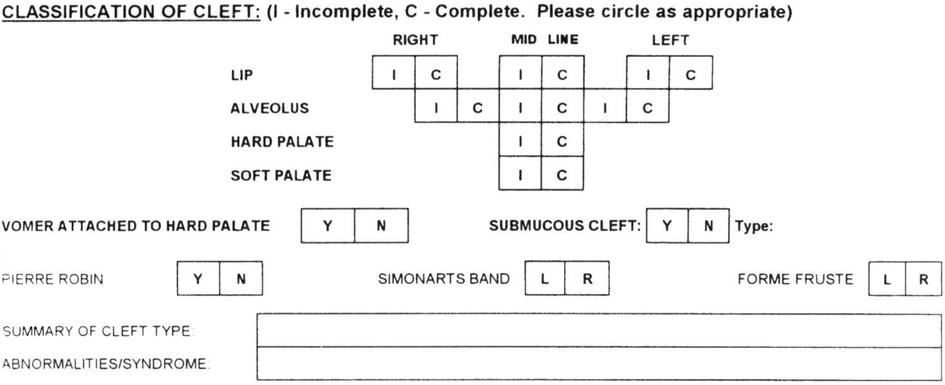

CLASSIFICATION OF CLEFT: (I - Incomplete, C - Complete. Please circle as appropriate)

	RIGHT		MID LINE		LEFT	
LIP	I	C	I	C	I	C
ALVEOLUS	I	C	I	C	I	C
HARD PALATE			I	C		
SOFT PALATE			I	C		

VOMER ATTACHED TO HARD PALATE | Y | N | SUBMUCOUS CLEFT: | Y | N | Type:

PIERRE ROBIN | Y | N | SIMONARTS BAND | L | R | FORME FRUSTE | L | R |

SUMMARY OF CLEFT TYPE:

ABNORMALITIES/SYNDROME:

Figure 2.4. CARE variation on the Striped Y classification of clefts. (Reproduced with permission of the Craniofacial Anomalies Register.)

understood; for example, 'an incomplete left-sided cleft of the lip with notching of the alveolus' is clearer and gives more detail than 'a left incomplete cleft of the primary palate'. 'A cleft of the soft palate and posterior third of the hard palate' is more informative than 'an incomplete cleft of the secondary palate'. However, when recording or reporting a series of cases, there is the need to compare one group or series with another. In some circumstances a very simple grouping is adequate. For example, with references to the two genetically distinct groups of cleft patient the abbreviations CL±P or CL(P) or simply CLP and CP are used. Sometimes the prefix 'U' (unilateral) or 'B' (bilateral) may be added. In context the meaning is clear in spite of the brevity. It is when more detail is required that the difficulties arise.

The need to build up computerized cleft databases, which are compatible between centres nationally and internationally, has been recognized and steps have already been taken to try to achieve this. Arguments will doubtless persist as to how much detail it is desirable to record, but this should not create problems providing there is general agreement on the basic minimum that is necessary. It seems likely that one of the modern variations of the Striped Y will become the generally accepted way of recording these data.

References

Berlin J (1971) Classification of cleft lip and palate and related craniofacial disorders. In: Grabb WC, Rosenstein SW, Bzoch KR (eds) Cleft Lip and Palate. Boston: Little Brown.

Davis JR, Ritchie HP (1922) Classification of congenital clefts of the lip and palate. Journal of the American Medical Association 79: 1323.

Davison JA, Mirlohi H, Rowsell AR (1998) Modified diagram of Friedman's symbolic representation of cleft lip and palate anomalies. British Journal of Plastic Surgery 51: 281–284.

Elsahy NI (1973) The modified striped Y. A systematic classification for cleft lip and palate. Cleft Palate Journal 10: 247–250.

Fogh-Anderson P (1942) Inheritance of Hare Lip and Cleft Palate. Copenhagen: Busck.

Friedman HI, Sayetta RB, Coston G, Hussey JR (1991) Symbolic representation of cleft lip and palate. Cleft Palate–Craniofacial Journal 28: 252–260.

Harkins CS, Berlin A, Harding R, Longacre JJ, Snodgrass R (1960) Report of the nomenclature committee of the American Cleft Palate Association. Cleft Palate Bulletin 10: 11.

International Confederation for Plastic and Reconstructive Surgery (1968) Cleft Palate nomenclature. Newsletter, March.

Kernahan DA (1971) The Striped Y – a symbolic classification for cleft lips and palates. Plastic and Reconstructive Surgery 47: 469.

Kernahan DA, Stark RB (1958) A new classification for cleft lip and cleft palate. Plastic and Reconstructive Surgery 22: 435.

McCabe PA (1966) A coding procedure for classification of cleft lip and cleft palate. Cleft Palate Journal 3: 383.

Millard DR (1976) Cleft Craft: the Evolution of its Surgery, vol. 1. Boston: Little Brown.

Pfeifer G (1964) In: Schuchardt K (ed.) Treatment of Patients with Clefts of Lip, Alveolus and Palate. Stuttgart: Thieme, pp. 225–226.

Schwartz S, Kapala JT, Rajchgot H, Roberts GL (1993) Accurate and systematic numerical recording system for the identification of various types of cleft of lip and maxillary clefts (RPL System). Cleft Palate–Craniofacial Journal 30: 330–332.

Spina V (1974) A proposed modification of the classification of cleft lip and cleft palate. Cleft Palate Journal 10: 251.

Veau V (1931) Division Palatine. Paris: Masson.

CHAPTER 3

Anatomy and Function

B.C. SOMMERLAD

Lip

Normal

The musculature of the lip is arranged as a circular ring of muscle, the orbicularis oris, interdigitating with the elevators and depressors of the lip and angles of the mouth and forming the modiolus with other cheek muscles at the corner of the mouth. In cross-section, the orbicularis is 'J' shaped, with the lower curve of the 'J' everting the lip and passing very close to the mucosa. Elsewhere, the mucosa is separated from the muscle by a thick layer of mucous glands. Superficially, the muscle is adherent to and partially inserted into the dermis. At the philtrum, the orbicularis decussates and is attached directly to the dermis on each side of the philtral columns (Briedis and Jackson, 1981). However, the exact anatomy of the philtrum is disputed.

The arterial supply of the upper lip is dominated by the labial arteries, which arise from the facial artery at the corner of the mouth and meet in the midline. Sensation of the upper lip is provided by the infra-orbital nerve laterally and branches of the long sphenopalatine nerve near the midline.

Cleft

In a complete unilateral cleft, the orbicularis sphincter is interrupted and muscle fibres turn upwards at the cleft to insert partly into its margin, with some fibres extending up towards the anterior nasal spine medially and the alar base laterally (Fára, 1981) (Figure 3.1). The labial vessels also pass upwards in the margins of the cleft.

In a complete bilateral cleft, there is no functional orbicularis muscle in the central prolabium and the main arterial supply of the prolabium is through branches of the midline paired long sphenopalatine vessels emerging beneath the columella.

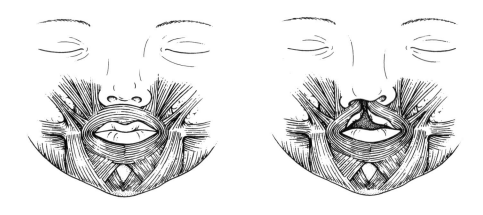

Figure 3.1. A schematic drawing of the lip musculature in a cleft compared with the normal (after Fára).

In incomplete clefts, there may be varying degrees of muscle and arterial continuity.

Nose

Normal

The nose is a pyramid, supported in the midline by the nasal septum, with the sides being formed by the nasal bones and nasal processes of the maxilla and frontal bone above, the upper lateral cartilages in the middle and the lower lateral (alar) cartilages below. The septum is made up of bone posteriorly (the vomer and the vertical plate of the ethmoid) and is cartilaginous anteriorly, attached at its base to the anterior maxillary spine.

The alar cartilages consist of domes supported by lateral and medial crura, with the medial crus extending into the columella. Their upper borders overlap the upper lateral cartilages.

Cleft

In complete unilateral clefts, the septum is deviated away from the midline and the lower cartilaginous septum and vomer are angled at up to 90 degrees from the vertical septum. The bases of the medial and lateral crura are displaced medially and laterally and the dome is slumped (Figure 12.6). A fold (plica) forms in the lining and the upper border of the alar cartilage may lie inside the upper lateral cartilage (Skoog, 1974). The nasal bones are broad and there may be a degree of hypertelorism.

Upper alveolus

Normal

The upper alveolus, with its contained toothbuds, is covered by attached gingiva, continuous with labial mucosa above and anteriorly and palatal mucoperiosteum posteriorly.

Cleft

Both medial (greater) and lateral (lesser) segments tend to be rotated outwards. The cleft would be expected, on an embryological basis, to occur between the lateral incisor tooth in the premaxilla and the canine in the lesser segment. However, supernumerary lateral incisors frequently occur lateral to the cleft site in both deciduous and permanent dentition. Neonatal teeth may appear and exfoliate, especially from the greater (medial) egment.

One of the great debates concerns the relative importance of hypoplasia and/or displacement in the cleft lip and alveolus.

Hard palate

Normal

The bony hard palate is formed by the palatal shelves of the maxilla anteriorly and by the horizontal plate of the palatine bones posteriorly, forming a midline posterior nasal spine at its posterior edge. Lateral to and above the palatal shelves are the vertically-orientated medial and lateral pterygoid plates, with the hamulus curving down, medially and posteriorly, from the medial pterygoid plate (Figure 3.2). In the midline, the nasal septum is attached to the hard palate along its length. On its oral side, the bone is covered by the mucoperiosteum of the hard palate, which is continuous with the gingiva of the alveolus anteriorly. On the nasal side, the hard palate is covered medially by the mucosa of the floor of the nose.

The blood supply is predominantly from the greater palatine arteries (and venae comitantes), which pass through the greater palatine foramen near the posterior border of the hard palate. They pass forwards, close to the bone, to join the branches of the paired long sphenopalatine arteries which emerge anteriorly through the incisive foramen.

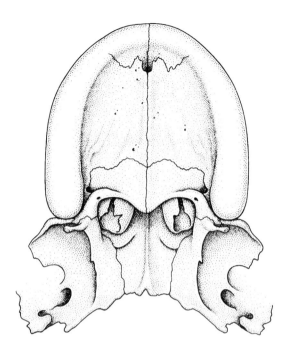

Figure 3.2. A view of the base of the skull, showing bones of the hard palate and the pterygoid hamulus extending downwards, backwards and medially from the pterygoid plate. More posteriorly, the site of origin of the levator and tensor palati muscles are seen.

Sensation is through the greater palatine and long sphenopalatine nerves, which follow the pattern of the arteries.

Cleft

Clefts of the lip and palate (CLP) disrupt the hard palate unilaterally or bilaterally to varying degrees. In unilateral clefts, the vomer is joined to the palatal shelf on the non-cleft side, although the angulation of the vomer means that it may be almost horizontal and appear part of the palate except for the more pink appearance of its covering mucosa. In complete bilateral clefts, the vomer remains unattached in the midline.

Complete clefts of the secondary palate (CP) extend forwards to the incisive foramen with incomplete clefts involving the hard palate to varying degrees. The bony defect may be much more extensive than the mucosal defect. In the classical submucous cleft palate (SMCP), there is a defect of the hard palate which may range from absence of the posterior nasal spine to V-shaped notching of the posterior border of the hard palate, to a significant bony defect.

Soft palate (velum)

Normal

The soft palate (velum) is attached to the hard palate anteriorly and to the pharynx laterally, and its free edge forms the uvula in the midline. The mucosa of the oral surface (and, to a lesser extent, of the nasal surface) is rich in mucous glands. Sandwiched between the oral and nasal mucosa is a complex arrangement of muscles and, anteriorly, the palatal aponeurosis. The fibrous aponeurosis is continuous with the tendon of the tensor veli palatani (the tensor), which passes down from the base of the skull (where it originates from the membranous portion of the Eustachian tube, the scaphoid fossa and the spine of the sphenoid bone) to pass around the pterygoid hamulus and fan out as the aponeurosis.

The tensor tendon is partially attached to the hamulus (in its anterior third) and excursion is limited perhaps to 5 mm. Some authorities recognize a separate but closely related muscle – the dilator tubae which rounds the middle third of the pterygoid hamulus without an insertion (Barsoumian et al., 1998). The aponeurosis is attached to the back of the hard palate, occupies the anterior one-third of the soft palate and is thick anteriorly and thins out posteriorly. The most oral (inferior) muscle of the soft palate is palatoglossus, a thin sheet of muscle arising from the oral surface of the back of the palatal aponeurosis and the region of the maxillary tuberosity, passing backwards and laterally to condense to form the anterior pillar of the fauces. Above this is the palatopharyngeus, which is a more substantial sheet of muscle within the velum, arising anteriorly from the maxillary tuberosity and the palatal aponeurosis, blending with the fibres of the levator. Some reports describe two heads within the velum, separated by the levator (Huang et al., 1998). Lateral to the velum, the muscle passes down (forming the posterior pillar of the fauces) to the pharyngeal aponeurosis and thyroid cartilage. Other fibres pass posteriorly to intermingle with the superior constrictor muscle.

The levator veli palatini (the levator) arises from the inferior surface of the petrous temporal bone and from the lower and medial part of the Eustachian tube cartilage, and passes downwards, forwards and medially to enter the velum and join with its fellow on the opposite side, occupying the middle 40% of the velum (Figure 3.3) and being related to the palatopharyngeus. Anteriorly, it is continuous with the thinned posterior edge of the palatal aponeurosis. Oral examination of the soft palate on production of the sound 'ah' (/ɑ/) reveals dimples, or points of maximum movement, which have been shown to correlate well with the insertion of the levator within the velum (Boorman and Sommerlad, 1985a). Above the levator palati lie the paired musculus uvulae muscles, attached to the posterior nasal spine anteriorly, passing into the uvula posteriorly and covered nasally (and especially laterally) by mucous glands (Boorman and Sommerlad, 1985b).

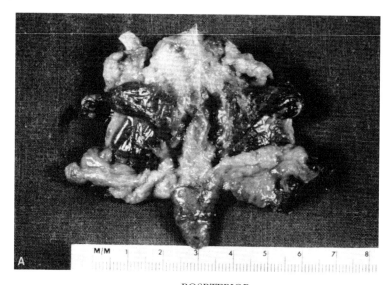

POSRTERIOR
NASAL
SPINE

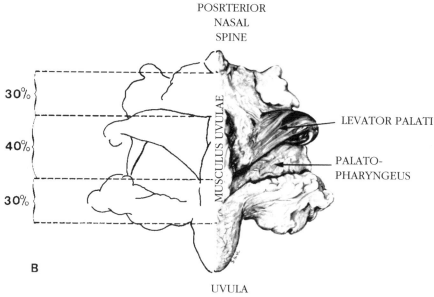

Figure 3.3. A cadaver dissection and explanatory diagram to show the muscles of the normal velum with the levator inserted in the middle 40% (Boorman and Sommerlad, 1985a). Reproduced from the British Journal of Plastic Surgery by permission of Harcourt Publishers Ltd.

The primary velar muscles (levator, palatopharyngeus and palatoglossus) form interlocking slings with the levators acting as elevators and the palatopharyngeus (in its inferior portion) and palatoglossus being depressors of the velum. All, however, act potentially to extend (lengthen) the soft palate and to narrow the pharynx. The horizontal component of palatopharyngeus and some fibres of the superior constrictor, which arise from the medial pterygoid plate and hamulus, form a muscular ring around the pharynx, and one or both form Passavant's ridge.

There has been much debate about whether the tensor (and/or dilator tubae) have a significant action on the velum. This could only happen if there is considerable movement of the tendon over the hamulus, and the majority view would appear to be that the tensor could have only a limited role, although the dilator tubae could play a more important part in tensing the palate through the aponeurosis. There has also been debate about the relative importance of the tensor (or dilator tubae) and the levator in Eustachian tube function (opening and closing).

The blood supply is rich, with branches from the lesser palatine, ascending palatine, ascending pharyngeal, tonsillar branches of the facial artery and dorsal lingual branches of the lingual artery – all direct or indirect branches of the external carotid artery. The all important levator palati is apparently supplied primarily from near its origin and vessels course along its length (Figure 3.4), although other vessels may also supply this and the other velar muscles (Mercer and MacCarthy, 1995).

The nerve supply of most of the palatal muscles is primarily from the pharyngeal plexus formed by branches of the ninth (glossopharyngeal) and tenth (vagus) cranial nerves. The pharyngeal plexus is situated within the muscle layers of the pharynx. However, it has been suggested that there may be some supply to the levator palati through the seventh nerve via the greater superficial petrosal nerve. The only velar muscles not supplied by the pharyngeal plexus are the tensor palati muscle (not strictly a palatal muscle), which is supplied by a motor branch of the fifth (trigeminal) nerve, and the musculus uvulae, which is said to be supplied by lesser palatine nerves (Broomhead, 1951).

The sensory supply is predominantly by the lesser palatine nerves, which emerge through multiple small foramina at the back of the hard palate with some overlap with glossopharyngeal sensory fibres laterally.

Cleft

The abnormal velar musculature in the cleft was first described by Veau (1931) and has been further amplified by Fára and Dvorak (1970) and Kriens (1969). The tensor, having passed around the hook of the

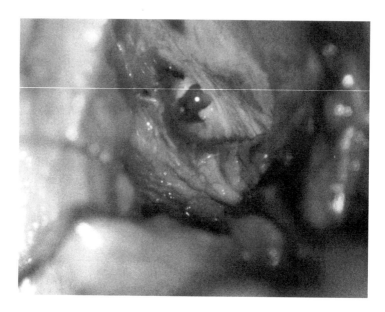

Figure 3.4. A view of the levator palati muscle through the operating microscope, showing vessels coursing along its length.

hamulus, forms a thick fibrous triangular insertion into the lateral part of the posterior edge of the hard palate. This is very different to the normal, thinner, expanded and presumably more elastic palatal aponeurosis (Figure 3.5). The levator, palatopharyngeus and palatoglossus, unable to meet in the midline, pass more anteriorly than in the normal to be inserted into the margins of the cleft, the oral and nasal mucosa, the abnormal palatal aponeurosis and into the back of the hard palate. Near the midline, the levator and palatopharyngeus fuse to form what Veau called 'the cleft muscle', but more laterally they are clearly separate.

The submucous cleft palate is best regarded as a spectrum rather than a clear subdivision between classic and occult, with varying degrees of anterior muscle orientation and diastasis (failure to join in the midline).

Pharynx

Normal

The opening between nose and mouth is formed by the velopharyngeal orifice, a sphincter, formed by velar and pharyngeal muscles at different levels. The upper fibres of the palatopharyngeus and the superior

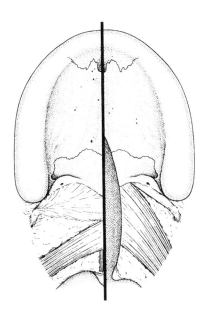

Figure 3.5. A diagram of the cleft muscular anatomy, with the anatomy of the cleft on the right side (with the abnormal triangular insertion of the tensor palati and the anterior insertion of the levator muscle) and the normal anatomy on the left (with the tensor tendon/palatal aponeurosis thinning posteriorly and occupying the anterior third of the velum and the levator in the middle third).

constrictor are the pharyngeal components of this sphincter. The superior constrictor is a sheet of muscle attached to the medial pterygoid plate, hamulus and the pterygomandibular ligament (raphe) anteriorly, and meeting its opposite number in the midline posteriorly. The horizontal component of palatopharyngeus lies within superior constrictor but is intermingled with it. It is attached by the pharyngobasilar fascia to the base of the skull superiorly, and lies on the pre-vertebral fascia.

Salpingopharyngeus arises from the cartilage of the Eustachian tube, forming what looks like an inverted 'J' prominence on the lateral pharyngeal wall with the long limb passing from behind the orifice downwards to the larynx.

The pharynx is supplied by the ascending pharyngeal artery and by other branches of the external carotid – branches from the lingual, facial and from the superior and inferior laryngeal arteries (Boorman and Freedlander, 1992). Venous drainage is largely into the internal jugular vein.

The nerve supply is from the pharyngeal plexus of nerves which is formed from branches of the vagus (tenth), glossopharyngeal (ninth) cranial nerves and the cervical sympathetic. The pharyngeal plexus lies on the lateral wall of the pharynx, mainly over the middle constrictor.

Cleft

The anatomy of the muscle wall of the pharynx is not obviously abnormal in the cleft, although the muscles may be hypoplastic in cleft-associated conditions such as velocardiofacial syndrome.

Anatomy – implications for surgery

(see also Watson, Chapter 12)

Hard palate repair

The greater palatine vessels and nerves are pre-eminent in the hard palate. Any incision in the hard palate may divide branches. Incisions lateral to the main neurovascular trunk may partially reduce the blood supply and denervate the lateral hard palate and alveolus, while incisions medially may compromise medial flaps. In addition, the greater palatine neurovascular bundle may be damaged as it leaves the foramen during attempts to mobilize it to facilitate closure in wide clefts. However, Demjen in Bratislava routinely divided the greater palatine bundle during palate repair, apparently without specific detrimental effect (Morris and Demjen, 1978).

Whether the apparent adverse effect of surgery on maxillary growth is due to denervation, devascularization, disturbance of periosteum or simply the restrictive effect of scars, is widely debated. In the current state of knowledge, it seems wise to minimize surgery on the hard palate and attempts to narrow the clefts (by presurgical orthopaedics or by early closure of the velum) are intended to allow minimal hard palate surgery. There is considerable evidence that pushback procedures (such as the Veau/Wardill/Kilner technique) are detrimental to growth. If relaxing incisions are necessary, it is unclear whether these are better made lateral (Von Langenbeck) or medial (Delaire/Pigott) to the greater palatine neurovascular bundle.

Surgical repair of the velum

The anterior, partly bony, insertions of the velar muscles in the cleft means that they must function, partially at least, isometrically. Attempted correction was first described by Braithwaite (1964) and further methods have been described. Kriens (1969) emphasized what he called 'the myofascial apparatus of the velopharyngeal area'. Furlow's technique (1986) depends on retro-displacement of muscle with mucosa (oral on one side and nasal on the other). Sommerlad et al. (1994a) separate the muscles en masse with the hypoplastic tensor/aponeurosis, from the posterior hard palate and from both oral and nasal mucosa, aiming to create a sling across the midline in at least the middle third of the velum.

Many repaired palates (and submucous cleft palates) fail to show the normal convexity of the middle of the velum as seen on nasopharyngoscopy, and may be concave or grooved centrally. Some believe this to be due to the absence or lack of action of musculus uvulae (Pigott, 1969; Lewin et al., 1980), while others doubt the importance of musculus uvulae – particularly in clefts (Boorman and Sommerlad, 1985b). Uniting the velar muscles beneath as much nasal mucosa and mucous glands as possible can produce a convexity approaching normal.

Surgery on the pharynx

An understanding of the anatomy of the pharyngeal muscles and their nerve and blood supply is important for a surgeon undertaking a pharyngoplasty. The widely-used midline pharyngeal flap cannot contain effective functional muscle because of the direction of the muscle fibres, and the viability of any pharyngeal flap obviously depends on the anatomy of the blood supply (Boorman and Freedlander, 1992). (See also Mercer and Pigott, Chapter 17.)

Function

Lip

Lip closure is necessary for the normal production of bilabial sounds. It requires a lip of adequate length and mobility, particularly for sounds such as 'oo'. Satisfactory function of the orbicularis oris muscle is therefore important. Lip depression, elevation and spread are all important for facial expression and depend on the levator and depressor muscles of angle of mouth and lip.

Nose

The nasal mucosa is important for humidifying inspired air and the nasal cavities act as resonators. Nasal airway obstruction is not uncommon in cleft patients and may be caused by septal deviation, enlargement of the turbinates and asymmetries of the nostrils with stenosis. This may produce hyponasality, or contribute to mixed nasality.

Velopharyngeal function

(see also Mercer and Pigott, Chapter 17)

Normal

The velopharyngeal sphincter

Earlier views of velopharyngeal function (based on oral observation and lateral X-rays) envisaged a primarily valvular mechanism in which the velum functions as an active flap valve with Passavant's ridge forming on the posterior pharyngeal wall only when necessary in velopharyngeal dysfunction (Calnan, 1957). Nasendoscopy, as developed by Pigott (1969), and multi-view videofluoroscopy (Skolnick et al., 1973) have demonstrated a much more complex mechanism, with both velum and pharynx being important in function. Closure patterns differ (a) between individuals, (b) between speech and swallowing, and (c) with different sounds – as follows:

(a) Between individuals.
    Closure patterns have been classified as coronal/sagittal/sphincteric (Golding-Kushner et al., 1990). This is a simplification of a spectrum of velar and pharyngeal movement.
(b) Between speech and swallowing.
    Closure of the velopharyngeal orifice to prevent nasal regurgitation during swallowing is a slower mechanism occurring at a lower level and over a longer distance than that which occurs with speech. Lateral pharyngeal wall movement is particularly important.
(c) Between different sounds.
    Endoscopy and videofluoroscopy have shown that patterns of movement of both velum and pharynx differ greatly with different sounds. For example, the sound 'eeh' (/i/) produces high velar lift and relatively little pharyngeal wall movement (a mainly valvular closure) while 'aah' (/a/) produces a more sphincteric pattern, with less velar lift and more lateral and posterior pharyngeal wall movement. Unfortunately, most observations have been based on the distorted images seen through the wide-angle lens of the nasendoscope, and attempts to quantify movement, even ratiometrically (Golding-Kushner et al., 1990) cannot be accurate. Videofluoroscopy has more mathematical validity (Birch et al., 1994), if performed under standardized conditions (Sommerlad et al., 1994b), but requires interpretation of superimposed images and involves some radiation exposure – however small. Non-radiating, non-distorting and three-dimensional imaging is required and real-time MRI scanning holds promise for the future.

Velar function

Despite the contribution of pharyngeal wall movement, velar function is crucial to velopharyngeal closure. Several aspects of velar function may be important:

(a) Size.
    The velum must be long and wide enough in its stretched state to physically occlude the orifice remaining after maximal pharyngeal wall movement.

(b) Extensibility.

Standardized lateral videofluoroscopy shows that the segment of velum between the back of the hard palate and the prominence produced by the levator insertion (the levator knee) extends maximally by 56% (Birch et al., 1994) (Figure 3.6). This probably depends on the elastic structure provided by the normal palatal aponeurosis in the anterior third of the velum, and on the mobile insertion of the velar muscles (especially the levator and probably palatopharyngeus) into this elastic membrane.

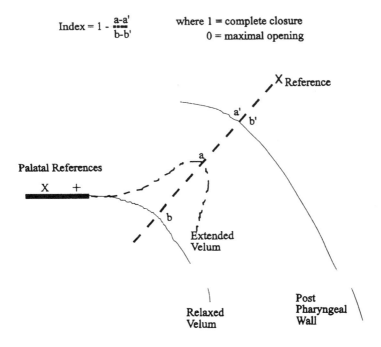

$$\text{Index} = 1 - \frac{a\text{-}a'}{b\text{-}b'} \qquad \text{where } 1 = \text{complete closure} \\ 0 = \text{maximal opening}$$

Figure 3.6. A diagram to show measurements of velar function in lateral videofluoroscopy.

(c) Velocity.

Velar movement must be rapid, with touch closure occurring in 100 msec, continuing to firm closure in 160 msec on the sound 'eeh' (/i/). Closure which occurs after a sound has been vocalized is ineffective in preventing nasal emission of air and hypernasality. Measurement of velocity has been relatively crude in the past, relying on frame-counting of standard videofluoroscopy (with a frame duration of 25 msec) (Figure 3.7).

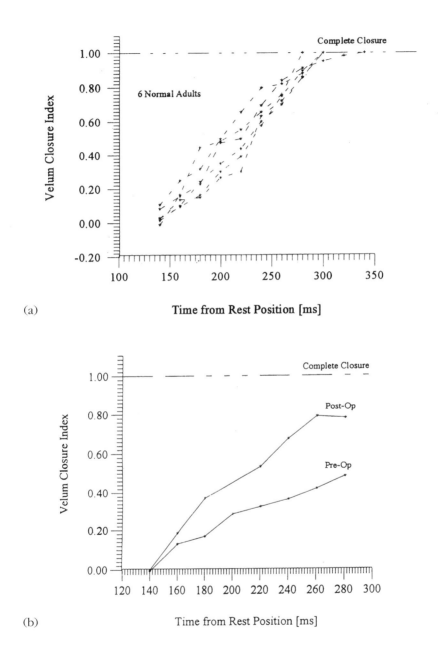

(a)

(b)

Figure 3.7. (a) graph to show the rate of elevation of the levator knee in six normal adults. (b) graph to show a repaired cleft with VPI before and after re-repair (Birch et al, 1999).

(d) Timing.

Delayed initiation of velar movement may have the same effect as appropriately initiated but slower movement. If closure occurs too late, nasal air emission and hypernasality will result.

(e) Lift.

In addition to extensibility, velar lift is necessary to some degree to achieve closure against the posterior pharyngeal wall, which slopes forwards.

(f) Velopharyngeal configuration.

Finally, the three-dimensional configuration of the part of the velum making (or attempting to make) contact and the posterior pharyngeal wall is important. The point of contact of the velum may be the levator knee or more posteriorly. The slope of the posterior pharyngeal wall is obviously important. Irregularity and asymmetry of the posterior pharyngeal wall, for example by adenoid tissue, may also result in velopharyngeal dysfunction.

This discussion has concentrated on the closing function of the velum, but opening is also important and little studied. Palatoglossus and the descending component of palatopharyngeus are the depressors of the velum but the relative contribution of gravity and active depression are not clear. Electromyography (EMG) studies have been used to try to elucidate the function of the different palatal muscles (Fritzell, 1979), but interpretation is difficult due to the uncertainty of placement of electrodes in very small and intimately related muscles.

Velopharyngeal dysfunction

Velopharyngeal dysfunction in the cleft patient may, therefore, be the result of any or a combination of abnormalities of velar dimensions, extensibility, velocity, timing, lift or velopharyngeal configuration. There may be a relationship between the size of the residual velopharyngeal defect and the degree of nasality (Warren, 1964) but this seems likely to be an oversimplification. The relatively inactive mechanism following posterior pharyngeal flap surgery may be more predictable than the more physiological mobile velopharyngeal orifice. It may be that small defects are associated with audible nasal emission and turbulence, while large defects are associated with hypernasal resonance.

Measurement of the size of the velopharyngeal orifice has proved difficult. X-rays are quantifiable but two-dimensional. Endoscopy introduces problems of lens distortion, parallax and interpretation of a three-dimensional orifice. Phototransducers have been used (Dalston, 1982; Moon and Lagu, 1987).

Simultaneous studies of voice, nasal and oral air flows and pressure (Warren et al., 1985) are proving interesting in measuring timing, but can only be correlated with the size of the velopharyngeal defect if this can be simultaneously measured by a non-invasive and accurate method. Unfortunately, this is not available at present. Real-time MRI scanning may provide the key.

Investigation of velopharyngeal function, therefore, requires endoscopy, multiview videofluoroscopy, air-flow/pressure/resistance measurements and, ideally, three-dimensional imaging. There is much to be learned.

Velar function in clefts

Between 5 and 50% of patients who have had cleft palate repairs exhibit velopharyngeal insufficiency. Lack of standardization of speech assessment and scoring methods makes comparison between patients, and especially between different cleft units and surgeons, of limited value (see Grunwell and Sell, Chapter 5). Results seem to be surgeon dependent, with rates varying between 0 and 44% among higher volume surgeons in a large UK-wide study (CSAG, 1998).

Early efforts to improve velopharyngeal closure were based on the concept that palate length was all important. Palate lengthening by V–Y pushback procedures have been unsuccessful in improving speech results. Lengthening of the soft palate by the double opposing Z-plasty technique of Furlow (1986) has produced some good results, but whether this is produced by lengthening or reorientation of muscles or both has yet to be resolved. Retro-displacement of uncorrected anteriorly directed cleft musculature has been shown to be of benefit as a secondary procedure (Sommerlad et al., 1994a) in reducing the speech consequences of velopharyngeal dysfunction.

Until all factors, such as velocity, timing, lift and velopharyngeal configuration are better understood, the treatment of velopharyngeal dysfunction in clefts will be inadequate.

Relationship between velopharyngeal and Eustachian dysfunction
(See also Lennox, Chapter 15.)

The increased incidence of secretory otitis media, glue ear and conductive hearing loss in cleft patients has long been recognized (Bluestone, 1978). Theories of causation abound. Continual contact of the Eustachian orifice with milk and food has been implicated. However, it seems likely that the abnormal anatomy of the levator and/or the tensor palati muscles is the most likely cause, by impairing Eustachian opening and closing. There is no convincing evidence that retropositioning the levator muscles into a more normal position improves Eustachian function. The insertion of ventilating tubes (grommets) as required remains the mainstay of treatment in infants and young children.

Function – implications for the surgery of velopharyngeal dysfunction

Phoneme-specific nasality, often associated with fricatives, is an abnormal articulatory mechanism which may occur despite normal velopharyngeal function with other sounds. Speech therapy is the appropriate treatment (see Sell and Grunwell, Chapter 16). Prosthetic support, with either palatal lifts or speech bulbs, is used in certain situations (see Sell and Grunwell, Chapter 16).

Surgical treatment

If disordered structure or function make velopharyngeal closure during speech impossible, surgery is the most usual treatment. This may involve secondary surgery to the palate, or pharyngeal surgery. The choice should depend on the results of velopharyngeal investigations (see Mercer and Pigott, Chapter 17).

Secondary velar surgery has been shown to be beneficial but not to correct velopharyngeal dysfunction in all patients (Sommerlad et al., 1994a). It does have the advantage that other management options remain open.

Pharyngeal surgery is an attempt to alter the velopharyngeal sphincter by narrowing the pharynx (in most pharyngoplasties), partially occluding the orifice (in posterior midline pharyngeal flap surgery), attempting to build up the posterior pharyngeal wall (in a classical Hynes pharyngoplasty), or producing an artificially low and partly functional sphincter (in the Orticochoea or sphincter pharyngoplasty) (see Mercer and Pigott, Chapter 17). Although potentially improving velopharyngeal closure, these procedures also limit velopharyngeal opening, reducing the size of the velopharyngeal orifice at rest. They may therefore result in nasal airway obstruction, snoring and possibly sleep apnoea.

However, until more accurate measurement of size, timing and configuration of the velopharyngeal defect and of the relative contribution of velar and pharyngeal dysfunction is possible, surgical decision-making will be unreliable.

References

Barsoumian R, Kuehn DP, Moon JB, Candy SW (1998) An anatomic study of the tensor veli palatini and dilator tubae muscles in relation to Eustachian tube in velar function. Cleft Palate–Craniofacial Journal 35: 101–110.

Birch M, Bhatt A, Sommerlad BC (1994) Image analysis of lateral velopharyngeal closure in cleft palate patients and normal palates. British Journal of Plastic Surgery 47: 400–405.

Birch MJ, Sommerlad BC, Jenn C (1999) A study of the measurement areas associated with the analysis of velopharyngeal measurements assessed from videofluoroscopy investigations. Cleft Palate-Craniofacial Journal 36 (6): 499–507.

Bluestone CD (1978) Eustachian tube obstruction in the infant with cleft palate. Annals of Otology, Rhinology and Laryngology 80 (Suppl 2): 1–30.

Boorman J, Freedlander E (1992) Surgical anatomy of the velum and pharynx. In: Recent Advances in Plastic Surgery 4. Edinburgh: Churchill Livingstone, Ch. 2, pp. 17–28.

Boorman JG, Sommerlad BC (1985a) Levator palati and palatal dimples – their anatomy, relationship and clinical significance. British Journal of Plastic Surgery 38: 326–332.

Boorman JG, Sommerlad BC (1985b) Musculus uvulae and levator palati: their anatomical and functional relationship in velopharyngeal closure. British Journal of Plastic Surgery 38: 333–338.

Braithwaite F (1964) Cleft palate repair. In: Gibson T (ed.) Modern Trends in Plastic Surgery I. London: Butterworth.

Briedis J, Jackson IT (1981) The anatomy of the philtrum: observations made on dissections in the normal lip. British Journal of Plastic Surgery 34(2): 128–132.

Broomhead IW (1951) The nerve supply of the muscles of the soft palate. British Journal of Plastic Surgery 4: 1–15.

Calnan I (1957) Modern views on Passavant's ridge. British Journal of Plastic Surgery 10: 89–113.

CSAG Report, Clinical Standards Advisory Group (1998) Cleft Lip and/or Palate. London: HMSO.

Dalston R (1982) Photodetector assessment of velopharyngeal activity. Cleft Palate–Craniofacial Journal 19: 1–8.

Fára M (1981) Functional anatomy of lip and palate and its application to cleft lip and palate surgery. In: Jackson IT (ed.) Recent Advances in Plastic Surgery 2. Edinburgh: Churchill Livingstone, pp. 145–163.

Fára M, Dvorak I (1970) Abnormal anatomy of the muscles of palatopharyngeal closure in cleft palates. Plastic and Reconstructive Surgery 46: 488–497.

Fritzell B (1979) Electromyography in the study of the velopharyngeal function – a review. Folia Phoniatrica 31(2): 93–102.

Furlow LT Jr (1986) Cleft palate repair by double opposing Z-plasty. Plastic and Reconstructive Surgery 78: 724–736.

Golding-Kushner KJ et al. (1990) Standardization for the reporting of nasopharyngoscopy and multiview videofluoroscopy: A report from an international working group. Cleft Palate–Craniofacial Journal 27: 33–347.

Huang MHS, Lee ST, Rajendran K (1998) Anatomic basis of cleft palate and velopharyngeal surgery: implications from a fresh cadaveric study. Plastic and Reconstructive Surgery 101: 613–627.

Kriens OB (1969) An anatomical approach to veloplasty. Plastic and Reconstructive Surgery 43: 29–41.

Lewin ML, Croft CV, Shprintzen RJ (1980) Velopharyngeal insufficiency due to hypoplasia of the musculus uvulae and occult submucous cleft palate. Plastic and Reconstructive Surgery 65(5): 585–591.

Mercer SG, MacCarthy P (1995) The arterial supply of the palate: implications for closure of cleft palates. Plastic and Reconstructive Surgery 96: 1038–1044.

Moon J, Lagu R (1987) Development of a second-generation phototransducer for the assessment of velopharyngeal activity. Cleft Palate–Craniofacial Journal 24: 240–243.

Morris H, Demjen S (1978) The Bratislava Project: Some Results of Cleft Palate Surgery. University of Iowa Press, p. 8.

Pigott RW (1969) The nasendoscopic appearance of the normal palatopharyngeal valve. Plastic and Reconstructive Surgery 43: 19.

Skolnick MC, McCall GN, Barnes MB (1973) The sphincteric mechanism of velopharyngeal closure. Cleft Palate–Craniofacial Journal 10: 286.

Skoog T (1974) Plastic Surgery: New methods and Refinements. Philadelphia: WB Saunders.

Sommerlad BC, Henley M, Birch M, Harland K, Moimen N, Boorman JG (1994a) Cleft palate re-repair – a clinical and radiographic study of 32 consecutive cases. British Journal of Plastic Surgery 47: 406–410.

Sommerlad BC, Rowland N, Harland K (1994b) Lateral videofluoroscopy – a modification to aid in velopharyngeal assessment and measurement. Cleft Palate–Craniofacial Journal 31: 134–135.

Veau V (1931) Division palatine. Paris: Masson & Cie.

Warren DW (1964) Velopharyngeal orifice size and upper pharyngeal pressure-flow patterns in normal speech. Plastic and Reconstructive Surgery 33: 148–162.

Warren DW, Dalston RM, Trier WC, Holder MB (1985) A pressure-flow technique for quantifying temporal patterns of palatal pharyngeal closure. Cleft Palate–Craniofacial Journal 22: 11–19.

CHAPTER 4

Facial Growth

M. MARS

Individuals with repaired clefts of the lip and/or palate do not present with normal facial appearance. In addition to obvious nasal deformities and lip scarring, such individuals demonstrate characteristic features of distorted facial growth.

The majority of clinicians dealing with this condition would concur with the following observation:

> That facial growth is often unsatisfactory and that these children present with aesthetic and functional problems that are difficult to overcome. These clinical findings are confirmed by virtually every comparative cephalometric study published. (Ross, 1990)

Normal growth of the face

At birth, the face is a very small proportion of the overall volume of the head; the cranium, eyes and orbits contributing to the major proportion. Facial growth from birth to maturity results in a reversal of these proportions (Figure 4.1). At birth, there is no maxillary antrum, no tuberosity, and the pterygoid plates are extremely small.

Facial growth occurs essentially by two related processes – displacement and remodelling. Displacement involves movement of whole bones or bony complexes away from one another at their junctions with one another. These junctions may be movable joints or sutures or synchondroses.

Osteogenic activity results in remodelling of a bone by deposition or resorptive processes. These result in overall enlargement and changes in shape.

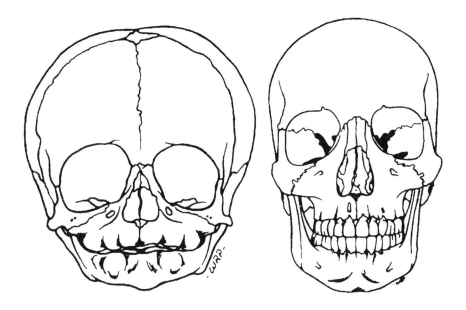

Figure 4.1. By enlarging the neonatal skull to match that of the adult, the marked differences between the two become evident. (From Enlow DH (1982) Handbook of Facial Growth, 2nd edn. Philadelphia: WB Saunders, p. 13.)

The maxilla

Static measurements of bony length, e.g. maxillary length, give only a partial account and explanation of maxillary growth because the position of the bone in space (its displacement) is critical to its contribution to overall facial harmony. Disturbed displacement of the maxilla results in abnormal facial form even if that maxilla is of normal proportions. A maxilla of normal length that has not been displaced downwards and forwards from the cranial base results in severe mid-face retrusion. Simultaneous remodelling results in subtle changes of shape and expansion of the maxilla with growth. Figures 4.2, 4.3 and 4.4 illustrate the relative contribution of displacement and remodelling resulting in facial growth changes.

The mandible

Many textbooks have simplistically and erroneously described mandibular growth as the gradual enlargement of a small mandible to a larger one of similar proportions (Figure 4.5).

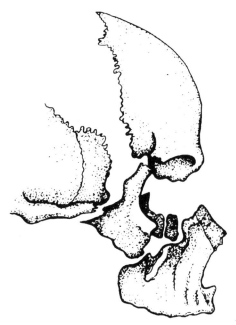

Figure 4.2. The separate bones of the maxillary complex are displaced away from one another and from the cranial base. Sutural bone growth simultaneously enlarges each bone by an amount that equals the displacement. (From McCarthy JG (1990) Plastic Surgery, Volume 4. WB Saunders, p. 2508.)

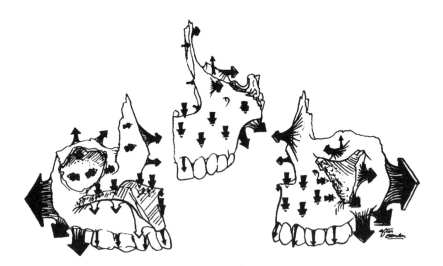

Figure 4.3. Remodelling growth in the maxilla: arrows penetrating the bone surface represent resorption; arrows leading away from the surface indicate fields of surface deposition. (From Enlow DH (1968) Human Face. New York: Harper and Row.)

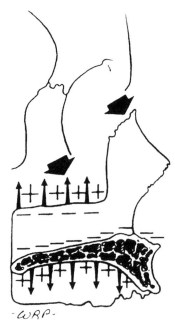

Figure 4.4. Palatal and orbital growth. (From Enlow DH (1982) Handbook of Facial Growth, 2nd edn. Philadelphia: WB Saunders. Reprinted by permission of Butterworth Heinemann Publishers, a division of Reed Educational and Professional Publishing Ltd.)

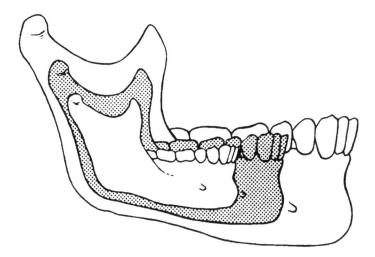

Figure 4.5. Enlargement of each individual bone in the face does not take place in the simplified manner shown here, but by extensive remodelling. (From Cohen B and Kramer IRN (1975) Scientific Foundations of Dentistry. London: William Heinemann Medical Books, p. 30.)

The whole mandible becomes displaced downwards and forwards from the cranial base, and remodelling (resorption and deposition) by osteoblastic and osteoclastic activity maintains a normal relationship of the condyle and ramus to one another. Growth of the alveolar process maintains dental contact of both the changing maxilla and mandible. The muscle attachments to the mandible result in significant changes to its overall shape at the angle where the masseter and medial pterygoid muscles are attached, and the condylar process, where the temporal and the lateral pterygoid muscles are attached.

Condylar growth was previously considered to be the main cartilagenous factor determining downwards and forward movement of the mandible – a primary growth site. This view is controversial and not generally accepted by most authorities at present. Mandibular growth is considered to be essentially similar to that of the maxilla, i.e. a process of displacement and remodelling.

Abnormal facial growth in cleft lip and palate

The causes of mid-face retrusion and poor facial growth in repaired cleft lip and palate subjects are poorly understood and the cause of much, often heated, debate: lip surgery, palatal surgery, early surgery to the hard palate, aggressive surgery and repeated surgery, the competence of the surgeon, as well as the timing and nature of surgery have all been separately implicated. At the other extreme, some authorities still claim that any growth disturbance is purely intrinsic and that surgery does no harm.

Maxillary retrusion (Figures 4.6 and 4.7), evident in a proportion of operated cleft lip and palate subjects in teenage years, is a well recognized phenomenon (Ross, 1986, 1987a, 1987b, 1987c, 1987d, 1987e, 1987f, 1987g). Such retrusion does not happen in all cases or to the same extent in every case. The need for maxillary advancement surgery has been reported as being of the order of 25% (Ross, 1986) or even up to 50% (Mars et al., 1987). Cross-centre studies show significant differences between participating centres with a range of severe maxillary retrusion from 10% to over 50% (Mars et al., 1992). A later study shows severe maxillary retrusion in one centre as low as 5% (Sommerlad et al., 1997). The debate between intrinsic and iatrogenic growth disturbance has continued for the past 80 years (Gillies and Fry, 1921). Additional arguments which permeate the literature are the separate effects of lip repair and palate repair on facial form and the vexed question of the timing of surgery, particularly to the palate.

The cause of abnormal facial morphology may be intrinsic, iatrogenic or functional (Ross and Johnston, 1972). Major differences of opinion regarding the relative importance of each of these three possible causes still exist.

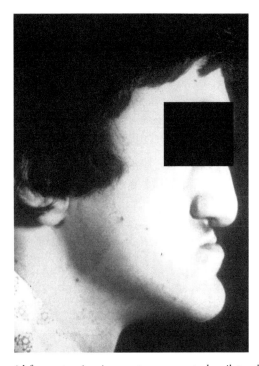

Figure 4.6. Severe mid-face retrusion in a mature, operated unilateral cleft lip and palate subject.

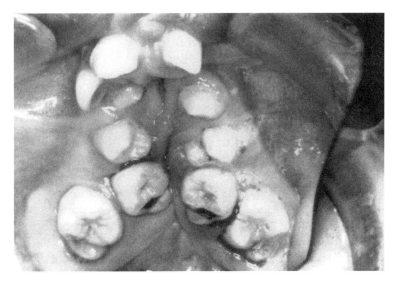

Figure 4.7. Gross maxillary arch contraction in a repaired unilateral cleft lip and palate subject.

The difficulties experienced by research workers in the field of cleft lip and palate are seen in the limitations of many of the studies that have been undertaken. These may be summarized as follows:

- Small sample size.
- Wide age distribution.
- A narrow age distribution of very young subjects.
- Mixtures of unoperated, partially operated, late operated and early operated subjects.
- Mixtures of subjects from different cleft types.
- Males and females grouped together.
- No controls on the normal population.

Unquestionably, the major problem is that of small sample size, which has been responsible for frequent inappropriate handling of the available data.

Sophisticated statistical and philosophical arguments are used to justify 'pooling' in order to increase sample size (Semb, 1991a; Brattstrom et al., 1991). Such 'pooling' can distort the results so that important differences are lost. Where growth changes on an annual basis are small but are incremental over the period of growth studied, the overall effect, particularly between pre- and post-pubertal individuals, is likely to be considerable.

Facial growth, especially mid-face growth, is often compromised in subjects with repaired cleft lip and palate. Many early authorities blamed palatal repair for mid-face growth problems (Graber, 1949; Slaughter and Brodie, 1949). Some authorities do not accept that growth disturbance is caused by surgery (Aduss, 1971), whilst lip surgery rather than palatal surgery is held responsible by others (Bardach, 1990; Hagerty et al., 1964). The timing of palatal repair is the main focus of some clinicians who claim that 'early' repair is responsible for poor mid-face growth. They advocate 'delayed' hard palate closure (Hotz et al., 1978; Schweckendiek, 1978). Their definitions of 'early' and 'delayed' vary considerably.

The nature of surgery itself has been blamed for disappointing results, especially 'traumatic assault on the palatal shelves' (Bill et al., 1956). They, in common with other investigators, blame lip repair for growth problems (Bardach, 1990). It has been suggested that the competence of the surgeon, rather than the surgery itself, might be the most important variable affecting facial growth outcome (Ross, 1990). There has been evidence to show that a high volume of patients with centralized care demonstrated the best facial growth in a cross-centre study (Shaw et al., 1992; Mars et al., 1992).

An excellent overall review of facial growth in cleft lip and palate, without detailed individual critical appraisal of papers, is that of R. Bruce Ross (in McCarthy, 1990). This is a broad and balanced account of the problem of facial growth in cleft lip with or without cleft palate. His main conclusions are:

- The intrinsic defect in an individual is mild except in the immediate area of the cleft.
- The potential for growth of the maxillary complex is adequate to produce harmonious skeletal relationships.
- The teeth and alveolar bone have the capacity to overcome deficiencies in the maxillary complex and produce a satisfactory occlusion.
- Surgery produces scar tissue that interferes with maxillary growth. It is not necessary that this should be a severe restriction. Any reduction in maxillary growth can be significant for children with cleft lip and palate.
- Surgery produces scar tissue in the palate that prevents the free adjustment of the teeth and causes distortion of the dental arch by deflecting the eruption of the teeth.
- Secondary changes in tongue position cause displacement and deformation of the mandible.
- Early repair of the alveolus, with or without bone grafting, is detrimental to facial growth.
- The most important variable in cleft palate surgery is the surgeon. The traditional techniques do not exert appreciably different influences on facial growth.
- The timing of hard palate repair within the first decade is not critical. There is no advantage in delaying repair for up to four to seven years.

The debate concerning the possible deleterious effects of surgery, the timing of palatal repair and the suggestion of delayed hard palate closure first arose nearly 80 years ago (Gillies and Fry, 1921). This is probably the earliest published account suggesting the potential deleterious effects of surgical closure in cleft palate subjects. The controversy has persisted to the present. They were forthright in their statements.

> All unoperated hard palate cases have normal occlusion of the non involved teeth. Nearly all operated hard palates have abnormal occlusion of the non involved teeth. In any case of malocclusion of the teeth in an operated palate such a serious defect may definitely be assigned to the results of the operation and would not have occurred had the hard palate been left alone. (Gillies and Fry, 1921)

These authors advocate closure of the soft palate and delayed closure of the hard palate with a prosthetic obturator placed until possible eventual surgical closure. Such a regimen has been enthusiastically and controversially carried out to the present day (Schweckendiek, 1978; Hotz et al.,

1978). Delayed hard palate closure was further recommended in other early papers (Rayner, 1925).

Adult unoperated cleft lip and palate studies

Adults with unoperated clefts of the lip and palate provide the ideal control group for investigators studying the natural history of facial growth and morphology in these subjects. The absence of surgical intervention provides an opportunity to study the outcome of facial growth, morphology and speech using an absolute comparative baseline. When this group is compared to conventionally operated subjects, an evaluation of the intrinsic versus the potential iatrogenic influences can be separately analysed. Withdrawal of surgery for research purposes would be unethical where such facilities are available. Likewise, assignment to surgical or non-surgical management programmes on a prospective random allocation basis could not be permitted. For these reasons, studies on the unoperated subject have been made on individuals from the developing world, where surgery may not be readily available.

The concept of studying unoperated clefts is not new. The most frequently quoted work is that of Ortiz-Monasterio et al. (1959, 1966, 1974). In the first of these, they claim that 'early surgery in the first few years of life and repeated and aggressive surgery will produce under-development of the maxilla'. Their impression is that a greater percentage of growth defects is produced in early palate closure (18–24 months): 'Even when treatment is performed by the most able hands'. Quoting Brodie (1941) Slaughter and Brodie (1949), Graber (1949) and Broadbent (1937), Ortiz-Monasterio et al. (1974) conclude that four-fifths of the total facial growth takes place in the first five years of life. Furthermore, they claim that patients operated on after five years of age have normal facial development. No evidence is provided to support this claim. It is claimed that in unoperated subjects forward growth of the maxilla is normal, or even greater than normal. These studies conclude that embryonic factors responsible for cleft lip and palate do not interfere with maxillary growth and that middle third facial growth defects are caused by early or repeated and aggressive surgery. Delayed palatal closure is recommended, preferably at five years coupled with an active speech therapy intervention programme. Sadly, the view that facial growth is four-fifths completed by five years has been perpetuated in the literature and in surgical protocols (Hotz, 1969). Whilst the absolute length and dimensions of the maxilla as an isolated bony complex are important, the position of this complex in its relation to the craniofacial form and in partic-ular the cranial base, from where it is propelled downwards and forwards, is of greater significance. The answer to the question as to why patients are experiencing growth problems in the post pubertal period, but often not in the pre-pubertal period, is because there is a lack of displacement of the maxilla from the cranial base, rather than failure of absolute growth of the maxilla. It is conceivable that pursuing the delayed palate surgery protocol may not only compromise speech but may still lead to poor facial growth (Ross, 1987e; Witzel et al., 1984).

In studies of large numbers of unoperated unilateral cleft lip and palate subjects from Sri Lanka (Mars and Houston, 1990; Mars, 1993), the following conclusions were drawn:

• Subjects with unoperated cleft lip and palate have the potential for normal facial growth. Indeed, because there is not an intact lip, maxillary growth is unrestrained and exuberant.
• Lip surgery in infancy, without palatal surgery, results in near normal facial growth with some retroclination of the upper incisor teeth.
• Palatal surgery in infancy has the potential to cause severe mid-face retrusion.
• The mandible in operated unilateral cleft lip and palate subjects is both smaller and retropositioned.

Figures 4.8a and 4.8b illustrate measurements for maxillary protrusion for four groups of Sri Lankan subjects: (1) normal healthy non clefts; (2) totally unoperated subjects (Figure 4.9); (3) subjects who had lip surgery but not palatal surgery in infancy; (4) subjects who had lip and palate surgery in infancy.

A study of similar design to the Sri Lankan project has been reported from Brazil (Capelozza et al., 1996). Quoting the earlier paper from Sri Lanka (Mars and Houston 1990), they point out that there is little difference in maxillary length between subjects who had had lip repair and those who had had lip and palate repair. They conclude, therefore, that lip surgery is responsible for mid-face retrusion, at least to an equal degree as palatal surgery. This paper selects just one parameter, maxillary length, as the basis for this conclusion, but ignores the major differences in all measures of maxillary protrusion and maxillary/mandibular relationships, which show dramatically better results for the 'lip surgery group' than for the 'lip and palate surgery group' in the Sri Lankan studies. Further, the results of the Goslon Yardstick analysis (Mars et al., 1987) clearly demonstrate that very few subjects who have had lip repair are assigned to groups 4 and 5 (the most severe maxillary retrusion requiring maxillary advancement osteotomy), whereas, 50% of those who have had lip and palate repair present in groups 4 and 5 (Mars and Houston, 1990).

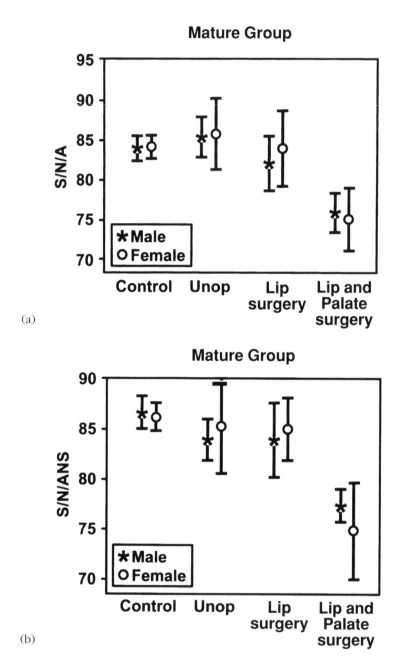

(a)

(b)

Figure 4.8. (a) The different measures for the value S/N/A, demonstrating excessive protrusion of the maxilla in unoperated subjects, and retrusion for those with lip and palate surgery in infancy. Those who have had lip repair only show only mild retrusion. (b) The value S/N/ANS, represents basal bone protrusion as opposed to dento-alveolar bone. Basal bone is unaffected by lip repair but is affected by lip and palate repair.

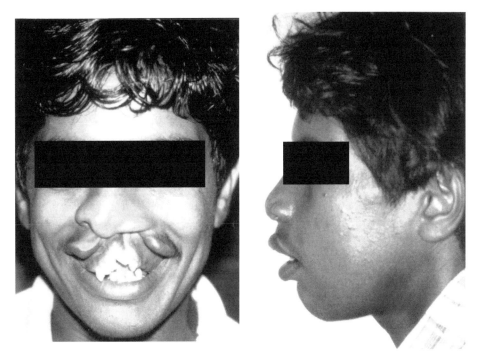

Figure 4.9. The full face and profile of an adult unoperated unilateral cleft lip and palate subject.

Clearly, the effect of lip repair on the dento-alveolar process can be considerable, but the effects at the basal bony maxilla are small. The precise absolute length of the maxilla, whilst important, should be considered in relation to its *position* in the facio-maxillary complex. It is clear that when palatal surgery is undertaken the downward and forward movement of the maxilla and its subsequent propulsion from the cranial base is compromised – and this is why many such patients demonstrate concave profiles. This disruption to the translocation of the maxilla from the cranial base is thought to be caused by bands of scar tissue created around the circum-maxillary sutures at palate repair (Figure 4.10).

Subsequent analysis of somatic growth of Sri Lankan patients has revealed that the onset of puberty is much later in normal Sri Lankans, as well as those with cleft lip and palate, than in Western populations (Balasuriya and Fernando, 1983; Habel et al., 1996). Small maxillae previously reported (Mars, 1990) in the Sri Lankan material may have resulted from the erroneous pooling of pre- and post-pubertal subjects into one group. In a subsequent study (Mars, 1993) it was shown that Sri Lankan boys could not be considered to be post-pubertal until 20 years of age, and girls until 18 years of age. The separation into pre- and post-pubertal groups

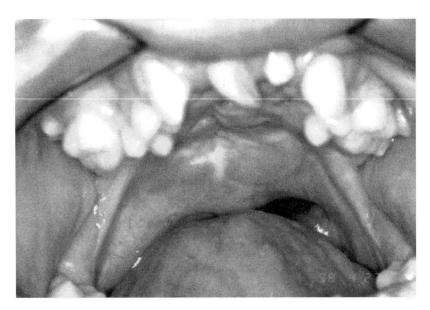

Figure 4.10. Bands of scar tissue in the maxilla.

based on these new ages has revealed significant and dramatic differences for somatic and facial growth dimensions, demonstrating continuing growth in the pre-pubertal groups who have a mean age of 15.5 years.

Figure 4.11 shows the differences in maxillary length for the pre- and post-pubertal groups. The considerable difference that further growth makes in the lip surgery group should be noted.

In general, the consensus relating to unoperated cleft lip and palate subjects suggests that they have the potential for near normal facial growth. Mid-face depth, the parameter of most concern, is not compromised in unoperated subjects. Whilst mid-face distortion does not occur in all cases of operated cleft lip and palate, when it does so, it is iatrogenic rather than intrinsic in origin.

The pubertal growth spurt

A significant feature of facial growth in repaired cleft and palate subjects is that the maxilla fails to grow at the same rate as the mandible during the adolescent growth spurt. Many children present with pleasing facial profiles and appearance at around ten years of age, but then display progressive mid-facial retrusion by the mid to late teens (Figures 4.12 and 4.13).

To date, it has not been possible to predict accurately which patients will develop mid-face retrusion during puberty. However, evidence of poor mid-face growth before puberty is indicative of a very poor outcome.

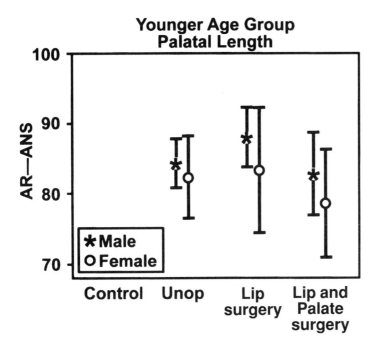

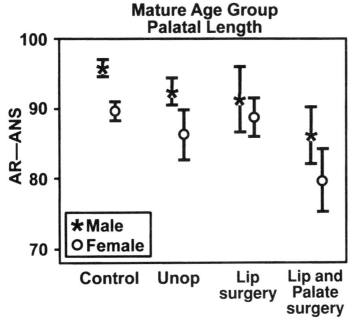

Figure 4.11. Maxillary length in pre- and post-pubertal Sri Lankan patients. Note the large change of those who have undergone lip surgery but not palatal surgery.

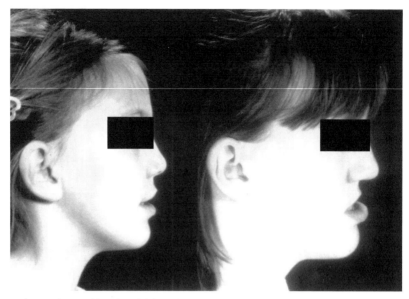

Figure 4.12. The profile of a child with repaired unilateral cleft lip and palate at 10 years of age, and at 16 years of age.

Age (years)

11.1   15.1   16.5

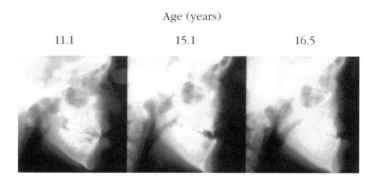

Figure 4.13. The lateral skull radiographs of the same child as in Figure 4.12 showing progressive concavity of the facial profile. Analysis shows that the maxilla has become 'stuck' on the cranial base.

Different cleft types

Most studies are undertaken on unilateral complete cleft palate subjects because these are the largest subgroup of cleft patients. Studies on bilateral cleft lip and palate subjects are few. They show an obvious tendency to premaxillary protrusion though, as in unilateral cleft lip and palate subjects, this protrusion decreases with age (Semb, 1991b).

Subjects with isolated cleft palate are often associated with syndromic conditions and results from potentially mixed cleft types should be cautiously interpreted. The classical Danish study remains the most reliable (Dahl, 1970). Operated subjects demonstrate both smaller mandibles and maxillae with high gonial angles and reduced posterior face heights.

Variability of outcome and cross-centre studies

Outcome studies between different centres have demonstrated considerable variation in the quality of results (Ross, 1987a, 1987b, 1987c, 1987d, 1987e, 1987f, 1987g; Mars et al., 1987; Shaw et al., 1992; Mars, 1993).

The first British cross-centre study introduced a new system of analysis, the Goslon Yardstick (Mars et al., 1987). This has subsequently been employed in the European cross-centre study (Mars et al., 1992 and the Clinical Standards Advisory Group (CSAG, 1998). This coarse, but reliable and robust yardstick displays the outcome of dental arch relationships in five groups: groups 1 and 2 being excellent or good; group 3, satisfactory; and groups 4 and 5 poor or very poor. The groupings correlate closely with cephalometric analyses and may be considered as a simple way of assessing and demonstrating facial growth outcome (Mars and Plint, 1985).

Figure 4.14 shows the Goslon graphs from the GOS Oslo study (Mars et al., 1987) relating to patients born between 1960 and 1970. Figure 4.15 shows the Goslon graphs for the Eurocleft Study together with the North Thames East recent study. It should be noted that patients in groups 4 and 5 require maxillary advancement osteotomies to restore facial harmony.

Clearly, future studies need to investigate the factors that lead either to good or to poor outcome. Whilst high volume centres do not guarantee good outcome, they do provide the means whereby such outcome can be monitored and assessed.

Growth and speech outcomes

Whilst consideration of facial growth outcome in cleft lip and palate patients has been the preoccupation of orthodontists, this has often been to the exclusion of other aspects of care, especially speech (Morris, 1990). Orthodontists and surgeons pursuing the goal of good facial growth have not infrequently advocated surgical protocols in which the potential for compromised speech has been ignored (Schweckendiek, 1978; Rayner, 1925; Witzel et al., 1984). It has been considered to be axiomatic that the goals of good speech and good facial growth are mutually exclusive. Speech and language therapists and orthodontists have appeared to be pulling their surgical colleagues from opposite poles. A recent study of

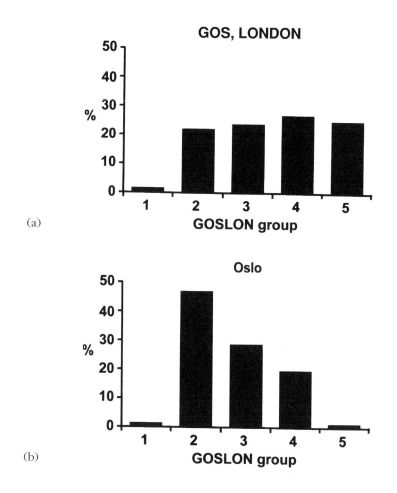

Figure 4.14. The Goslon grouping of an historic sample from (a) Great Ormond Street (GOS) London, and (b) Oslo. Subjects in groups 4 and 5 are candidates for mid-face advancement surgery, whereas subjects in groups 1 and 2 showed good facial growth.

outcome for North East Thames (Sommerlad et al., 1997) has demonstrated that it is possible to achieve both good speech and good facial growth. In this study palatal surgery is undertaken before one year of age, but crucially involves a minimal dissection and incision procedure in which periosteal flaps are elevated only minimally from bone. It would seem that the nature of surgery and the skill of the operator, not the precise timing of surgery, are the important factors determining the outcome of facial growth. The classical Wardill–Kilner pushback procedure now seems to be obsolescent if not obsolete.

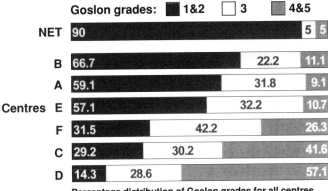

Figure 4.15. The Goslon outcome scores for six European centres and Northeast Thames.

The results of speech studies from the Sri Lankan Cleft Lip and Palate Project clearly demonstrate that when palatal surgery is delayed, certainly after three years of age, then speech is likely to be impaired and that even after repair this is likely to be permanently compromised (Sell et al., 1990; Sell, 1992; Nayak, 1996).

The Goslon Yardstick and speech outcome of delayed surgery are displayed in Figures 4.16 and 4.17. These clearly demonstrate an inverse relationship for speech and growth outcomes in delayed palate repair where good growth but poor speech results. In the overall rehabilitation of patients, according priority to either good speech or good facial growth is likely to result in overall failure for the patient.

Longitudinal facial growth studies

The value of longitudinal growth studies is demonstrated from two centres in Scandinavia (Enemark et al., 1990; Semb, 1991a). It is especially interesting to note that both centres have large samples of consecutively treated patients – a reflection of the value of centralized care for cleft lip and palate patients in Denmark and Norway (Shaw et al., 1992).

In the first of these papers 57 complete unilateral cleft lip and palate subjects operated upon in infancy, were followed longitudinally from birth to 21 years of age. Cephalometry was performed at ages 5, 8, 12, 16 and 21 years. Enemark states, 'None of our patients demonstrated a normal growth pattern'.

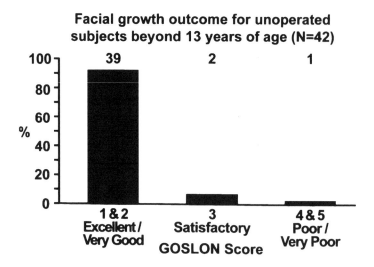

Figure 4.16.

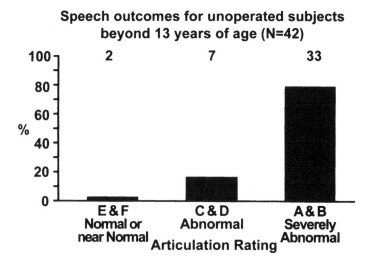

Figure 4.17.

Figures 4.16 and 4.17. The Goslon and articulation ratings showing the inverse relationship of the quality of facial growth outcome and speech outcome for unoperated Sri Lankan unilateral cleft lip and palate subjects.

A reduction of maxillary protrusion of 7 degrees measured by S/N/A, and 4 degrees measured by S/N/ANS, was noted from 5 to 21 years of age (angular measurements from the cranial base to points on the anterior of the maxilla; ANS, the anterior nasal spine, is a basal bone structure, whilst the A point is related to the dentition). This paper (Enemark et al., 1990) demonstrates the differing effects of lip and palate surgery at the dento-alveolar level (around A) and the basal level (around ANS), the A point showing more deleterious retrusion with age than the latter (Figure 4.18).

In a commentary on the above paper (Aduss, 1990), this problem is addressed: 'In short, A is not a good landmark for assessing craniofacial growth in patients with complete unilateral cleft lip and palate'.

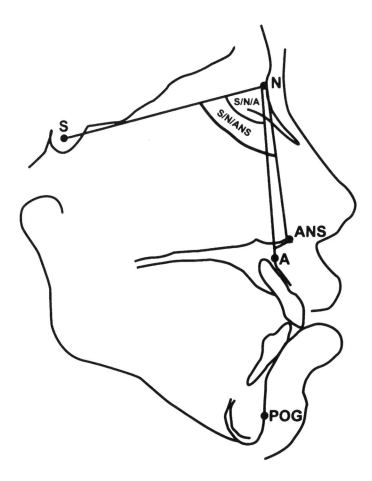

Figure 4.18. A linear diagram displaying the measures S/N/A and S/N/ANS, and bony chin point pogonion.

The facial growth study using the Oslo archive (Semb, 1991a) is quite outstanding in its sheer size and thoroughness: 257 patients, with yearly lateral skull radiographs in approximately 130 subjects (a tribute to the late Professor Olav Bergland).

The results conform to those of previous cephalometric descriptions for individuals with unilateral cleft lip and palate: a short, retrusive maxilla, and vertical elongation of the anterior face (even though the upper face is shorter), a retrusive mandible and a reduction in posterior face height is noted.

The raw data for males and females are presented separately, but are also pooled and presented as a total for the whole sample. It is considered that facial form is essentially the same in both sexes but that males are larger than females. This pooling has obscured several important differences between the sexes during the pubertal growth phase, which become evident when the raw data for the separate sexes are scrutinized. The decreasing values of S/N/ANS and S/N/A reach their minima at 16 years of age for boys but at 12 years for girls. The increasing values for N/A/PG likewise reach their maxima at 16 years of age for boys but at 12 years for girls. Clearly, females are suffering the adverse growth effects of surgery earlier than males, but males do continue to deteriorate to a greater extent and for a longer period than females. These findings are in conformity with somatic growth studies relating to the different onset of pubertal growth spurts in boys and girls (Eveleth, 1975; Eveleth and Tanner, 1990), support the separate study of males and females, especially during a period of pubertal growth which has different potential and different onset and termination in males and females. The clinical significance of such sexual dimorphism is of considerable importance because orthodontic treatment often commences during the pubertal period, and the need for maxillary osteotomy in some patients needs to be related to the termination of facial growth.

Summary

Facial growth is an extremely complex subject. The precise processes are still poorly understood and facial growth prediction remains unreliable and imprecise. Facial growth in cleft lip and palate subjects is unquestionably disturbed. Whilst there is an intrinsic defect, surgery itself contributes to further disruption. There is evidence that minimally invasive surgery produces less disturbance to facial growth than historical techniques which are now obsolescent. Careful measurements of outcome from fewer high volume centres should provide insights into the factors producing the best results.

References

Aduss H (1971) Craniofacial growth in complete unilateral cleft lip and palate. Angle Orthodontist 41: 202–213.

Aduss H (1990) Commentary on evaluation of unilateral cleft lip and palate treatment: long term results (Enemark et al). Cleft Palate Journal 27: 361.

Balasuriya S, Fernando MA (1983) Age at menarche in three districts in Sri Lanka. Ceylon Medical Journal 28: 227–231.

Bardach J (1990) Research revisited: the influence of cleft lip repair on facial growth. Cleft Palate Journal 27: 76–78.

Bill AH, Moore AW, Coe HE (1956) The time of choice for repair of cleft palate in relation to the type of surgical repair and its effect on bony growth of the face. Plastic and Reconstructive Surgery 18: 469–473.

Brattstrom V, McWilliam J, Semb G (1991) Cephalometric scaling methodology in limited samples. European Journal of Orthodontics 13: 157–160.

Broadbent BM (1937) Face of normal child. Angle Orthodontist 7: 183–208.

Brodie AG (1941) Behaviour of normal and abnormal facial growth patterns. American Journal of Orthodontics 27: 633–647.

Capelozza FL, Normando AD, da Silva FOG (1996) Isolated influences of lip and palate surgery on facial growth: comparison of operated and unoperated male adults with UCLP. Cleft Palate–Craniofacial Journal 33: 51-56.

CSAG Report – Clinical Standards Advisory Group (1998) Cleft Lip and Palate. London: HMSO.

Dahl E (1970) Craniofacial morphology in congenital clefts of the lip and palate. Acta Odontologica Scandinavica 28 (Suppl. 57): 11.

Enemark H, Bolund S, Jorgensen I (1990) Evaluation of unilateral cleft lip and palate treatment: long term results. Cleft Palate Journal 27: 354–361.

Eveleth PB (1975) Differences between ethnic groups in sex dimorphism of adult height. Annals of Human Biology 2: 35–39.

Eveleth PB, Tanner JM (1990) Worldwide Variation in Human Growth. Cambridge: Cambridge University Press.

Gillies HD, Fry KW (1921) A new principle in the surgical treatment of congenital cleft palate and its mechanical counterpart. British Medical Journal i: 335–338.

Graber TM (1949) A cephalometric analysis of the developmental pattern and facial morphology in cleft palate. Angle Orthodontist 19: 91–97.

Habel A, Sell D, Mars M (1996) Management of cleft lip and palate. Archives of Disease in Childhood 74(4): 360–366.

Hagerty RF, Andrews EB, Hill M, Calcote C, Karesh S, Lifschiz J, Swindler D (1964) Dental arch collapse in cleft palate. Angle Orthodontist 34: 25–35.

Hotz RP (1969) The role of orthodontics in treatment management of cleft lip and palate. Cleft Palate Journal 7: 371–379.

Hotz MM, Gnoinski WM, Nussbaumer H, Kistler E (1978) Early maxillary orthopedics in CLP cases: guidelines for surgery. Cleft Palate Journal 15: 405–411.

Mars M (1993) PhD, The effects of surgery on facial growth and morphology in Sri Lankan unilateral cleft lip and palate subjects. University of London.

Mars M, Houston WJB (1990) A preliminary study of facial growth and morphology in unoperated male unilateral cleft lip and palate subjects over 13 years of age. Cleft Palate Journal 27: 7–10.

Mars M, Plint DA (1985) Correlation of Goslon Yardstick results and cephalometric analysis. Fifth International Congress on Cleft Palate and Related Craniofacial Anomalies, Monaco.

Mars M, Plint DA, Houston WJB, Bergland O, Semb G (1987) The Goslon Yardstick: a new system of assessing dental arch relationships in children with unilateral clefts of the lip and palate. Cleft Palate Journal 24: 314–322.

Mars M, Asher-McDade C, Brattstrom V, Dahl E, McWilliam J, Molsted K, Plint DA, Prahl-Andersen B, Semb G, Shaw, The RPS (1992) A six-centre international study of treatment outcome in patients with clefts of the lip and palate: Part 3, dental arch relationships. Cleft Palate Journal 29: 405–408.

McCarthy JG (ed.) (1990) Plastic Surgery: Vol. 4, Cleft Lip and Palate and Cranio Facial Anomalies, Ch. 49. Philadelphia: WB Saunders.

Morris HL (1990) Surgery, speech and growth. Paper presented at the First International Meeting of the Craniofacial Society of Great Britain, 1983. In: Huddart A, Ferguson M (eds) Cleft Lip and Palate: Long-term Results and Future Prospects. Manchester: Manchester University Press, pp. 420–429.

Nayak J (1996) A systematic study correlating speech results of Sri Lankan unilateral cleft lip and palate participants (aged 10–13) with timing of surgery. MSc, University of London.

Ortiz-Monasterio F, Rebeil AF, Valderrama M, Cruz R (1959) Cephalometric measurements on adult patients with nonoperated cleft palates. Plastic and Reconstructive Surgery 24: 53–61.

Ortiz-Monasterio F, Serrano A, Barrera G and Rodriguez-Hoffman H (1966) A study of untreated adult cleft palate patients. Plastic and Reconstructive Surgery 38: 36–41.

Ortiz-Monasterio F, Olmedo A, Trigos I, Yudovich M, Velazquez M, Fuente-del-Campo A (1974) Final results from the delayed treatment of patients with clefts of the lip and palate. Scandinavian Journal of Plastic and Reconstructive Surgery 8: 109–115.

Rayner HH (1925) The operative treatment of cleft palate. Lancet i: 816.

Ross RB (1986) Growth prediction in cleft lip and palate. Transactions of the British Craniofacial Society International Conference.

Ross RB (1987a) Treatment variables affecting facial growth in complete unilateral cleft lip and palate: Part 1. Cleft Palate Journal 24: 5–23.

Ross RB (1987b) Treatment variables affecting facial growth in complete unilateral cleft lip palate: Part 2, Presurgical orthopedics. Cleft Palate Journal 24: 24–32.

Ross RB (1987c) Treatment variables affecting facial growth in complete unilateral cleft lip palate: Part 3, Alveolar repair and bone grafting. Cleft Palate Journal 24: 33–44.

Ross RB (1987d) Treatment variables affecting facial growth in complete unilateral cleft lip palate: Part 4, Cleft lip repair. Cleft Palate Journal 24: 45–53.

Ross RB (1987e) Treatment variables affecting facial growth in complete unilateral cleft lip palate: Part 5, Timing of cleft palate repair. Cleft Palate Journal 24: 54–63.

Ross RB (1987f) Treatment variables affecting facial growth in complete unilateral cleft lip palate: Part 6, Techniques of cleft palate repair. Cleft Palate Journal 24: 64–70.

Ross RB (1987g) Treatment variables affecting facial growth in complete unilateral cleft lip palate: Part 7, An overview. Cleft Palate Journal 24: 71–77.

Ross RB (1990) In: McCarthy JG (ed.) Plastic Surgery: Vol. 4, Cleft Lip and Palate and Craniofacial Anomalies. Philadelphia: WB Saunders, Ch. 49, pp. 2553–2580.

Ross RB, Johnston MC (1972) Cleft Lip and Palate. Baltimore: Williams & Wilkins.

Schweckendiek W (1978) Primary veloplasty: long term results without maxillary deformity. A twenty-five year report. Cleft Palate Journal 15: 268–274.

Sell D (1992) Speech in Sri Lankan cleft palates subjects with delayed palatoplasty. PhD thesis, De Montfort University.

Sell D, Grunwell P, Mars M (1990) Preliminary speech results in a subgroup of unoperated Sri Lankan cleft lip and adolescents following late palatal surgery. Cleft Palate Journal 27: 162–168.

Semb G (1991a) A study of facial growth in patients with unilateral cleft lip and palate treated by the Oslo CLP team. Cleft Palate Journal 28: 1–21.

Semb G (1991b) A study of facial growth in patients with bilateral cleft lip and palate treated by the Oslo CLP team. Cleft Palate Journal 28: 22–39.

Shaw WC, Asher-McDade C, Brattstrom V, Dahl E, Mars M, McWilliam J, Molsted K, Plint, DA, Prahl-Andersen B, Semb G, The RPS (1992) A six-centre international study of treatment outcome in patients with clefts of the lip and palate: Part 1, Principles and study design. Cleft Palate Journal 29: 393–397.

Slaughter WB, Brodie AG (1949) Facial clefts and their surgical management. Plastic and Reconstructive Surgery 4: 311–332.

Sommerlad B et al. (1997) Facial growth outcomes for the North East Thames (St Andrews) cleft lip and palate centre, a comparison with the Eurocleft results using the Goslon Yardstick. Proceedings of the Craniofacial Society of Great Britain.

Witzel MA, Salyer K, Ross RB (1984) Delayed hard palate closure: the philosophy revisited. Cleft Palate Journal 21: 263–269.

CHAPTER 5

Speech and Cleft Palate/ Velopharyngeal Anomalies

P. GRUNWELL AND D.A. SELL

Introduction

Initial attempts at cleft palate closure focused on the anatomical closure of the cleft and were associated with very unsatisfactory speech results, facial growth and dentition. From around 1925 onwards, there was a shift to an interest in outcome, as understanding of the anatomical and functional requirements for speech increased, and the risks of surgery decreased with the advent of antibiotics, transfusions and anaesthesia. Speech performance then became one of the criteria by which the operative procedure was judged, the other being facial growth (see Mars, Chapter 4), especially in relation to the timing and nature of primary surgery (see Watson, Chapter 12). In the past the evaluation of speech outcome has not always drawn upon appropriate expertise, as emphasized by Jackson et al. (1983): "the main contributions that have revolutionized cleft palate surgery over the years more often than not do not contain representatives from the speech world". Fortunately, more recently this situation has changed and speech and language therapists are accepted as equal and valued members of the interdisciplinary team (Sommerlad et al., 1996; Sandy et al., 1998; Mars et al., 1990; Eurocleft Speech Group, 1993, 2000; Scancleft, work in progress).

Speech is an important and still controversial outcome at several stages in the management of cleft lip and palate from birth to maturity. There are still many different surgical regimes with different timing and sequences of palate closure and inconclusive evidence with regard to speech outcome (see Watson, Chapter 12). The importance of the emerging pattern of speech development and the preventative role of speech and language therapy during this period have recently been recognized (LeBlanc, 1996; see Russell and Harding, Chapter 14). Furthermore speech is the primary outcome measure for velopharyngeal management (see Mercer and Pigott,

Chapter 17), and there remains controversy over the effects of maxillary advancement on speech production (see Lello, Chapter 21, and Sell and Grunwell, Chapter 16).

In recognizing the primary importance of speech, this chapter begins with an overview of the incidence of speech problems, followed by a description of some of the difficulties in measuring speech outcome which probably account in part for the large variation in prevalence/incidence figures. Nevertheless there are some common findings, which recur in the literature, and these are briefly summarized. This is followed by a discussion of the physical production of speech in the context of speech motor control and an introduction to a phonetic and linguistic framework for approaching speech disorders associated with cleft palate/velopharyngeal anomalies. Although traditionally, the medical model has been employed, focusing on structure and function, such an approach does not take account of the structure and function of spoken language. The two approaches used together usefully inform each other. This section is followed by a description of the characteristics of cleft palate speech from a phonetic perspective, which leads into a discussion of the speech patterns that have been observed by different authorities. Finally there is a discussion of the aetiology of speech difficulties in the context of cleft palate/velopharyngeal anomalies.

Incidence of speech problems

Differing figures are quoted for the incidence/prevalence of speech problems. In part this reflects changes in practice, such as the timing of palate surgery, but a major drawback has been the many and differing approaches to the measurement of speech. For example, Spreistersbach et al. (1973) estimated that 50% of children with cleft palate repairs develop normal speech spontaneously, 25% require speech and language therapy and 25% need secondary velopharyngeal surgery. Although not explicitly stated, it is highly likely that this latter group would also require speech therapy intervention. More recently Hall and Golding-Kushner (1989) stated that approximately 80% of children born with cleft lip and palate who have surgery before the age of 18 months develop speech that does not require any type of therapeutic intervention. Witzel (1991), in contrast, stated that following palate repair about 25% of cleft lip and palate patients develop normal speech spontaneously, but the remaining 75% require episodes of speech therapy throughout childhood and adolescence to achieve acceptable speech production.

The incidence of velopharyngeal insufficiency following primary palate repair varies across studies from 5 to 40% (McWilliams et al., 1990; Enderby and Emerson, 1995), reflecting either actual differences in treatment outcome or differences in methodology and assessment techniques. Morris (1973) and Spreistersbach et al. (1973) reported the incidence of velopharyngeal incompetence as 25%. More recently Peterson-Falzone (1990) described a prevalence of 16% of velopharyngeal insufficiency as the current average reported by centres, although she also stated that it could be as high as 40% when applying a strict criterion of normal speech. Often hyponasality, inaudible nasal escape, or inconsistent audible nasal escape/hypernasality have been categorized as normal outcomes. Even more recently both the Eurocleft Speech Study of children with unilateral cleft lip and palate aged between 11 and 14 years (Eurocleft Speech Group, 1993) and the United Kingdom national CSAG UCLP study (age range 5–6 and 11–12 years of age) found that approximately 27% of patients had hypernasality following primary surgery (CSAG Report, 1998; Sandy et al., 1998).

With regard to the need for speech and language therapy intervention, studies report similar findings. Two-thirds of children with cleft palate repairs are estimated to receive speech therapy (Dalston, 1990; Albery and Grunwell, 1993; Sell et al., 2000). Hall and Golding-Kushner (1989) stated that 20% had severe problems for whom 'the road to normal speech is long and arduous', requiring long-term speech therapy intervention. They found that approximately two thirds of patients required therapy, which is almost identical to the findings of Dalston (1990).

Methodological issues

Some of the variation in prevalence figures is in part attributable to the wide-ranging speech methodologies used, making detailed comparison of the results of different studies of cleft palate speech difficult, if not invalid. Details of patient characteristics have in the past been unclear or unspecified. At the extreme, for example, unrepaired and repaired subjects have been studied as one group (Spreistersbach et al., 1956; Spreistersbach and Powers, 1959; Byrne et al., 1961; Skoog, 1965). Some studies report results in which all cleft palate children in one centre are included, whereas in others only children with speech problems are included. Some of the other methodological flaws include the lack of specification of age at surgery (Morris, 1973), and at assessment, and the reporting of results with mixed cleft types. Furthermore, the reporting of results at different times postoperatively makes comparison between studies difficult as maturation and/or therapy intervention may have taken place. In several studies professionals other than speech and language therapists have reported speech results, with no evidence of inter- and intra-assessor reliability (Moll, 1968). Even when the speech and language therapist carried out the assessment, listener reliability studies were not always carried out (Greene, 1960). There has been wide variation in the types of speech samples studied. Data have been collected and analysed in different formats, e.g. audiotape recordings, video-tape recordings, live recordings using detailed phonetic transcription (Grunwell, 1993). Different stimuli have been used to elicit responses and different criteria to score responses. Indeed one of the most fundamental methodological problems has been the lack of an acceptable framework for measuring speech, such that no single framework has been agreed and used across studies (McComb, 1989). Even the parameters of speech, which are agreed upon as essential, do not have universally accepted approaches. For example, the parameter of hypernasality may be rated in one study on a three-point scale and by a six-point scale in another study, again making comparisons between studies difficult. Furthermore, a comparison of specific articulation characteristics is difficult when errors are interpreted differently. For example, palatal plosives are classified as compensatory errors in the American literature, anterior errors in the UK literature and retracted errors in the Swedish literature, making the interpretation and comparison of different studies again very difficult (Trost, 1981; Harding et al., 1997; Sell, Harding and Grunwell 1994, 1999; Lohmander-Agerskov 1996).

Common findings

Early studies by speech and language therapists/pathologists reported on the nature of cleft palate speech. These studies were almost exclusively presented in a traditional phonetic framework of error analysis now recognized as rather limited (Grunwell, 1987; see Sell and Grunwell, Chapter 16). Another shortcoming of these studies was the tendency to attribute all artic-ulatory disturbances to velopharyngeal insufficiency. The fact that other factors, for example the developmental dimension of speech, might influence performance was frequently overlooked. Since 1960, however, Morris (1981) reports an increase in awareness of the range of factors that may influence speech outcome.

Despite the many methodological issues described there are some commonly recurring findings that have stood the test of time:

- Individuals with cleft palate are at high risk of disordered articulation (Spreistersbach et al., 1956; Counihan, 1960; Morris, 1962; Bzoch, 1965; Philips and Harrison, 1969; Fletcher, 1978; Van Demark et al., 1979).
- The nature of disordered articulation is heterogeneous in presentation (Moll, 1968; Spreistersbach et al., 1961; Riski and Delong, 1984; Philips and Harrison, 1969).

- Plosives /pb td kg/, fricatives /fv sz ʃ/ and affricates /tʃ ʤ/ have been found to be more often affected than the other phonetic classes of nasals /m n ŋ/ and glides /j/ and /w/ (Bzoch, 1965; Spreistersbach et al., 1956; Counihan, 1960; Moll, 1968; Van Demark, 1969; Philips and Harrison, 1969). These are the so-called 'pressure consonants' which are particularly vulnerable when there is velopharyngeal dysfunction (VPD) or velopharyngeal insufficiency (VPI).
- One common finding is the tendency for anterior tongue placements to be shifted backwards in speakers with cleft palate (Brooks et al., 1965, 1966; Morley, 1970; Lawrence and Phillips, 1975; Trost, 1981).
- Articulation improves with advancing age although the rate of improvement slows after ten years of age (Van Demark, 1969, 1979; Harding and Grunwell, 1993; CSAG Report, 1998).
- Severity of speech problems has been shown to increase with severity of cleft type (Morley, 1970; Moll, 1968; Fletcher, 1978; Riski and Delong, 1984; McWilliams et al., 1990; Karling et al., 1993; Albery and Grunwell, 1993).

Normal speech production

In normal speech production the processes of phonation, resonance and articulation are intimately related. The action of the velopharyngeal sphincter ensures that these processes are produced effectively. If the velopharyngeal sphincter is dysfunctional, then this can have adverse consequences for phonation, resonance and articulation (Stengelhofen, 1989; McWilliams et al., 1990; Wyatt et al., 1996). Indeed Warren (1986) describes a finely balanced speech regulating system: deviant articulatory gestures, such as pharyngeal fricative and glottal stop, may develop in an attempt to satisfy the requirements of a regulating system.

Equally any anatomical or physiological disturbances in these processes can have linguistic consequences for an individual. Disturbances in articulation and resonance, in particular, may result in failures to signal significant differences between speech sounds, thus resulting in both phonetic and phonological disorders. This in turn may lead to failures to communicate adequately, which may result in a breakdown in communication and an inability to elicit reciprocal reinforcing and enhancing responses from the listener. For a child in the early stages of language development, this cycle of failure can be potentially very damaging, not only to speech development but also to lexical and grammatical development (see Russell and Harding, Chapter 14).

The phonetic and phonologic perspective

Until relatively recently all articulation disorders including 'cleft palate speech' were described from an articulatory and phonetic perspective (see

further below). Since the 1970s phonological principles have been introduced to the study of disordered speech. Therefore a contemporary
perspective on speech and language in individuals with cleft
palate/velopharyngeal anomalies needs to be set in a phonetic
and linguistic developmental framework. Phonology is concerned with
evaluating an individual's ability to signal differences in meaning. In
other words the term articulation refers to the peripheral motor activity
whereas phonology refers to the speaker's knowledge of the sound
system and the rules that govern it. Stoel-Gammon and Dunn (1985) state
that:

> Phonology refers to the organization and classification of speech sounds that
> occur as contrastive units within a language, as well as speech perception and
> production, cognitive and motor aspects of speech.

Crystal (1981) underlined how important it is to use both phonetic and
phonological principles in the study of the speech of cleft palate children:

> ... in order to determine the extent to which an adequate phonological system is
> being obscured by purely phonetic deviance, or whether there is in addition an
> underlying disturbance of a phonological type; if the latter, whether it is
> something unique to the cleft palate condition, or a manifestation of some
> general pattern of delay.

A child with a phonetic deviance or delay has difficulty in physically articu-
lating certain consonants in the language. He/she is unable to, or does not,
articulate certain sounds. A phonetic deviance affecting the child's ability to
signal meaning differences results in a phonological deficit. For example,
backing of alveolar consonants, a typical speech cleft type characteristic,
results in the loss of contrasts between /t/ and /k/, and /d/ and /g/ (see
Russell and Harding, Chapter 14). There is also the possibility that a child is
aware of the need to signal phonological differences (i.e. is phonologically
'able') but is physically unable to achieve the appropriate articulatory
and/or resonatory position (i.e. is phonetically 'disabled') (see Hewlett,
1990). This may result in the child actively endeavouring to produce atypical
speech sounds, or 'compensatory articulations' (Trost 1981; see further
below) which render speech obtrusive and do not necessarily achieve the
intended function of making speech intelligible. Indeed, this also applies to
obligatory errors described by Golding-Kushner (1995) (see below). Harris
and Cottam (1985) explain the deviant phonological patterns associated
with this condition as 'natural to the extent that they are attributable to
external phenomena'. Thus the characteristics of cleft palate speech may
phonetically be a natural result of the condition whilst being developmentally and phonologically abnormal. The diagnosis of phonetic and phono-

logical delay or deviance, and developmental characteristics of a child's speech and their relationship to each other, should be attempted using principles of phonological and phonetic analysis (Grunwell, 1985; Trost-Cardamone and Bernthal, 1993) (see Russell and Harding, Chapter 14).

The characteristics of cleft palate speech

The term 'cleft palate speech' has been used to describe an increasing range of phenomena as understanding of the speech characteristics associated with this condition has grown. These include *abnormal nasal resonance, abnormal nasal airflow* and *altered laryngeal voice quality, nasal or facial grimace* and *atypical consonant production* (McWilliams et al., 1990; Bzoch, 1979; Trost-Cardamone, 1990; Sell et al., 1994, 1999; Wyatt et al., 1996).

Abnormal nasal resonance typically describes excessive nasal resonance, *hypernasality*, which is particularly noticeable on vowels and glides/approximants (Sell et al., 1994, 1999). There may also be inadequate nasal resonance, known as *hyponasality*, which may be observable on target nasals. It should be noted that hypernasality and hyponasality can co-occur resulting in mixed nasality. Indeed nasality is a complex phenomenon, and other types do exist, such as cul-de-sac nasality (McWilliams et al., 1990) and potato-in-the-mouth (Henningsson, 1988). *Abnormal nasal airflow, nasal emission*, involves inaudible or, more commonly, audible airflow from the nose during the production of target sounds that in their normal production require velopharyngeal closure and oral airflow only. *Nasal turbulence* is another form of abnormal nasal airflow, a distracting nasal 'noise' which accompanies consonant production, and has been variously described as nasal snort, nasal rustle and nasal friction. It is thought to occur where there is a small constriction in the nasopharynx, which creates the distinctive turbulent fricative sound. The target pressure consonants are particularly susceptible to abnormal nasal airflow. *Nasal or facial grimace* occurs when speakers attempt to inhibit airflow through the nose by constricting the nares and sometimes other facial muscles. This is viewed as unconscious compensatory behaviour developed to prevent the nasal emission of air, and is often indicative of anatomical limitations. Although it has no direct effect on speech production, this speech-related behaviour might adversely affect the communication process because it is visually distracting.

Phonation is at risk; the altered laryngeal voice qualities that are often associated with cleft palate speech are hoarseness and reduced volume (D'Antonio et al., 1988; Lewis et al., 1993). The CSAG data showed an incidence of 29% dysphonia in the five-year-old cohort and 17% in the twelve-year-old cohort. It is commonly hypothesized that the speaker uses excessive laryngeal valve action, resulting in laryngeal constriction to compensate for inadequate velopharyngeal closure (McWilliams et al., 1969; Bzoch, 1979; Witzel, 1991). However, voice disorders are probably multifactorial, and may also relate to increased respiratory force and raised fundamental frequency to compensate for lowered intensity, abnormal laryngeal configurations during glottal sound production, tongue retraction and rigidity, and persisting learned compensations after surgical correction of VPI. In addition, psychological factors, personality traits, vocal abuse and misuse, faulty learning and imitation may all be significant. The commonest laryngeal pathology reported is vocal cord nodules (McWilliams et al., 1969; D'Antonio et al., 1988).

The understanding of *consonant production* has grown considerably since the 1960s. In 1968, Moll described the speech sound articulation of individuals with cleft palate as nasal distortions of fricatives and plosives, frequent use of glottal stop substitutions, and general inaccuracy of sound articulation. In 1972, Subtelny et al. emphasized how 'cleft palate speech' was made up of various attributes (articulation errors, nasal air escape, lack of intelligibility, nasality, and phonation) and each needed to be separately assessed. This was subsequently reinforced by Dalston et al. (1988). Much of the research at this time concentrated on the velopharyngeal mechanism and the nasality aspect of the speech disorder. For example, Edwards (1980) wrote that 'cleft palate speech' provided a shorthand term that implied a syndrome of speech disability characterized by hypernasal resonance with pharyngeal and glottal realizations of many sounds. The restricted nature of this definition is now well-recognized. Bzoch (1979) described the characteristics of 'cleft palate speech' in a traditional error framework with the aetiological factors that accounted for them. The characteristics that he listed included: laryngeal and pharyngeal substitution errors of articulation for target consonant sounds; distortion of consonant sounds due to audible nasal emission; lisping and other articulatory distortions related directly to dental or occlusal abnormalities; articulatory deviations related to loss of hearing acuity. Stengelhofen (1989) summarized the potential range of phonetic problems associated with cleft palate as: changes in breath direction; inadequacy of breath support because of air waste; weakened fricatives, plosives and affricates; audible nasal emission; tendency for contacts to be towards the back of the oral cavity; preponderance of laminal contacts and imprecise tongue tip movements; use of double articulations; secondary articulations such as pharyngealization and velarization; frequent use of glottal stop; fricatives backed to velar, pharyngeal or glottal place of articulation. This is one of the most phonetically detailed descriptions, prior to Grunwell (1993).

Contribution from instrumentation

Understanding of the speech anomalies associated with this condition has been further informed by videofluoroscopy, nasopharyngoscopy and electropalatography (EPG) (Witzel and Stringer, 1990; Moon, 1993; Shprintzen and Bardach, 1995; Hardcastle et al., 1989a). Electropalatography has been used extensively within the field of cleft palate (Michi et al., 1986; Gibbon and Hardcastle, 1989; Hardcastle et al., 1989b; Yamashita and Michi, 1991; Yamashita et al., 1992). There are several features that have been found to cluster together, in particular excessive and more posterior tongue–palate contact. Examples include lateralized articulations, particularly of targets /sz, ʃ, ʤ/, palatal and velar places of articulation for alveolar targets and double articulations (Hardcastle et al., 1989b; Gibbon and Hardcastle, 1989; Michi et al., 1986; Yamashita and Michi, 1991; Dent et al., 1992). Double articulations may involve a bilabial or alveolar closure occurring simultaneously with complete velar closure. Another type of double articulation error pattern involves complete velar constriction co-occurring with nasopharyngeal fricatives (Gibbon and Hardcastle, 1989). Speakers with cleft palate may have a pervasive pattern of abnormal velar contact which occurs during production of a whole range of consonants, but which has more perceptually detectable consequences for some sounds than others. Dent et al. (1992) hypothesize that sometimes double articulations develop out of a frank backed velar placement which is then later superimposed with additional labial or alveolar articulation, often as a result of therapy. They suggest that the presence of retracted articulations, especially to velar for labial and alveolar targets, at an early stage of speech development could indicate that the child is at risk for developing this type of double articulation at a later stage of speech development. Some of the findings from EPG have informed the recent introduction of the concept of speech cleft type characteristics by Harding and Grunwell (1996). These characteristics include dentalization, lateralization/lateral articulation, palatalization/palatal articulation, double articulation, backing to velar or uvular, pharyngeal articulation, glottal articulation, active nasal fricatives, weakened/nasalized consonants, nasal realizations of plosives or fricatives, absent pressure consonants, and gliding of fricatives/affricates. The reader is also referred to Sell et al. (1994, 1999) (see Sell and Grunwell, Chapter 16).

The difficulty of differentiating the pharyngeal and laryngeal fricative on the basis of auditory impression alone was identified by Brown et al. (1990) and Kawano et al. (1997). Based on multiview videofluoroscopy and nasopharyngoscopy, they found that pharyngeal fricatives and affricates were often reclassified as laryngeal fricatives. They observed a narrowing of the vocal tract, by the posterior positioning of the epiglottis, and elevation of the arytenoid cartilages. Frication was produced in the constriction between the epiglottis and the arytenoids, thus resulting in a laryngeal, rather than pharyngeal, place of articulation. Brown et al. (1990) also observed that the base of the tongue moved posteriorly and inferiorly, making contact with the epiglottis, and causing the epiglottis to move posteriorly. They also observed similar articulatory gestures at the level of the larynx during affricates and plosives, resulting in the identification of the new categories of laryngeal affricate and laryngeal plosive. The articulatory posture for the laryngeal plosive involved posterior–inferior lingual movement against the epiglottis, which in turn contacted the posterior pharyngeal wall and the elevated arytenoids to create a plosive. Golding-Kushner (1995) appropriately questioned the significance of these phonetic distinctions in therapy, since the focus of therapy is on how to produce the target sound correctly and not on the error. Therapy principles and techniques are often the same regardless of whether the erroneous place of articulation is laryngeal or pharyngeal.

Speech patterns

Other authorities have described overall patterns of speech encompassing the phenomena that could be disordered. In 1970, Morley described two types of speech pattern. The first was identified as an intelligible speech pattern characterized by correct place of articulation, with nasal emission and consonant weakness resulting from lack of intra-oral air pressure. The second pattern, though usually unintelligible, was characterized by nasal escape, nasal snort, glottal stops, pharyngeal fricatives, nasal grimace, and other articulatory substitutions. Hoch et al. (1986) subsequently developed this to include also a pattern in which the correct placement of oral articulators occurs, but the plosive/fricative manner of articulation is affected by velopharyngeal insufficiency such that plosives are realized as nasal consonants and fricatives as nasal fricatives.

Trost-Cardamone (1990) like Bzoch (1979, 1989), categorized cleft palate misarticulations with respect to underlying causes, particularly focusing on velopharyngeal dysfunction. Trost-Cardamone's Category One misarticulations are structurally based and include such features as audible nasal emission, weakness of manner of articulation for plosives, fricatives and affricates, and excessive hypernasality of vowels, liquids and glides. Category Two misarticulations are compensatory substitutions, coarticulations, and atypical backed articulations. Category One and Two misarticulations can coexist. Harding and Grunwell (1998) used the active/passive distinction first proposed by Hutters and Bronsted (1987) in a rather similar way to the Trost-Cardamone (1990) categories. Their active processes are similar to Trost-Cardamone's Category Two misarticulations and are defined by Harding and Grunwell 'as alternative articulations thought to have been actively generated to establish the necessary phonemic distinctions between consonant targets'. An example of an active process affecting the pronunciation of target /d/ is 'backing' to [g]. Passive processes (Trost-Cardamone's Category One misarticulations) involve 'no alteration of the articulatory placement for the intended consonant but are accompanied by nasal air flow or are realized as the nasal equivalent'. Continuing the example above, an example of a passive process affecting the pronunciation of target /d/ is the production of target /d/ as [n].

Hutters and Brondsted (1987) hypothesized that the speech characteristics are dependent on the strategy adopted by each individual speaker. The speech cleft type characteristics of dentalization, lateralization/lateral articulation, palatalization/palatal articulation, double articulation, backing to velar or uvular, pharyngeal articulation, glottal articulation and active nasal fricatives usually represent realizations that are produced as active alternatives to the target consonants. In contrast, the speech cleft type characteristics of weakened/nasalized consonants, nasal realizations of plosives or fricatives, absent pressure consonants, and gliding of fricatives/affricates are usually the consequences of velopharyngeal dysfunction or less commonly fistulae (Harding and Grunwell, 1996; Sell et al., 1994, 1999).

Trost (1981) popularized the use of the term 'compensatory articulation' although in fact Morris (1968) first used the term. Morley (1970) used the term 'compensatory adjustments' subsequently referred to as 'gross substitutions' by Bzoch (1979). Trost-Cardamone (1990) proposed the theory that in attempting to match perceptual speech models, two options were available to a speaker with velopharyngeal dysfunction. The first was to accept the inability to produce high-pressure sounds and use a restricted phonetic inventory limited to nasals, glides and liquids. The second was to reject the inability to produce high-pressure sounds and develop compensatory or 'adaptive' strategies in order to accomplish speech pressure-valving resulting in compensatory articulation (Warren, 1986). In effect, compensatory articulations developed out of the speaker's attempts to 'valve the articulation' where success is more likely. This may be either below the level of the impaired velopharyngeal mechanism, or in the area of the palatal defect mechanism so that the tongue is used to occlude the cleft or fistula, or alternatively, the tongue is used as a 'lingual assist' to occlude the velopharyngeal port, causing inevitable backing for many speech sounds. In addition, Trost-Cardamone and Bernthal (1993) also suggest that the development of backed articulations may be the consequence of early chronic hearing loss associated with otitis media effusion.

Golding-Kushner (1995) has subsequently drawn the distinction between compensatory, obligatory, developmental articulation errors, and compensatory adaptations. Compensatory articulation errors refer to that group of errors which are usually associated with the structural anomaly of VPI. Following successful surgery or prosthetic management of the defect, although resonance may be normal, these compensatory articulation errors tend to persist (Trost, 1981), involving incorrect place of articulation, and can usually only be corrected by speech therapy intervention. Obligatory errors result directly from an anatomical defect. They are not amenable to therapy, and often self correct when the underlying structural anomaly is corrected. For example, the incorrect realizations of /b d/ as their nasal equivalents [m n] spontaneously correct to [b d] following secondary velopharyngeal management. Compensatory adaptations, alternatively, include errors that are the closest possible approximation to a sound in the presence of an anatomical deviation, for example, the use of a reversed labiodental fricative for a dento-labial fricative often associated with a class III malocclusion (see Semb and Shaw, Chapter 19). These articulation placement errors may or may not resolve spontaneously when the anatomical deviation is corrected but may be a reasonable functional compensation sometimes until the correct placement can be taught. Developmental errors refer to those errors that would be considered appropriate at an earlier stage of development.

All the above descriptions provide an overall impression of the phonetic properties and patterns that may be present in 'cleft palate speech'. They do not, however, provide a systematic framework in which to evaluate, in phonetic detail, the individual characteristics of different parameters of cleft palate speech. Trost-Cardamone and Bernthal (1993) advocate such a framework and GOS.SP.ASS.98 (Sell et al.,1994, 1999) provides it (see Sell and Grunwell, Chapter 16).

Aetiological factors

The aetiology of speech disorders is often multifactorial and complex (McWilliams et al., 1990). As LeBlanc (1996) points out, the speech assessment should provide information on how the multiple factors of causation interact to cause disordered speech and identify those factors that can be modified, and the appropriate sequence to do so, to achieve speech potential. The GOS.SP.ASS.98 framework meets such a requirement. Causes of speech disorders may be any one or more of the examples given in Table 5.1.

Persistent speech disorders are also found in which the aetiology is unclear. The nature of surgery, timing of palate repair, surgical skill, or the availability, quality and amount of speech therapy may all influence speech. For example, it has been suggested that the delayed hard palate repair

Table 5.1. Causes of speech disorders

Aetiological Factors	Examples	Further information
Abnormal oronasal structure and/or function	Past or present VPI; nasal airway deviations; hearing and ENT problems; oronasal fistulae	See Mercer and Pigott, Chapter 17; Lennox, Chapter 15; Watson, Chapter 18
Abnormal orofacial structure and growth	Dental, occlusal factors, maxillary collapse	See Semb and Shaw, Chapter 19; Mars, Chapter 4
Abnormal neuromotor development	Abnormal learned neuromotor patterns (Bzoch, 1979); developmental (Grunwell, 1987); learning or neurological factors	See Sell and Grunwell, Chapter 16; Russell and Harding, Chapter 14
Abnormal or disturbed psychosocial development	Social, environmental, emotional factors	see Bradbury, Chapter 23

technique has contributed to the development of velar and backed articulation. Very delayed palatal closure into adulthood is associated with severely disordered speech (Sell, 1992). Diminished sensation resulting from scar tissue in the alveolar region following surgery or from the presence of a dental plate has been suggested as a significant aetiological factor (Fletcher, 1978). There is controversy as to the effect of fistulae on speech, with some authorities maintaining that they always result in speech disorders (Isberg and Henningsson, 1987; Le Blanc and Shprintzen, 1994) and others suggesting that this is not always the case (Clark et al., 1992; Harding and Grunwell, 1993). Furthermore, although it was once considered that there was a direct relationship between the size and location of a fistula, and speech symptoms, there is recent evidence to suggest a far more complex relationship (Clark et al., 1992). Cleft type is also significant. McWilliams et al. (1990) attributed the differences between groups with complete cleft lip and palate and groups with cleft palate only to dental problems, maxillary collapse, and protrusion of the premaxilla associated with clefting of the alveolus. Spreistersbach et al. (1961, 1964) reported that the speech results of the cleft palate only group were less favourable than those of the complete cleft lip and palate group, often in association with other congenital deformities. Recent studies have added new dimensions to the influence of syndromes on speech outcomes (see Lees, Chapter 6).

This brief review clearly demonstrates that there are multiple structural and non-structural factors which may interact and cause speech disorders. When one part of the vocal tract structure is changed, the control system for the speech structures may be adjusted to adapt to the changes in order to achieve the intended perceptual consequences. Perceptually appropriate speech may be produced, even though the movement patterns may be different from those used by normal speakers.

Conclusion

This chapter has confirmed the central role of speech pathology associated with cleft palate and velopharyngeal anomalies. The incidence of speech disorders and the position of speech as an important outcome measure have been described. Current understanding of cleft palate speech, issues regarding its measurement and aetiological factors have been summarized. In conclusion, this chapter has set the scene for the subsequent chapters on speech development and early intervention by Russell and Harding (see Chapter 14) and speech assessment and therapy in the older patient by Sell and Grunwell (see Chapter 16).

References

Albery E, Grunwell P (1993) Consonant articulation in different types of cleft lip and palate. In: Grunwell P (ed.) Analysing Cleft Palate Speech. London: Whurr, pp. 83–110.

Brooks AR, Shelton RL, Youngstrom KA (1965) Compensatory tongue–palate–posterior pharyngeal wall relationships in cleft palate. Journal of Speech and Hearing Disorders 30: 166–173.

Brooks R, Shelton RL, Youngstrom KA (1966) Tongue–palate contact in persons with palate defects. Journal of Speech and Hearing Disorders 31: 15–25.

Brown SL, Laskin R, Margar-Bacal F, Witzel MA, Bedder-Manley C (1990) The laryngeal fricative in cleft palate speech: description and diagnosis. Paper presented at the American Cleft Palate–Craniofacial Association Meeting, Missouri.

Byrne MC, Shelton RL, Diedrich WM (1961) Articulation skill, physical management and classification of children with cleft palate. Journal of Speech and Hearing Disorders 26: 326–333.

Bzoch KR (1965) Articulatory proficiency and error patterns of preschool cleft palate and normal children. Cleft Palate Journal 2: 340–349.

Bzoch KR (1979) Measurement and assessment of categorical aspects of language, voice and speech disorders. In: Bzoch KR (ed.) Communicative Disorders Related to Cleft Lip and Palate. Boston: Little, Brown and Company, pp. 161–191 (2nd edn 1989).

Clark DE, D'Antonio LL, Liu JR, Welch TB (1992) Radiographic demonstration of oronasal fistulas in patients with cleft palate with the use of barium sulfate contrast. Oral Surgery, Oral Medicine, and Oral Pathology 74: 661–670.

Counihan DT (1960) Articulation skills of adolescents and adults with cleft palates. Cleft Palate Journal 25: 181–187.

Crystal D (1981) Clinical Linguistics. Vienna: Springer Verlag. p. 193.

CSAG Report – Clinical Standards Advisory Group (1998) Cleft Lip and/or Palate. London: HMSO.

D'Antonio LL, Muntz H, Providence M, Marsh J (1988) Laryngeal/voice findings in patients with velopharyngeal dysfunction. Laryngoscope 98: 432.

Dalston RM (1990) Communication skills of children with cleft lip and palate: a status report. In: Bardach J, Morris HL (eds) Multidisciplinary Management of Cleft Lip and Palate. Philadelphia: Saunders, pp. 746–749.

Dalston RM, Marsh JL, Vig KW, Witzel MA, Bumstead MA (1988) Minimal standards for reporting the results of surgery on patients with cleft lip, cleft palate or both: a proposal. Cleft Palate Journal 25: 3–7.

Dent H, Gibbon F, Hardcastle W (1992) Inhibiting an abnormal lingual pattern in a cleft palate child using electropalatography (EPG). In: Lahey MM, Kallen JL (eds) Interdisciplinary Perspectives in Speech and Language Pathology. Dublin: School of Speech and Language Studies, pp. 211–221.

Edwards M (1980) Speech and language disability. In: Edwards M, Watson ACH (eds) Advances in the Management of Cleft Palate. Edinburgh: Churchill Livingstone, pp. 83–96.

Enderby P, Emerson J (1995) Cleft palate. In: Enderby P, Emerson J (eds) Speech and Language Therapy: Does it Work? London: Whurr, pp. 58–83.

Eurocleft Speech Group: Grunwell P, Brondsted K, Henningsson G, Jansonius K, Karling J, Meijer M, Ording U, Sell D, Wyatt R, Vermeij-Zieverink E (1993) Cleft palate speech in a European perspective: Eurocleft Speech Project. In: Grunwell P (ed.) Analysing Cleft Palate Speech. London: Whurr, pp. 142–165.

Eurocleft Speech Group (Grunwell P, Bronsted K, Henningsson G, Jansonius K, Karling J, Meijer M, Ording U, Wyatt R, Vermeij-Zieverink E, Sell D) (2000) A six-centre international study of treatment outcomes in patients with clefts of the lip and palate. Scandinavian J. of Plastic Reconstr Hand Surger 34 (3): 1–11.

Fletcher SG (1978) Diagnosing Speech Disorders from Cleft Palate. New York: Grune and Stratton.

Gibbon F, Hardcastle W (1989) Deviant articulation in a cleft palate child following late repair of the hard palate: a description and remediation procedure using electropalatography (EPG). Clinical Linguistics and Phonetics 3: 93–110.

Golding-Kushner K (1995) Treatment of articulation and resonance disorders associated with cleft palate and VPI. In: Shprintzen RJ, Bardach J (eds) Cleft Palate Speech Management. A Multidisciplinary Approach. St Louis: Mosby. pp. 327–349.

Golding-Kushner KJ, Argamaso RV, Cotton RT, Grames LM, Henningsson G, Jones DL, Karnell MP, Klaiman PG, Lewin ML, Marsh JL, McCall GN, McGrath CO, Muntz HR, Nevdahl MT, Rakoff SJ, Shprintzen RJ, Sidoti EJ, Vallino LD, Volk M, William WN, Witzel MA, Dixon Wood VL, Ysunsa A (1990) Standardization for the reporting of nasopharyngoscopy and multiview videofluoroscopy: a report from an international working group. Cleft Palate Journal 27: 337–348.

Greene MCL (1960) Speech analysis of 263 cleft palate cases. Journal of Speech and Hearing Disorders 25: 43–48.

Grunwell P (1985) Phonological Assessment of Child Speech. Windsor: NFER-Nelson.

Grunwell P (1987) Clinical Phonology, 2nd edn. London: Croom Helm.

Grunwell P (1993) Analysing Cleft Palate Speech. London: Whurr.

Hall C, Golding-Kushner, KJ (1989) Long-term follow-up of 500 patients after palate repair performed prior to 18 months of age. Paper presented at Sixth International Congress on Cleft Palate and Related Craniofacial Anomalies, Jerusalem, Israel.

Hardcastle W, Jones W, Knight C, Trudgeon A, Calder G (1989a) New developments in electropalatography: a state-of-the-art report. Clinical Linguistics and Phonetics 3: 1–38.

Hardcastle W, Morgan-Barry R, Nunn M (1989b) Instrumental articulatory phonetics in assessment and remediation: case studies with the electroplatograph. In: Stengelhofen J (ed.) Cleft Palate: The Nature and Remediation of Communication Problems. Edinburgh: Churchill Livingstone, pp. 136–164.

Harding A, Grunwell P (1993) Relationship between speech and timing of hard palate repair. In: Grunwell P (ed.) Analysing Cleft Palate Speech. London: Whurr, pp. 48–81.

Harding A, Grunwell P (1996) Cleft palate speech characteristics: a literature review. European Journal of Disorders of Communication 31: 331–358.

Harding A, Harland K, Razzell R (1997) Cleft Audit Protocol for Speech (CAPS). Available from Speech/Language Therapy Department, St Andrews Plastic Surgery Centre, Broomfield, Chelmsford, Essex.

Harding A, Grunwell P (1998) Active versus passive cleft-type speech characteristics: implications for surgery and therapy. International Journal of Language and Communication Disorders 33: 329–352.

Harris J, Cottam P (1985) Phonetic features and phonological features in speech assessment. British Journal of Disorders of Communication 20: 61–80.

Henningsson G (1988) Impairment of velopharyngeal function in patients with hypernasal speech. A clinical and cineradiographic study. PhD thesis, Department of Logopedics and Phoniatrics and Department of Oral Radiology, Karolinska Institutet, Stockholm, Sweden.

Hewlett N (1990) Processes of development and production. In: Grunwell P. Developmental Speech Disorders. Edinburgh: Churchill Livingstone, pp. 15–38.

Hoch L, Golding-Kushner K, Sadewitz VL, Shprintzen RJ (1986) Speech Therapy. Seminars in Speech and Language 7: 311–323.

Hutters B, Bronsted K (1987) Strategies in cleft palate speech – with special reference to Danish. Cleft Palate Journal 24: 126–136.

Isberg AM, Henningsson G (1987) Influence of palatal fistulas on speech and resonance. Folia Phoniatrica 39: 183–191.

Jackson I, McLellan G and Scheker LR (1983) Primary veloplasty or primary palatoplasty: some preliminary findings. Plastic and Reconstructive Surgery 72: 153–157.

Karling J, Larson O, Leanderson R, Henningsson G (1993) Speech in unilateral and bilateral cleft palate patients from Stockholm. Cleft Palate–Craniofacial Journal 30: 73–77.

Kawano M, Isshiki N, Honjo I, Kojima H, Kurata K, Tanokuchi F, Kido N, Isobe M (1997) Recent progress in treating patients with cleft palate. Folia Phoniatrica Logopedica 49: 117–138.

Lawrence CW, Philips BJ (1975) A telefluoroscopic study of lingual contacts made by persons with palatal defects. Cleft Palate Journal 12: 85–94.

LeBlanc EM, Shprintzen RJ (1994) Speech and the maxillofacial complex. A structural-functional perspective for diagnosis and management. In: Kaban LD (ed.) Oral and Maxillofacial Surgery Clinics of North America 6: 113–120.

LeBlanc EM (1996) Fundamental principles in the speech management of cleft lip and palate. In: Cleft Lip and Palate with an Introduction to Other Craniofacial Anomalies Perspectives in Management. San Diego: Singular, pp. 75–84.

Lewis J, Andreassen M, Leeper H, Macrae D (1993) Vocal characteristics of children with cleft lip/palate and associated velopharyngeal incompetence. Journal of Otolaryngology 22: 113–117.

Lohmander-Agerskov A (1996) Speech in children with cleft lip and palate treated with delayed closure of the hard palate. PhD thesis, Goteborg, Sweden.

Mars M, Lamabadasuriya S, James DRJ (1990) The Sri Lankan Cleft Lip and Palate Project: The unoperated cleft lip and palate. Cleft Palate Journal 27: 3–6.

McComb H (1989) Cleft lip and palate: new directions for research. Cleft Palate Journal 26: 145–147.

McWilliams BJ (1990) The long-term speech results of primary and secondary surgical correction of palatal clefts. In: Bardach J, Morris HL (eds) Multidisciplinary Management of Cleft Lip and Palate. Philadelphia: Saunders, pp. 815–819.

McWilliams B, Bluestone C, Musgrave CD (1969) Diagnostic implications of vocal cord nodules in children with cleft palate. Laryngoscope 79: 2072.

McWilliams BJ, Morris HL, Shelton RL (1990) Cleft Palate Speech, 2nd edn. Philadelphia: BC Decker.

Michi K, Suzuki N, Yamashita Y, Imai S (1986) Visual training and correction of articulation disorders by use of dynamic palatography: serial observation in a case of a cleft palate. Journal of Speech and Hearing Disorders 51: 226-238.

Moll KL (1968) Speech characteristics of individuals with cleft lip and palate. In: Spreistersbach DC, Sherman D (eds) Cleft Palate and Communication. New York: Academic Press, pp. 61–118.

Moon JB (1993) Evaluation of velopharyngeal function. In: Moller KT, Starr CD (eds) Cleft Palate Interdisciplinary Issues and Treatment. Austin, TX: Pro-ed, pp. 251–306.

Morley ME (1970) Cleft Palate and Speech, 7th edn. Baltimore: Williams & Wilkins.

Morris HL (1962) Communication skills of children with cleft lips and palates. Journal of Speech and Hearing Research 5: 79–90.

Morris HL (1968) Etiological bases for speech problems. In: Spreistersbach DC, Sherman D (eds) Cleft Palate and Communication. New York: Academic Press, pp. 119–168.

Morris HL (1973) Velopharyngeal competence and primary cleft palate surgery, 1960–1971: a critical review. Cleft Palate Journal 10: 62–71.

Morris HL (1981) The child with cleft lip and palate: 20 years of progress. International Journal of Pediatric Otorhinolaryngology 3: 93–99.

Peterson-Falzone SJ (1990) A cross-sectional analysis of speech results following palatal closure. In: Bardach J, Morris HL (eds) Multidisciplinary Management of Cleft Lip and Palate. Philadelphia: Saunders, pp. 750–757.

Philips BJ, Harrison RJ (1969) Articulation patterns of preschool cleft palate children. Cleft Palate Journal 6: 245–253.

Riski JE, Delong E (1984) Articulation development in children with cleft lip/palate. Cleft Palate Journal 21: 57–64.

Sandy J, Williams A, Mildinhall S, Murphy T, Bearn D, Shaw B, Sell D, Devlin B, Murray J (1998) The Clinical Standards Advisory Group (CSAG) Cleft Lip and Palate Study. British Journal of Orthodontics 25: 21–30.

Sell D (1992) Speech in Sri Lankan cleft palate subjects with delayed palatoplasty. Unpublished PhD, De Montfort University.

Sell D, Harding A, Grunwell P (1994) GOS.SP.ASS. A screening assessment of cleft palate speech. European Journal of Disorders of Communication 29: 1–15.

Sell D, Harding A, Grunwell P (1999) Revised GOS.SP.ASS (98): Speech assessment for children with cleft palate and/or velopharyngeal dysfunction. International Journal of Disorders of Communication 34: 17–33.

Sell D, Grunwell P, Mildinhall S, Murphy T, Cornish TC, Williams A, Bearn D, Shaw WC, Murray J, Sandy J. (2000) Cleft lip and palate care in the United Kingdom (UK) – The Clinical Standards Advisory Group (CSAG) Study. Part 3 – Speech outcomes. Submitted to Cleft Palate–Craniofacial Journal (in press).

Shprintzen RJ, Bardach J (1995) Instrumental assessment of velopharyngeal valving. In: Cleft Palate Speech Management. A Multidisciplinary Approach. St Louis: Mosby, pp. 221–256.

Skoog T (1965) The pharyngeal flap operation in cleft palate. British Journal of Plastic Surgery 18: 265–282.

Sommerlad BC, Di Biase D, Harland K, Lake R, Moss J, Williams et al. (1996) An 'extended' audit of complete bony unilateral cleft lip and palate patients aged 5–6 and 8–11. Paper presented at the annual meeting of the Craniofacial Society of Great Britain, London.

Spreistersbach DC, Powers G. (1959) Articulation skills, velopharyngeal closure and oral breath pressure of children with cleft palates. Journal of Speech and Hearing Research 2: 318–325.

Spreistersbach DC, Darley FL, Rouse V (1956) Articulation of a group of children with cleft lips and palates. Journal of Speech and Hearing Disorders 21: 436–445.

Spreistersbach DC, Moll KL and Morris HL (1961) Subject classification and articulation of speakers with cleft palates. Journal of Speech and Hearing Research 4: 362–372.

Spreistersbach DC, Moll KL, Morris HL (1964) Heterogeneity of the cleft palate population and research designs. Cleft Palate Journal 1: 210–216.

Spreistersbach DC, Dickson DR, Fraser FC, Horowitz SL, McWilliams BJ, Paradise J, Randall P (1973) Clinical research in cleft lip and cleft palate: the state of the art. Cleft Palate Journal 10: 113–165.

Stengelhofen J (1989) Cleft Palate: The Nature and Remediation of Communication Problems. Edinburgh: Churchill Livingstone.

Stoel-Gammon C and Dunn C (1985) Normal and Disordered Phonology in Children. Austin, TX: Pro-Ed.

Subtelny JD, Van Hattum RJ, Myers BB (1972) Ratings and measures of cleft palate speech. Cleft Palate Journal 9: 18–27.

Trost JE (1981) Articulatory additions to the classical description of the speech of persons with cleft palate. Cleft Palate Journal 18: 193–203.

Trost-Cardamone JE (1990) The development of speech: assessing cleft palate misarticulations. In: Kernahan DA, Rosenstein SN (eds) Cleft Lip and Palate: A System of Management. Baltimore: Williams & Wilkins.

Trost-Cardamone JE, Bernthal JE (1993) Articulation assessment procedures and treatment decisions. In: Moller KT, Starr CD (eds) Cleft Palate Interdisciplinary Issues and Treatment. Austin, TX: Pro-ed, pp. 307–336.

Van Demark DR (1969) Consistency of articulation of subjects with cleft palate. Cleft Palate Journal 6: 254–262.

Van Demark DR, Morris HL, Vandehaar C (1979) Patterns of articulation abilities in speakers with cleft palate. Cleft Palate Journal 16: 230–239.

Warren DM (1986) Compensatory speech behaviours in individuals with cleft palate: a regulatory control phenomenon. Cleft Palate Journal 23: 251–260.

Witzel MA (1991) Speech evaluation and treatment. Oral and Maxillofacial Surgery Clinics of North America 3: 501–516.

Witzel MA, Stringer DA (1990) Methods of assessing velopharyngeal function. In: Bardach J, Morris HL (eds) Multidisciplinary Management of Cleft Lip and Palate. Philadelphia: Saunders, pp. 763–775.

Wyatt R, Sell D, Russell A, Harland K, Albery E (1996) Cleft palate speech dissected: a review of current knowledge and analysis. British Journal of Plastic Surgery 49: 143–149.

Yamashita Y, Michi K (1991) Misarticulation caused by abnormal lingual-palatal contact in patients with cleft palate with adequate velopharyngeal function. Cleft Palate–Craniofacial Journal 28: 360–366.

Yamashita Y, Michi K, Imai S, Suzuki N, Yoshida H (1992) Electropalatographic investigation of abnormal lingual-palatal contact patterns in cleft palate patients. Clinical Linguistics and Phonetics 6: 210–217.

CHAPTER 6

Genetics of Cleft Lip and Palate

M. LEES

Orofacial clefting is the most common congenital craniofacial malformation. In the majority of cases, the cleft will be the only defect, but clefts of the lip and palate may also be found in association with other congenital anomalies, and may occur as part of a well-defined syndrome. The clinical geneticist has an important role in the diagnosis, management and counselling of patients with clefts and their families.

This chapter aims to cover the basics of genetics as applied to facial clefting. The first section discusses the genetic basis of non-syndromic cleft lip and/or palate. Later sections deal with cases of clefting associated with other anomalies, including clefts secondary to environmental exposures, single-gene disorders and chromosomal aberrations. The main clinical features of some of the more common clefting syndromes are described.

Non-syndromic cleft lip and palate

A cleft is termed 'non-syndromic' where the affected individual has no other physical problems, or any evidence of delay in motor or cognitive development. It is important to determine the presence of any other anomalies or factors predisposing to clefting, such as maternal drug ingestion, as these will have a significant influence on the overall management of the child, in addition to genetic counselling issues. A detailed family history is required to establish whether there may be other family members with a cleft lip, cleft palate or both, or indeed a history of other anomalies, which may give a clue as to the aetiology of the cleft. The pregnancy history may identify factors thought to predispose an individual to being born with a cleft lip and/or palate (CL/P). A number of drugs taken by the mother during pregnancy, such as phenytoin, are associated with CL/P (see below). Other maternal environmental exposures may also result in a cleft in the child. A detailed clinical examination, noting any dysmorphic features and other structural anomalies in addition to an assessment of growth and development, will help establish whether the cleft is non-syndromic. This can be determined by a paediatrician with an interest in clefting. If dysmorphic features or additional anomalies are identified, or there are concerns regarding development, referral to a clinical geneticist is appropriate for consideration of a possible underlying diagnosis. Further investigation may be required at this stage.

Aetiology

Non-syndromic CL/P (NSCL/P) is thought to be a complex or multifactorial trait. Both environmental and genetic factors are involved (Murray, 1995). There is no evidence for classic Mendelian inheritance attributable to any single gene. Other examples of human disorders showing multifactorial inheritance are insulin-dependent diabetes mellitus, hypertension and congenital heart disease. The evidence for a genetic predisposition to NSCL/P comes from family and twin studies. Although most cases of NSCL/P occur as a one-off within a family, a positive family history is obtained in around 26% of cases (Hagberg et al., 1998). The chance of a sibling of a child with CL/P also being affected is around 30–40 times the risk in the general population. Monozygotic twins (identical, and therefore sharing the same genes) are far more likely to be concordant for CL/P (where either both are affected or both unaffected), than dizygotic twins, who share only half of their genes in common. Mitchell and Risch (1992) found the concordance rate in monozygotic twins to be 25–40%, and in dizygotic twins 3–6%.

The normal developmental processes resulting in formation of the face are largely genetically determined, and a number of genes have been identified as playing a particular role in the development of the lip and palate. Structural and regulatory genes involved in cell–cell adhesion, production of intercellular matrices, programmed cell death, cell transformation and neural crest cell migration may all play a role in the aetiology of clefting (see Watson, Chapter 1). The number of genes already determined to be important in facial development emphasizes the underlying complexity of the genetic contribution to CL/P (Schutte and Murray, 1999). Any of these genes may contribute to the genetic susceptibility, interacting both with each other and with undetermined environmental factors. Studies support a role for transforming growth factor-alpha and a gene located on chromosome 6p23-24 (Murray, 1995), and further contributing genes will be identified with time. By identifying susceptibility genes, light will be shed on the cause of clefts, and progress may be made towards identifying any preventable factors.

CL/P versus cleft palate only (CPO)

Cleft palate as an isolated finding is both genetically and embryologically distinct from cleft lip with or without cleft palate. Primary and secondary palatal defects rarely occur in members of the same family, other than in a few rare monogenic syndromes, the most common of which is the van der Woude syndrome. This suggests that the major causative genes for non-syndromic CL/P differ from those resulting in cleft palate only, although these defects may share one or two susceptibility genes of smaller effect.

Genetic counselling

Genetic counselling forms part of the overall management of a child with an orofacial cleft. Although corrective surgery combined with multidisciplinary specialized management often gives an excellent overall result, parents may want to know the genetic risks of having further children with the same problem. Before giving recurrence risks, one must be confident that a syndromic basis has been excluded. One particularly important condition to exclude is the dominantly inherited van der Woude syndrome (Van der Woude, 1954), as it closely mimics NSCL/P with the additional presence of lower lip pits (see below). The lower lip must be specifically examined in both the affected individual and parents, and if lip pits were identified in either parent, the recurrence risk would increase. Recurrence risks for NSCL/P are currently based on empirical figures, where the estimate of risk is based on observed data rather than calculated from theoretical predictions. Examination of close family members to exclude cleft microforms such as a forme fruste cleft lip, submucous cleft palate or bifid uvula is necessary. The risk for siblings born of unaffected parents increases from approximately 4% after one affected child, to 10% after two affected children (Curtis et al., 1961). If one parent is affected the risk to further children after one affected child is around 10% (Table 6.1). Jorde et al. (1995) calculated the risks to first-, second- and third-degree relatives as 4%, 0.7% and 0.3%, respectively. Once the probabilities of a recurrence have been outlined, possible ways of modifying this risk need to be discussed.

Predictors of risk

A number of studies have attempted to determine which characteristics provide the best predictor of recurrence risk to siblings of individuals with CL/P (Mitchell and Risch, 1993). They found that the severity of the proband's defect (specifically the extent of the lip defect, as opposed to palatal involvement) was a significant predictor of sibling recurrence. A positive family history was also found to be a significant predictor. After adjusting for family history effects, the risk to siblings of probands with

Table 6.1. Genetic risks of CL/P to relatives in the absence of a defined syndrome or Mendelian pattern (Harper, 1998)

Relationship to index case	Cleft lip with or without cleft palate (%)	Cleft palate alone(%)
Sibs (overall risk)	4.0	1.8
Sib (no other affected members)	2.2	
Sib (2 affected sibs)	10	8
Sib and affected parent	10	
Children	4.3	3
Second-degree relatives	0.6	
Third-degree relatives	0.3	
General population	0.1	0.04

bilateral defects was found to be twice the risk to siblings of probands with unilateral defects. The sex of the proband was not found to be a significant predictor.

X-linked cleft palate

When cleft palate is not part of a syndrome, recurrence risks are small (around 2%). There is, however, an X-linked type, found predominantly in Iceland and British Columbia, where there are large families with many affected members. Ankyloglossia (tongue-tie) was the only additional feature (Bjornsson et al., 1989).

Environmental factors

It has been recognized for some time that teratogens play a role in the aetiology of CL/P. Recognized teratogens include specific drugs such as phenytoin, methotrexate and sodium valproate (amongst others), alcohol (Munger et al., 1996), cigarette smoking (Khoury et al., 1989), and more recently pesticides such as dioxin (Garcia et al., 1999). Maternal epilepsy is associated with an increased risk of non-syndromic CL/P and, to a lesser extent, CPO. The risk is increased when the mother is taking anticonvulsant medication during pregnancy.

At present it is difficult to identify teratogens that may have a weak effect on the development of a facial cleft. Once the genetic contribution has been elucidated, however, the role of the environment may become easier to define, and the study of gene–environment interactions will identify possible preventable factors in those at risk of having a child with a cleft.

Folic acid

Preliminary data suggest that folic acid and multivitamin supplementation may play a role in the reduction of the incidence of CL/P (Czeizel, 1998), but further studies are required for validation. At present there are no guidelines on the recommended dose required for the prevention of a recurrence of CL/P.

Associated anomalies

Although CL/P occurs most frequently as an isolated anomaly, it is well recognized that it may be associated with other congenital defects. Recent studies have suggested that the incidence of additional anomalies varies between 21% (Milerad et al., 1997) and 38% (Tolarova and Cervenka, 1998). Malformations of the upper or lower limbs or the vertebral column are the most common associated anomalies, accounting for 33% of all associated defects, with malformations in the cardiovascular system accounting for around 24%. Cases with associated malformations are more likely to have combined cleft lip and palate or cleft palate only, rather than a cleft lip alone. Around 15% of all associated malformations are multiple (Milerad et al., 1997), and include cases that may be divided into recognized syndromes, chromosomal anomalies (e.g. trisomy 13, 18 and 21), and teratogens. Chromosome analysis should be carried out on cases with additional anomalies. The incidence of chromosome defects varies depending on the severity and type of the associated anomalies in addition to the type of facial anomaly; for example, with a midline CL/P (which accounts for less than 1% of all CL/P) the incidence of chromosomal anomalies is as high as 52% (Nyberg et al., 1995). Deletions or duplications in every chromosome arm have been associated with clefts (Brewer et al., 1998), suggesting that many genes are involved in facial development, and that cleft lip and palate can be a common end-point when normal facial development is disrupted.

Syndromes with orofacial clefting

There are over 400 syndromes listed in the London Dysmorphology Database which include cleft lip and/or cleft palate as a feature (Winter and Baraitser, 1998). Some of these are due to a single-gene disorder and therefore follow Mendelian inheritance. In this section the clinical features of some of the more commonly seen syndromes are outlined (Table 6.2).

Van der Woude syndrome (VDWS)

Van der Woude syndrome (VDWS) is an autosomal dominant condition where cleft lip and/or cleft palate is found in association with pits of the

Table 6.2. Some of the more common syndromes associated with CL/P

Chromosomal
Trisomy 13
Trisomy 18
Velocardiofacial syndrome (22q11 deletion)

Non-Mendelian
Pierre Robin sequence
CHARGE association
Goldenhar syndrome

Mendelian disorders
Ectrodactyly–ectodermal dysplasia–clefting syndrome (AD)
Gorlin syndrome (AD)
Oto-palato-digital syndrome (XL)
Oral-facial-digital syndrome (XL)
Smith–Lemli–Opitz syndrome (AR)
Stickler syndrome (AD)
Treacher Collins syndrome (AD)
Van der Woude syndrome (AD)

Unknown
de Lange syndrome
Kabuki syndrome

Teratogenic
Fetal alcohol syndrome
Fetal phenytoin syndrome
Fetal valproate syndrome

AD, autosomal dominant; AR, autosomal recessive; XL, X-linked inheritance.

lower lip, and was first described by Anne van der Woude in 1954 (van der Woude, 1954) (Figure 6.1). With the exception of the lip pits (and hypodontia seen in some gene carriers), this syndrome is phenotypically identical to NSCLP, and between 1% and 2% of cases of CL/P are thought to have VDWS, making it an important condition to exclude when cleft recurrence risks are being discussed (Ranta and Rintala, 1983). VDWS is one of the rare single-gene disorders where clefts of the primary and secondary palate are linked with a unitary cause, suggesting that a very early stage of embryogenesis is being affected. The diagnosis should be considered in families where a cleft lip is seen in one family member and a cleft palate in another. The condition shows reduced penetrance, where not all gene carriers will have any signs of the condition, and variable expressivity, where the severity of the condition varies. Eighty per cent of gene carriers have lip pits or symmetrical elevations, located on either side of the midline of the lower lip close to the vermilion border, and around 50% have clefts (one-third cleft palate alone and two-thirds cleft lip with or without cleft palate). Hypodontia (fewer than the normal number of teeth) is present in 10–20% of gene carriers. There are no other craniofacial anomalies, and the syndrome is associated with normal intelligence.

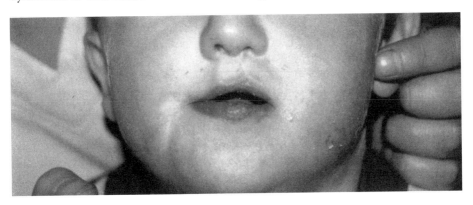

Figure 6.1. Van der Woude syndrome: lower lip pit seen in child with repaired cleft.

Although the gene has not been cloned, it has been located to a small region on chromosome 1q32.

Pierre Robin complex

The Pierre Robin sequence or complex is a common condition involving a combination of micrognathia (small chin) and glossoptosis (protruding tongue), with or without cleft palate. Respiratory distress may complicate the neonatal period. This sequence may occur alone or as part of a number of other conditions, many of which are genetically determined. The most frequently associated syndromes are Stickler syndrome (which may account for up to 35% of Pierre Robin cases) and velocardiofacial syndrome (around 11%).

Stickler syndrome

Stickler syndrome is an extremely variable autosomal dominant connective tissue disorder, first described by Stickler et al. in 1965. The variable findings of Stickler syndrome are greater between families rather than within families (possibly due to genetic heterogeneity of the condition), and can lead to diagnostic difficulties. The clinical manifestations can be divided into three main groups – those involving the eyes, the joints and the facial appearance (Temple, 1989). At birth the only features may be those of Pierre Robin sequence (cleft palate, micrognathia and glossoptosis). Cleft palate or lesser degrees of clefting such as bifid uvula can occur without micrognathia, and sometimes a high-arched palate may be the only manifestation. The facial appearance at birth results from mid-face hypoplasia, associated with a flat nasal bridge, anteverted nares and prominent eyes (Figure 6.2). These features usually improve with age. Myopia (usually present at birth) is generally severe but progression is minimal. Retinal changes can occur independently of myopia, and degeneration may progress to retinal detachment. Blindness may follow if the detachment is extensive. Joint problems, if present, are again variable, with prominent joints and hyperextensibility at birth, pain and stiffness in childhood, and early onset osteoarthritis in adulthood. Vertebral clefts and flaring of the metaphyses of the long bones may be seen radiologically in the neonatal period. As the child grows older these features become normal, although a mild epiphyseal dysplasia may develop. Height is generally normal. Sensorineural deafness can be present, in addition to a conductive element secondary to the cleft palate.

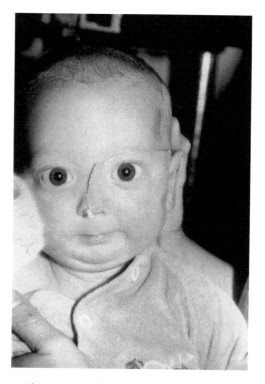

Figure 6.2. Stickler syndrome: prominent eyes and a flat nasal bridge seen in a child with Stickler syndrome.

The diagnosis at present is made clinically, and should be considered in any family with a history of dominant cleft palate or myopia. A skeletal survey in the neonatal period may be helpful. Any child with Pierre Robin association should have careful ophthalmic follow-up to exclude signs of Stickler syndrome, and so prevent complications arising from retinal detachment. The diagnosis is also important from a counselling point of view.

Mutations in several collagen genes have been identified in families with Stickler syndrome. Mutations in the alpha 1 chain of type 2 collagen (COL2A1) have been reported in some cases. Mutations in the alpha 2 chain of type 11 collagen gene on chromosome 6 have been identified in other families where the eye anomalies are not present, and it is likely that the different causative genes (genetic heterogeneity) account for some of the clinical variability between Stickler families (Snead and Yates, 1999).

Velocardiofacial syndrome

Velocardiofacial syndrome (VCFS) is one of the most common syndromes associated with a cleft palate without a cleft lip (although a cleft lip can occur), and the incidence has been estimated to be as high as 1 in 2000 live births (R. Shprintzen, personal communication). This variable syndrome combines cleft palate (often submucous cleft palate or velopharyngeal insufficiency), with cardiac anomalies, an unusual facial appearance, and learning difficulties (Figure 6.3). Velopharyngeal dysfunction or insufficiency (VPI) is found in around 30% of cases, with submucous cleft palate in 15% and an overt cleft palate in 11% (McDonald McGinn et al., 1997) (see Mercer and Pigott, Chapter 17). A cleft lip has been reported in around 2%. The face is long with a prominent nose and a squared-off nasal tip, narrow palpebral fissures, 'hooded' eyelids and a small mouth. The ears are often small with attached ear lobes. Fingers are long and hyperextensible. Nearly 80% of cases have cardiac defects, the most common being tetralogy of Fallot, interrupted aortic arch, ventricular septal defects and truncus arteriosus. Learning difficulties, when present, are often mild, but may be moderate or severe. Defects of the immune system, particularly of T-cell production, are common but rarely cause significant problems. Other recognized associations include hypocalcaemia, structural renal anomalies, ocular abnormalities, short stature and joint problems. Adults with VCFS may develop psychiatric problems (Shprintzen et al., 1992).

VCFS results from a microdeletion on chromosome 22q11, detected by fluorescent *in situ* hybridization (FISH). About 10–20% of affected individuals will have a parent who also carries the deletion. There is considerable overlap with DiGeorge syndrome, in which the majority of cases also have 22q11 deletions. DiGeorge syndrome is characterized by a conotruncal cardiac anomaly, most commonly an interrupted aortic arch or truncus arteriosus, and aplasia or hypoplasia of the thymus and parathyroid glands, with some mild facial features.

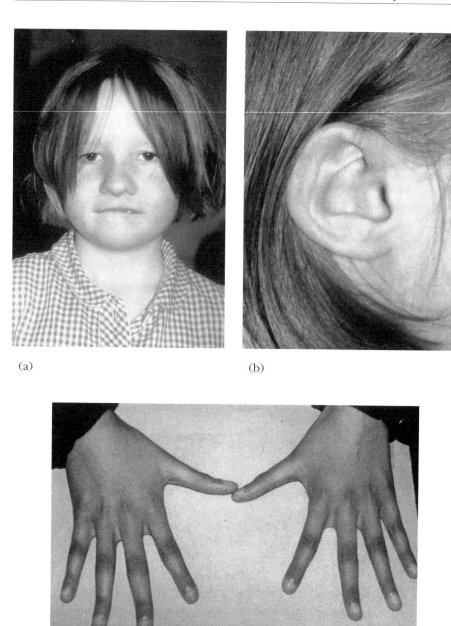

(a)   (b)

(c)

Figure 6.3. Velocardiofacial syndrome. (a) Characteristic face of a child with velocardio-facial syndrome, with a prominent nose, and squared-off nasal tip. The palpebral fissures are narrow. (b) Small ear with attached lobe. (c) Long thin fingers.

The diagnosis of VCFS should be considered in all children with VPI or a submucous cleft palate, particularly when an additional feature of the syndrome is present.

CHARGE association

The acronym CHARGE refers to a cluster of malformations including coloboma of iris or retina, heart defects, atresia of the choanae, retardation of growth and development, genital anomalies (micropenis and undescended testes), and ear abnormalities (usually simple and protruding) with or without or deafness (sensorineural, conductive or both). Developmental problems are variable, ranging from very mild delay associated with normal schooling to severe mental retardation. Additional anomalies including central nervous system malformations, facial palsy or asymmetry and renal malformations have also been reported. Cleft lip with or without cleft palate has been reported in 17% of cases (Tellier et al., 1998). To make a diagnosis four of the major criteria need to be present, and one should be either choanal atresia or a coloboma.

Most cases are sporadic, but rare familial cases have been reported. There is an association with increased paternal age at the time of conception. Although the cause remains unknown, CHARGE syndrome may be due to a *de novo* dominant mutation, or to a hitherto undetected chromosomal abnormality.

EEC syndrome

The three cardinal features of the EEC syndrome are ectrodactyly, ectodermal dysplasia and clefting (Roelfsema and Cobben, 1996). Ectrodactyly – or split hand/foot – occurs in over 80% of gene carriers, and may be accompanied by syndactyly (where the digits are joined) and oligodactyly (missing digits) (Figure 6.4). The ectodermal part of this syndrome involves the hair, teeth and nails. The hair is sparse, fair and dry and the eyebrows and eyelashes are often absent. The teeth are small and may be partially formed, and hypodontia and anodontia occur. The nails are thin, brittle and ridged. Facial clefting, affecting the lip and/or palate, occurs in nearly 70% of affected individuals. Tear duct abnormalities are common.

The EEC syndrome is inherited as an autosomal dominant condition, with a highly variable expression and reduced penetrance. All the features are very variable and extreme care must be taken in examining and counselling parents of an apparently isolated case. The gene for this condition has recently been identified as the p63 gene on chromosome 3q.

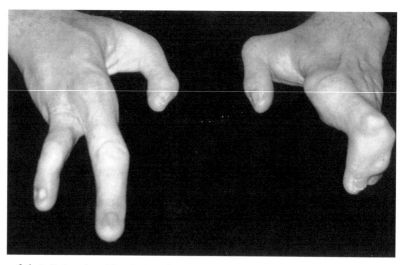

Figure 6.4. Split hands with missing digits in a patient with EEC syndrome.

Treacher Collins syndrome

This is a very variable autosomal dominant condition, named after E. Treacher Collins, who described the essential components of the condition in 1900 (Treacher Collins, 1900). The main features affect the face symmetrically, and consist of malformed external ears, often with associated external auditory canal defects and anomalies of the middle ear ossicles with resultant conductive hearing loss, hypoplasia of the facial bones, particularly of the mandible and zygomatic arch, downslanting palpebral fissures with notched defects of the lower eyelid with a lack of eyelashes medial to this, and a cleft palate (Dixon, 1995) (Figure 6.5). Sensorineural deafness may also occur. Intelligence is usually normal. Although autosomal dominant inheritance is well established, expression of the gene is extremely variable, even within the same family. Some patients are so mildly affected that it is hard to make a diagnosis, making genetic counselling difficult. In around 40% of cases there is a previous family history, with the remaining 60% having arisen as a new event in that family. The gene, located on 5q31-5q33, was isolated in 1996, and has been named Treacle (Dixon, 1996).

Kabuki syndrome

In this syndrome learning difficulties are associated with a characteristic face and short stature. The main diagnostic feature, reminiscent of the make-up worn by actors in Kabuki theatre (after which the condition is named), is eversion of the lateral third of the lower eyelid together with long palpebral fissures (Figure 6.6). Affected individuals also have a broad

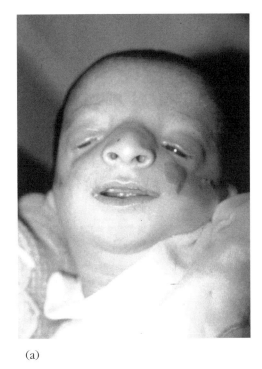

(a)

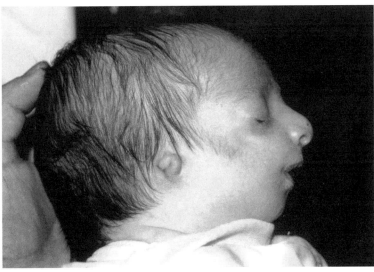

(b)

Figure 6.5. Treacher Collins syndrome. (a) Face of a child with Treacher Collins syndrome, showing symmetrical hypoplasia of the facial bones and downslanting palpebral fissures. (b) Small malformed external ear.

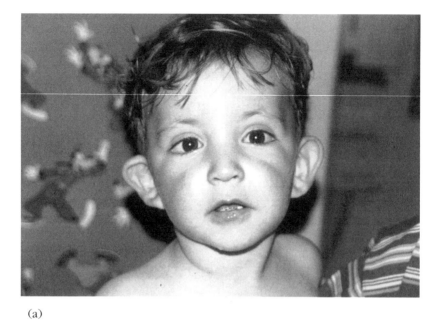

(a)

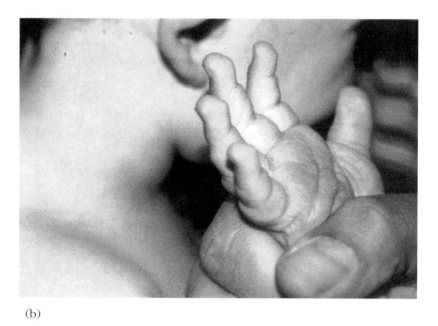

(b)

Figure 6.6. Kabuki syndrome. (a) Characteristic face of a child with Kabuki syndrome. This patient also has lower lip pits. (b) Pads of tissue seen on the finger tips.

nasal tip, prominent ear lobes and a cleft or high-arched palate (seen in around 40% of cases) (Philip et al., 1992). The fifth finger is short and there is persistence of the fetal finger pads (soft tissue pads found on the finger tips). Breast development may occur early in females. Congenital heart defects occur in about 50% of cases, and renal anomalies in 40–50%. Several cases with pits in the lower lip have been reported.

Most cases of Kabuki syndrome are sporadic, although dominant inheritance has occasionally been reported.

Oral-facial-digital syndrome

There are a number of different types of oral-facial-digital syndrome (OFD) (Toriello, 1993). The most common, OFD I, is characterized by a midline cleft or notch of the upper lip with cleft of the alveolar ridge and palate, multiple oral frenula, and a lobulated tongue. Facially, the nasal root is broad, and the nares narrow. The fingers and toes may be short with some skin webbing. Associated anomalies include polycystic kidneys, and structural central nervous system defects which may result in learning difficulties.

OFD I is an X-linked condition, seen in females. The gene is lethal in males, who are thought to die *in utero*.

Oto-palatal-digital syndrome type I

This syndrome comprises conductive deafness (as a result of abnormalities of the bones of the middle ear), cleft palate and a characteristic face. The overall impression is said to be of 'pugilistic' facies and this may become more marked with age (Dudding et al., 1967). The ends of the thumbs and big toes are flattened, and skin webbing of the digits is often seen. The appearance in the feet is particularly characteristic, with a large gap between the first and second toes, a short big toe, and lateral curvature of the toes.

The condition is X-linked, and is more severe in males, although females may show mild signs.

Smith–Lemli–Opitz syndrome

Smith–Lemli–Opitz syndrome (SLO) is an autosomal recessive disorder, associated with distinct facial features and developmental delay, and is due to a disorder of cholesterol biosynthesis. Clinical features are variable but include microcephaly with bi-temporal narrowing, ptosis, anteverted nostrils, prominent lateral palatine ridges and micrognathia (Ryan et al., 1998). A cleft palate may be present. There is significant syndactyly of the second and third toes. Hypospadias and a hypoplastic scrotum are often seen in males.

The diagnosis is confirmed by the finding of raised levels of plasma 7-dehydrocholesterol (7-DHC). Mutations in the 7-dehydrocholesterol reductase gene have been reported.

Goldenhar syndrome

This condition affects the face bilaterally, but asymmetrically. The ear is small, often with preauricular ear tags in a line between the front of the ear and the side of the mouth, which is wide (Feingold and Baum, 1978). An epibulbar dermoid is necessary for the diagnosis. If this is absent, and both sides of the face are affected, the term first and second branchial arch syndrome is preferable. Where the face is affected only on one side without an epibulbar dermoid, the term hemifacial microsomia is used (Cohen et al., 1989). Anomalies of the cervical vertebrae are common, and cardiac defects may occur.

Goldenhar syndrome is usually sporadic, but familial cases have been reported.

Basal cell naevus syndrome (Gorlin syndrome)

Gorlin syndrome, also known as naevoid basal cell carcinoma syndrome, is characterized by the development of jaw cysts in the first decade of life and basal cell carcinomas after puberty, particularly on the face and neck (Gorlin and Sedano, 1971). Other skin manifestations include pits on the palms and soles. CL/P is present in around 5% of cases. Rib anomalies are common, as is kyphoscoliosis.

The causative gene has been identified (Johnson et al., 1996).

Apert syndrome

Apert syndrome is a rare but distinct craniosynostosis syndrome, estimated to have a birth prevalence of about 1 in 65 000. Craniosynostosis, or premature fusion of the bones of the skull, results in an unusual head shape, with prominent eyes, beaked nose, and a high or cleft palate. The hands are characteristic, with fusion of digits 2–5 and sometimes including the thumb – the so-called mitten hand – and the toes are similarly affected (Cohen and Kreiborg, 1993).

Apert syndrome is due to mutations in the fibroblast growth factor receptor gene FGFR2.

Summary

Any child born with a cleft lip and/or cleft palate should be examined carefully to exclude associated anomalies which may have implications for the health of the child, and also to provide information that may be helpful in assessing any genetic risks for further children. The causes of clefts are complex, and involve both genetic and environmental factors. Identification of these factors will lead to more accurate genetic counselling, and the possibility of preventative measures.

References

Bjornsson A, Arnason A, Tippet P (1989) X-linked cleft palate and ankyloglossia in an Icelandic family. Cleft Palate Journal 26: 3–8.

Brewer C, Holloway S, Zawalnyski P, Schinzel A, Fitzpatrick D (1998) A chromosomal deletion map of human malformations. American Journal of Human Genetics 63: 1153–1159.

Cohen MM Jr, Rollnick BR, Kaye CI (1989) Oculoauriculovertebral spectrum: an updated critique. Cleft Palate J 26: 276–286.

Cohen MM Jr, Kreiborg S (1993) An updated paediatric perspective on the Apert syndrome. American Journal of Diseases of Children 147: 989–993.

Curtis E, Fraser F, Warburton D (1961) Congenital cleft lip and palate: risk figures for counselling. American Journal of Diseases of Children 102: 853–857.

Czeizel A (1998) Periconceptional folic acid containing multivitamin supplementation. European Journal of Obstetrics, Gynecology and Reproductive Biology 78(2): 151–161.

Dixon M (1995) Treacher Collins syndrome. Journal of Medical Genetics 32: 806–808.

Dixon M (1996) Treacher Collins syndrome. Human Molecular Genetics 5: 1391–1396.

Dudding B, Gorlin R, Langer L (1967) The oto-palato-digital syndrome. A new symptom-complex consisting of deafness, dwarfism, cleft palate, characteristic facies, and a generalized bone dysplasia. American Journal of Diseases of Children 113: 214–221.

Feingold M, Baum J (1978) Goldenhar's syndrome. American Journal of Diseases of Children 132: 135–136.

Garcia A, Fletcher T, Benavides F, Orts E (1999) Parental agricultural work and selected congenital malformations. American Journal of Epidemiology 149: 64–74.

Gorlin RJ, Sedano HO (1971) The multiple nevoid basal cell carcinoma syndrome revisited. BDOAS 7(8): 140–148.

Hagberg C, Larson O, Milerad J (1998) Incidence of cleft lip and palate and risks of additional malformations. Cleft Palate–Craniofacial Journal 35(1): 40–45.

Harper P (1998) Oral and craniofacial disorders. In: Practical Genetic Counselling. Oxford: Butterworth-Heinemann. Fifth edition p. 211.

Johnson RL, Epstein EH Jr, Scott MP, Rothman AL, Xie J, Goodrich LV, Bare JW, Bonifas JM, Quinn AG, Myers RM, Cox DR (1996) Human homolog of patched, a candidate gene for the basal nevus syndrome. Science 272: 1668–1671.

Jorde L, Carey J, White R (1995) Medical Genetics. St Louis: Mosby.

Khoury M, Gomez-Fariel M, Mulinare J (1989) Does maternal cigarette smoking during pregnancy cause cleft lip and palate in offspring? American Journal of Diseases of Children 143: 333–337.

McDonald McGinn D, LaRossa D, Goldmuntz E, Sullivan K, Eicher P, Gerdes M, Moss E, Wang P, Solot C, Schultz P, Lynch D (1997) The 22q11.2 deletion: Screening, diagnostic workup, and outcome of results; Report on 181 patients. Genetic Testing 1: 99–108.

Milerad J, Larson O, Hagberg C, Ideberg M (1997) Associated malformations in infants with cleft lip and palate: a prospective, population-based study. Pediatrics 100(2): 180–186.

Mitchell LE, Risch N (1992) Mode of inheritance of nonsyndromic cleft lip with or without cleft palate: a reanalysis. American Journal of Human Genetics 51(2): 323–332.

Mitchell LE, Risch N (1993) Correlates of genetic risk for non-syndromic cleft lip with or without cleft palate. Clinical Genetics 43(5): 255–260.

Munger R, Romitti PA, Daack-Hirsch S, Burns TL, Murray JC, Hanson J (1996) Maternal alcohol use and risk of orofacial cleft birth defects. Teratology 54: 27–33.

Murray J (1995) Face facts: genes, environment, and clefts. American Journal of Human Genetics 57: 227–232.

Nyberg D, Sickler G, Hegge F, Kramer D, Kropp R (1995) Fetal cleft lip with and without cleft palate: US classification and correlation with outcome. Radiology 195: 677–684.

Philip N, Meinecke P, David A (1992) Kabuki make-up (Niikawa-Kuroki) syndrome: a study of 16 non-Japanese cases. Clinical Dysmorphology 1: 63–77.

Ranta R, Rintala A (1983) Correlations between microforms of the van der Woude syndrome and cleft palate. Cleft Palate Journal 20: 158–162.

Roelfsema N, Cobben J (1996) The EEC syndrome: a literature study. Clinical Dysmorphology 5: 115–127.

Ryan A, Bartlett K, Clayton P, Eaton S, Mills L, Donnai D, Winter RM, Burn J (1998) Smith–Lemli–Opitz syndrome: a variable clinical and biochemical phenotype. Journal of Medical Genetics 35: 558–565.

Schutte B, Murray J (1999) The many faces and factors of orofacial clefts. Human Molecular Genetics 8(10 Review): 1853–1859.

Shprintzen R, Goldberg R, Golding-Kushner K, Marion RW (1992) Late-onset psychosis in the velo-cardio-facial syndrome. American Journal of Medical Genetics 42: 41–42.

Snead, M, Yates J (1999) Clinical and molecular genetics of Stickler syndrome. Journal of Medical Genetics 36(5): 353–359.

Stickler G, Belau P, Farrel FJ (1965) Hereditary progressive arthro-ophthalmology. Mayo Clinic Proceedings 40: 433–455.

Tellier A.-L, Cormier-Daire V, Abadie V, Amiel J, Sigaudy S, Bonnet D, De Lonlay-Debeney P, Morrisseau-Durand M, Hubert P, Michel J, Jan D, Dollfus H, Baumann C, Labrune P, Lacombe D, Philip N, Lemerrer M, Briard M, Munnich A, Lyonnet, S (1998) CHARGE syndrome: Report of 47 cases and review. American Journal of Medical Genetics 76: 402–409.

Temple I (1989) Stickler's syndrome. Journal of Medical Genetics 26: 119–126.

Tolarova M, Cervenka J (1998) Classification and birth prevalence of orofacial clefts. American Journal of Medical Genetics 75(2): 126–137.

Toriello H (1993) Oral-facial-digital syndromes. Clinical Dysmorphology 2: 95–105.

Treacher Collins E (1900) Cases with symmetrical congenital notches in the outer part of each lid and defective development of the malar bones. Trans Ophthalmol Soc UK 20: 190–2.

van der Woude A (1954) Fistula labii inferioris congenita and its association with cleft lip and palate. American Journal of Human Genetics 6: 244–256.

Winter R, Baraitser M (1998) London Dysmorphology Database. Oxford: Oxford University Press.

PART II
MANAGEMENT OF THE INFANT AND YOUNG CHILD WITH A CLEFT LIP AND/OR PALATE

CHAPTER 7

Abnormalities of the Fetal Lip and Palate: Sonographic Diagnosis

L.S. CHITTY AND D.R. GRIFFIN

Examination of the fetal face

The outline of the fetal face is recognizable sonographically late in the first trimester and, particularly if using transvaginal ultrasound, abnormalities may be identified by 12–14 weeks. However, examination of the fetal face is difficult at this stage in pregnancy and it is more usual to examine the face at around 18–22 weeks. Examination later in pregnancy may be difficult, particularly when trying to visualize the palate, as shadowing from surrounding bony structures may obscure the view.

Three views are used to examine the face (Figure 7.1) – the axial, coronal and sagittal. In the axial plane the orbits and nasal bones, lenses, mandible (Figure 7.2), palate and tooth buds (Figure 7.3) and lips (Figure 7.4) may all be visualized at different levels. In the coronal plane the upper and lower lips and nose may be seen (Figure 7.5), and at a higher level the cheeks, eyelids, lenses and forehead. Visualization of the mouth opening is often useful to define the integrity of the upper lip (Figure 7.6). The sagittal view demonstrates the fetal profile (Figure 7.7) and is useful when examining the chin, forehead and nasal bridge. There are charts documenting the normal ranges for a variety of bony parts that may be of use in diagnosing abnormalities of the fetal face. These include the mandible (Chitty and Altman, 1993a), orbital diameters (Chitty and Altman, 1993b).

Sonographic diagnosis of cleft lip and palate

Unilateral (Figure 7.8), bilateral (Figure 7.9) and midline (Figure 7.10) clefts of the lip and/or palate may be detected using prenatal ultrasound. Abnormalities of the palate are best seen in the axial view (Figure 7.11a), whereas those of the lip are often best seen in the coronal plane (Figure 7.8a), although examination of the axial (Figures 7.8b and 7.11b) and sagittal planes (Figures 7.8c and 7.9b) is also helpful. Clefts of the soft palate are not amenable to prenatal detection and small clefts of the hard palate alone are often not detected with ultrasound, as the palate is difficult to examine in detail due to shadowing from surrounding bony structures.

Prenatal screening for cleft lip and palate

In the UK the majority of women are offered a fetal anomaly scan at 18–20 weeks gestation. This scan is designed to check the number of fetuses present, to confirm viability and, in an increasing number of units, to detect fetal abnormalities. Detection rates for abnormalities overall vary from place to place depending on the local protocol (i.e. which parts are routinely examined), the skill of the sonographer, gestational age at the time of screening and time allowed for scanning (Chitty, 1995). In some units, time constraints prevent routine examination of the fetal face. Even when the face is routinely examined only around 40% of clefts of the lip and palate are detected in the absence of other gross fetal abnormalities (i.e. 'isolated clefts') (Chitty, 1995). This relatively poor detection rate is a reflection of the fact that fetal position often prevents good visualization of the face, and that the hands and umbilical cord often lie immediately in front of the face *in utero*. When scanning a fetus at low risk for a facial cleft it is often not possible to allow sufficient time in the routine clinic to wait for the fetus to move.

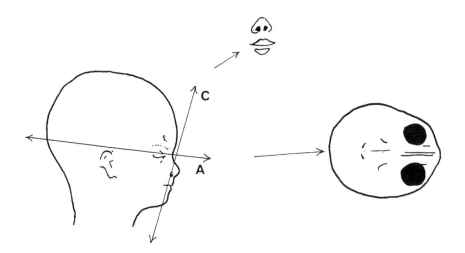

Figure 7.1. Diagram showing the scanning planes used for examination of the fetal face, coronal (C) and axial (A) planes. The profile view shows the sagittal plane.

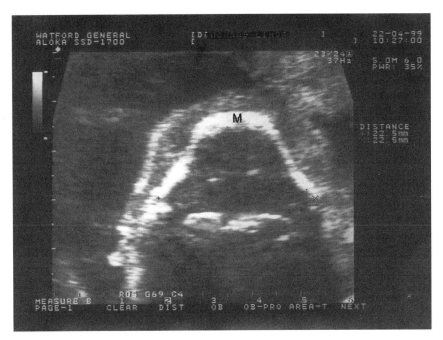

Figure 7.2. Axial view through the fetal head, demonstrating the mandible (M) with head in the occipital posterior position so that the rami are viewed symmetrically.

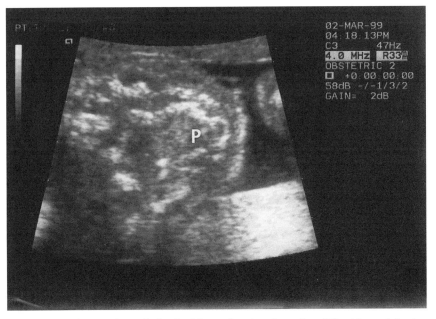

Figure 7.3. Axial view through the fetal face, showing the palate (P) with tooth buds and tongue visible.

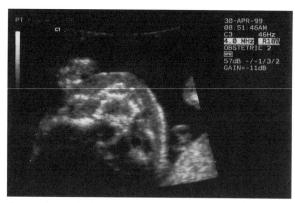

Figure 7.4. Axial view through the fetal face demonstrating the integrity of the upper lip in a normal fetus.

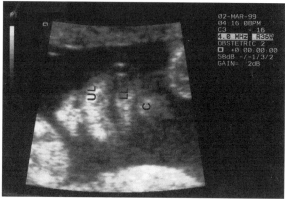

Figure 7.5. Coronal view of the face demonstrating the nostrils, upper (UL) and lower lip (LL) and chin (C).

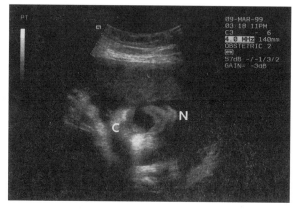

Figure 7.6. Coronal view of the face with the lips open. Note how the integrity of the upper lip is demonstrated with the mouth open. The nose (N) and chin (C) are labelled to aid orientation.

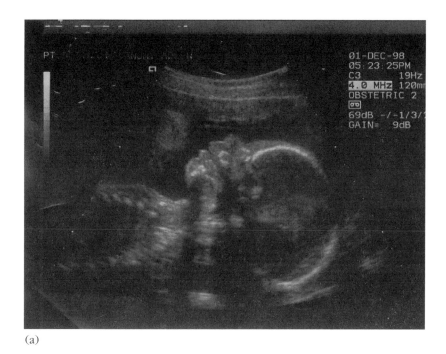

(a)

(b)

Figure 7.7. Sagittal view of the fetal face showing the profile. (a) Normal profile, (b) fetus with micrognathia, unilateral cleft lip and trisomy 18.

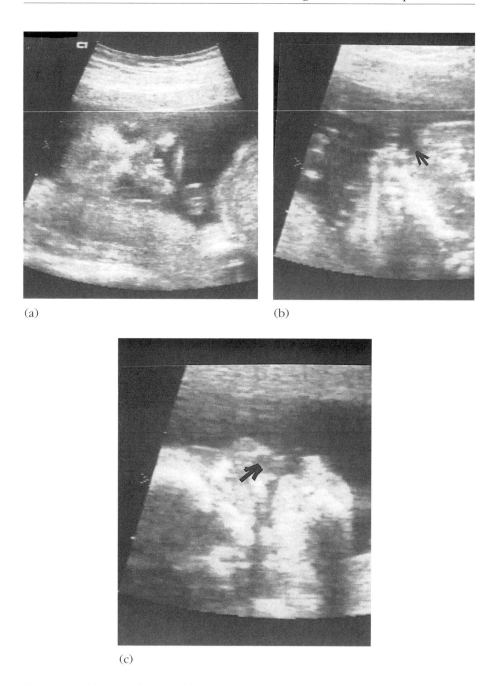

(a)

(b)

(c)

Figure 7.8. (a) Coronal view of the face showing a unilateral cleft of the lip (cranium to left, chin to the right). Note how examination in the axial plane (b) and parasagittal plane (c) can also be useful in defining the cleft lip (b, c) and palate (b). The cleft is marked by the arrow.

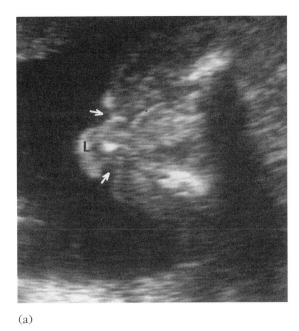

(a)

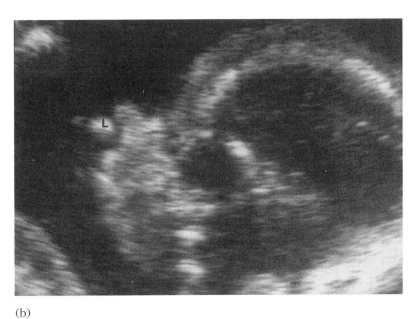

(b)

Figure 7.9. (a) Axial view demonstrating a bilateral cleft lip with the parasagittal view (b) showing the abnormal appearance of the median portion of lip (prolabium) (L). The arrows mark the clefts in the lip.

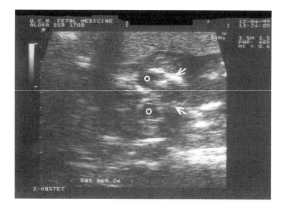

Figure 7.10. Coronal view of a fetus at 13 weeks gestation showing a large median cleft lip. The borders of the cleft are marked by arrows and orbits (o).

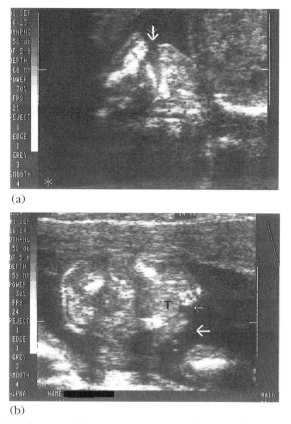

(a)

(b)

Figure 7.11. (a) Axial view of the palate showing cleft marked by the arrow. (b) Shows how the cleft lip, marked by the arrow, can also be defined in this plane with the tongue (T) inside the mouth. Note the asymmetry in the mandibular rami shown in (a) in this fetus with a diagnosis of hemifacial microsomia.

In women at known increased risk because of a family history, detection rates are better as these women are often referred for a detailed anomaly scan in a tertiary unit. In contrast to the routine anomaly scan, which is usually performed by a radiographer or midwife, a medically qualified sonographer trained in the examination of the abnormal fetus performs these scans in most cases. More time is allowed and, if the face cannot be visualized, the scan will be repeated on another occasion if required.

In families where there is a history of cleft lip and palate in a previous child or other relative, referral for a detailed scan can be very helpful. The majority of parents will be reassured that their baby does not have a cleft lip. In cases where an abnormality is detected, parents usually find the prior warning helpful as it allows time for them to come to terms with the need for postnatal surgery. Under these circumstances, parents find it very useful to have a prenatal meeting with members of the team who will be caring for their child after birth (see Bradbury and Bannister, Chapter 8).

Management of pregnancy following the detection of a cleft lip and palate

Having identified a cleft lip prenatally, it is important to examine the rest of the face carefully in order to detect abnormalities that may alter the prognosis. It is usually the cleft of the lip that is identified first as the lips are more readily visualized. Further examination of the palate can often reveal the associated cleft (Figure 7.11a) and the sagittal view may demonstrate a degree of micrognathia (Figure 7.7b). In the case shown in Figure 7.11, detailed examination of the face revealed the presence of an abnormal ear on one side and asymmetry of the mandible (Figure 7.11b) together with a midline cleft of the palate (Figure 7.11a) in a fetus with hemifacial microsomia.

In fetal life, facial clefts are often associated with other structural abnormalities or chromosomal abnormalities such as trisomy 13 or 18. Indeed, it is often the detection of anomalies outside the face that leads to a more detailed examination, at which time the cleft lip may be detected. One of the more common prenatal associations with facial clefts is holoprosencephaly, which may be associated with a range of midline fetal facial anomalies ranging from hypertelorism or a median facial cleft (Figure 7.10) to a single nostril or proboscis.

Careful examination of the rest of the fetus should be performed to exclude the presence of other structural abnormalities. Fetal karyotyping should be discussed, particularly if there are associated sonographic abnormalities or other risk factors present such as increased maternal age. In a fetus with an isolated facial cleft and no other risk factor, the chance of the karyotype being abnormal is very small (Snijders et al., 1996).

It is extremely important that, after the presence of other problems has been excluded, parents should be referred to the local cleft lip and palate team for detailed discussion regarding prognosis and postnatal management.

Parents will have questions regarding the cosmetic and functional results of surgery. They may have worries about breast feeding and speech development. Such questions are best answered by the team who will manage the baby postnatally as management may vary between units and technological advances may alter practice. It may be helpful for a member of the team to be present at the time of scanning, but, as this can be difficult to arrange, hard copy of scan images together with a detailed description of the abnormality will be of help to the person counselling the parents. In the presence of a severe cleft it can be difficult to define the extent of the lesion prenatally as the usual landmarks are often distorted. In such cases, and in any other than a simple lesion, it is useful for the sonographer to discuss the findings directly with the member of the cleft lip and palate team who will be counselling the parents.

It must also be remembered that fetal ultrasound cannot detect all abnormalities. Subtle abnormalities that may be associated with an underlying genetic syndrome may not be identified prenatally. There are around 400 syndromes that have cleft lip and/or palate as features (Winter and Baraitser, 1998 see Lees, Chapter 6)). Parents should be warned that, although a cleft is likely to be an isolated abnormality, a small residual risk remains of other problems being identified after birth (Milerad et al., 1997).

Conclusions

Modern technology now permits the diagnosis of many abnormalities prior to birth. Increasingly, anomalies of the fetal face are being detected prenatally. The management of a pregnancy complicated by a fetal facial cleft should include a detailed anomaly scan and discussion of karyotyping. As with many other abnormalities, involvement of the paediatric team at an early stage is essential for parents to gain a proper understanding of the nature and implications of the lesion and the potential for cosmetic and functional correction.

References

Chitty LS (1995) Ultrasound screening for fetal abnormalities. Prenatal Diagnosis 15: 1241–1257.

Chitty LS, Altman DG (1993a) Measurement of the fetal mandible – feasibility and construction of a centile chart. Prenatal Diagnosis 13: 749–756.

Chitty LS, Altman DG (1993b) Fetal Biometry. In: Meire H, Cosgrove K, Dewbury K (eds) Clinical Ultrasound. Vol. 3, Obstetrics and Gynaecology. Edinburgh: Churchill Livingstone, pp. 513–595.

Milerad J, Larson O, Hagberg C, Ideberg M (1997) Associated malformations in infants with cleft lip and palate: A prospective, population based study. Pediatrics 100: 180–186.

Snijders RJM, Farrias M, Von Kaisenberg C, Nicolaides KH (1996) Fetal abnormalities. In: Snijders RJM, Nicolaides KH (eds) Ultrasound Markers for Fetal Chromosomal Defects. New York: Parthenon Publishing Group, pp. 19–21.

Winter RM, Baraitser M (1998) London Dysmorphology Database. Oxford Medical Databases.

CHAPTER 8

Prenatal, Perinatal and Postnatal Counselling

E. Bradbury and P. Bannister

Children are born into families, into dynasties with a history stretching back over the generations and a future stretching ahead through further generations. The new baby is observed for physical resemblances which mark the child as being within the world of the family. The birth of a baby with a cleft can disrupt this process. An unrepaired cleft lip alters the appearance of the face, and problems relating to feeding may cause the baby to be more difficult and fractious, with his or her own personality masked by this early behaviour. As the child grows, and if there is a cleft palate, speech may be different from other family members. In addition, the future of the baby may seem to be compromised by long-term treatment and unknown social and psychological consequences.

When a baby is born with a cleft, parents go through a period of adjustment as they struggle to come to terms with their baby and to let go of the fantasized hopes for the whole baby that they were expecting. This process has been described as akin to bereavement, and parents' responses can be understood in terms of adjustment to loss (Solnit and Stark, 1962). Others have seen it as a threat to self-esteem, the damaged child being a projection of the parents' own feelings of inferiority (Mintzer et al., 1984).

In recent years, technological improvements in prenatal screening have meant that babies with clefts are increasingly being identified in the womb (see Chitty and Griffin, Chapter 7). This poses a new challenge to those who counsel parents. In this chapter, we will look at the problems parents face at diagnosis and its aftermath, and the ways in which counselling can help them to adjust to their baby and move forward in their lives.

Prenatal counselling

When the growing fetus in the womb has been identified as having a cleft, the parents will have to go through the process of adjustment in an atmos-

117

phere of uncertainty. They will not know exactly what their baby will look like and struggle to cope with images of a fantasized imperfect child. There are often conflicting images of the anticipated child: the concept of a chubby wholeness vies with the unknown.

Most people have never seen an unrepaired cleft, and find it hard to imagine. Pictures of babies with clefts can help this process, but because of uncertainties in the diagnostic process, there should be several different pictures which would allow the parents to gain an approximate image without being too specific.

One important task for the counsellor at this stage is to allow the parents to gain some understanding of what it means to have a cleft and thus gain mastery as they are able to explore their own responses and those of others. In addition, it is important to help parents understand the physical implications of a cleft and the likely course of treatment. There is sometimes confusion if parents are given faulty information by someone unfamiliar with clefts. For example, one family was told that it was likely that the baby would be blind, others have been told of associated anomalies that the baby might have, even when the statistical chances of this happening are very small. Parents then become unnecessarily alarmed and distressed. Once the baby has been born treatment is managed by the cleft team (Royal College of Surgeons, 1995). At the time of prenatal diagnosis, there is often very little support for the parents and the future remains uncertain. Being told of potential associated anomalies and then left to cope with the pregnancy can be very stressful.

It is important that parents gain knowledge from an experienced member of the cleft team. The question of termination often arises at such times, either explicitly or implicitly. Parents who have been unnecessarily alarmed and who are not given support may see termination as the only reasonable option.

Thus prenatal diagnosis can have a disruptive effect on parental adjustment. However, when handled well, it can help that process. It gives the family the opportunity to work through much of their distress before the baby is born. It allows all members of the family to be prepared, including siblings and grandparents. Whilst the pregnancy may be more difficult emotionally, the birth is a more positive experience and attachment between mother and baby is not disrupted by the shock of seeing the unexpected unrepaired cleft.

The principles of good prenatal counselling are:

• Parents should be given accurate information by someone with experience of clefts.

- The time from diagnosis to support should be as brief as possible.
- Parents should have early contact with members of the cleft team.
- All members of the family should be given the opportunity to express their concerns and their emotional responses.
- They should all be helped to prepare for the birth by having a clear view of how the baby is likely to look.
- Any discussion of termination should begin with the parents on the basis of accurate information.

Perinatal counselling

Most babies with clefts are born without any warning of the cleft. The sight of the unrepaired cleft can be very shocking and the process of parental adjustment follows an uneven course. Some parents adjust immediately and can accept their baby unconditionally. Others take time and, for some, the adjustment never fully takes place. They will still cry about it in clinic when the child is much older (Bradbury and Hewison, 1994). Children may grow up with a sense of shame, unable to talk about the cleft with their parents, who have never come to terms with it. The importance of early attachment between parent and child has been well established (Bowlby, 1965).

It is important that parents receive experienced counselling when the baby is born. In the UK the parental support group CLAPA often makes early contact (see Davies, Chapter 24), and whilst this helps parents feel less alone, it is not a substitute for skilled professional care. Some parents do have great difficulty adjusting to the cleft and find it difficult to accept their child. This may be expressed as emotional distancing from the baby, but it may also be expressed as a defensive over-protectiveness as the parent strives to cope with negative feelings and a sense of personal incompetence. Problems with adjustment may be masked by the physical needs of the new baby, and whilst the distraught mother is easy to identify and help, it is not so easy to recognize the angry or depressed mother, nor the one who withdraws into an introspective depressive state.

In addition, the emotional needs of the father may not be recognized, nor those of the wider family. Research has shown that one of the most significant factors to affect parental adjustment is the response of grandparents (Bradbury and Hewison, 1994).

Skilled and experienced counselling is needed to assess the family situation and to offer appropriate help. A specialist nurse/counsellor, who sees all families of children with clefts, has a vital role to play in helping with a whole range of problems including feeding, support through the early months and surgery. He or she is particularly well placed to recognize hidden problems and to know when to refer on to other mental health services where appropriate. In addition, this type of intervention is likely to be more acceptable to many families who may feel distrustful of seeing a psychologist. Close links between the nurse/counsellor and the psychologist attached to the cleft team ensures that the most appropriate care can be offered.

The principles of good perinatal counselling are:

- All families should have access to experienced counselling.
- Early assessment of problems is important.
- The needs of all family members should be recognized.
- Strengths should be emphasized rather than weaknesses.
- Parents should be empowered to gain mastery through interaction with professionals and access to relevant information.

Postnatal counselling

Once the early trauma is passed, there remains the need to offer a counselling service which is responsive to individual need. No two families are the same and the ways in which they cope are a factor of their history, their current life situation and the level of social support they receive from family and friends. The counsellor needs to assess the family situation in an empathetic and non-judgemental way, offering longer-term support with issues such as coping with feeding and the child's hospitalization for surgery where appropriate. The cleft becomes a risk factor, rendering both child and parents more vulnerable and less able to cope with other difficulties. For example, a parent who is struggling to overcome alcohol addiction may find that the event of the cleft is just one stress too many, and resume drinking.

Social and family support is particularly important, and the counsellor can help by encouraging this support, facilitating communication and sharing of responsibilities and referring on to agencies such as Relate or social services where appropriate.

It is particularly important for the counsellor to find ways of empowering the family to move forward without long-term dependency on professionals. Ways of developing this work have been described in more detail elsewhere (Bradbury, 1996; Lansdown et al., 1997).

Early indications of potential difficulty in adjustment and acceptance include social avoidance, the refusal to take and display baby photos, minimal interaction between mother and baby with very little non-essential holding and cuddling. It may also be expressed as anger against professionals as parents seek an outlet for their distress, or as an intense preoccupation with treatment and with feeding issues, the two becoming intertwined as parents feel under pressure to increase their baby's weight in preparation for surgery.

Parents sometimes feel de-skilled and incompetent because of problems with feeding, because of the intervention of professionals and because of perceptions of guilt. Counselling should focus on strengths rather than weaknesses, achievement rather than problems, and should encourage parents to feel empowered so that they can truly care for their children. The counsellor should not act as intermediary between the parents and the professionals, but enable parents to gain mastery over the situation through information, encouragement and support.

Principles of good postnatal counselling are:

- Individual needs should be assessed in a non-judgemental way.
- Communication should be encouraged between family members.
- Social and family support should be mobilized where it is lacking.
- If necessary, other agencies should be contacted to help deal with particular problems.
- Long-term dependency on the counsellor should be avoided and normalization of family life should be encouraged.

Conclusions

Having a baby with a cleft is stressful for many parents. It is a time when they are particularly vulnerable to feelings of distress as they adjust to this situation which has changed their lives. Early counselling plays a crucial role in identifying needs and offering appropriate help (Bradbury, 1997). This counselling should be skilled and experienced, with the aim of encouraging the family to adjust to the baby and to move forward as a family without the need for long-term dependency on professionals.

References

Bowlby S (1965) Child Care and the Growth of Maternal Love. London: Penguin.

Bradbury ET (1996) Counselling People with Disfigurement. Leicester: British Psychological Society.

Bradbury ET (1997) Cleft lip and palate surgery, the need for individual and family counselling. [Editorial] British Journal of Hospital Medicine 57(8): 366–367.

Bradbury ET, Hewison J (1994) Early prenatal responses to visible congenital disfigurement. Child Care, Health and Development 20: 251–266.

Lansdown R, Rumsey N, Bradbury ET, Carr A, Partridge J (eds) (1997)Visibly Different. Oxford: Butterworth-Heinemann.

Mintzer DM, Als H, Tronick EZ, Brazelton TB (1984) Parenting a child with a birth defect: the regulation of self esteem. Zero-to-three 5(5): 1–2, 4–8.

Royal College of Surgeons of England (1995) The Treatment of Cleft Lip and Palate: a Parents' Guide. London.

Solnit A, Stark MH (1962) Mourning and the birth of a defective child. Psychoanalytic Study of the Child 16: 9–24.

CHAPTER 9

The Role of the Paediatrician

A. HABEL

Introduction

Active participation of paediatricians in the cleft lip and palate (CLP) team was pioneered in Edinburgh in the 1960s by Drillien et al (1966), yet this presence remains a rarity. In the USA the situation is marginally better, with a few participating paediatricians (Kaufman, 1991). A forceful impetus to their inclusion is made in the Clinical Standards Advisory Group's Report on Cleft Lip and Palate services (CSAG, 1998). It recommends that each UK centre should have one or two paediatricians with a major time commitment in the cleft team. The special skills of paediatricians bring the following expertise to a family-focused team:

- A knowledge of the processes of development from embryo to maturity and how malformation and resultant therapeutic interventions may impact on growth and function. Three-quarters of the fetuses with clefts detected antenatally have additional malformations (see below).
- A whole child perspective, free of the need to focus exclusively on the surgery, speech, orthodontics or hearing problems.
- Familiarity with genetic issues in order that appropriate referral is made to a geneticist (CSAG, 1998). Such families can receive more specialized investigative and counselling facilities.
- Special skills in:
  (a) Working with families.
  (b) Liaison with social services over housing, disability living allowance, the provision of family aid workers where the caring load is overwhelming, and with regard to child protection issues.
  (c) Developing community links, especially through the recent introduction in the UK of Ambulatory Paediatricians, and Home Care

Paediatric Nursing teams. Together they bring high quality care to the child's own home. Hospital stay may be reduced or even prevented. Examples relevant to this population include the management of feeding difficulties in infants with clefts, gastrostomy care in those unable to feed long term, and care of a tracheostomy or nasopharyngeal tube in the Pierre Robin sequence.

(d) Medically related issues in the educational setting, both in normal and special schools. In addition to liaising with school teachers, school nurses and educational psychologists, the paediatrician has a pivotal role in investigating concerns raised by abnormal behaviour, bullying, impaired concentration, suspected seizures, and facilitating a child's full involvement in school life.

(e) Psychological issues. For example, the paediatrician is able to determine whether abdominal pain in a schoolchild with a cleft has an organic or functional basis. The paediatrician should have an understanding of how personal and family function is affected by clefting, and familiarity in working with child guidance teams.

The paediatrician acts as adviser to the team on:

- The timing of surgery. Typical situations to assess include where the infant is failing to thrive, or when asthma is poorly controlled. Advice is often sought on the timing of routine vaccinations, in particular whether delay is appropriate due to intercurrent illness.
- Whether, prior to surgery, there is a need to screen for underlying defects such as congenital heart disease.
- Family concerns raised by a team member. For example, the speech and language therapist may observe a lack of appropriate family interaction. This abnormal behaviour could be due to emotional withdrawal from depression or child abuse. The paediatrician can determine whether concerns justify onward referral.

Timetable for paediatricians

The reader is referred to Table 9.1 for a summary of the nature and timing of the paediatrician's involvement.

Antenatal

Improved ultrasound scanning between 1991 and 1995 increased the detection rate of isolated clefts from a quarter to a half of those identified at birth (Nicolaides, 1996). Nicolaides also observed that other ultrasound abnormalities were found in 75% of all clefts detected antenatally in his

Table 9.1. Timetable and agenda of paediatric contacts

Contingent on the severity of associated abnormalities and the involvement of tertiary centres.

Antenatal
Obstetric consultation regarding ultrasound scan: refer to team.

At birth
1. Diagnosis.
2. Initial assessment: associated malformations.
3. Special Care Baby Unit (SCBU): avoid unless airway problems or other abnormalities require active help. The infant should stay with mother unless feeding problem is major, e.g. danger of aspiration pneumonia.
4. CLP team referral.
5. Feeding.

Four weeks
Weight, head circumference, vaccination advice, initial genetic assessment, begin parental counselling.

Six months
Length, weight, head circumference, development, stress and its sequelae.

Preschool surveillance
Growth monitoring (height and weight), developmental delays, psychological issues that are likely to manifest, and anticipatory guidance. Ages one and a half years, three and a half years, five years.

School age concerns
7–10 years: height, schooling, emotional adjustment.

Adolescent issues for the paediatrician
13 years: delay in puberty, relationships.
16+ years: genetic counselling, job/continuing education plans, relationships.

practice. An apparently isolated cleft palate on antenatal ultrasound is, however, also compatible with Stickler syndrome or the velocardiofacial (VCF) spectrum (see genetics below), highlighting the need for caution when counselling antenatally. The finding of a facial cleft on antenatal ultrasound is therefore increasingly likely to involve the paediatrician in discussion about the presence and management of associated anomalies and the place of birth if there is a major surgical heart or gut abnormality. *In utero* surgery for clefts should not be considered until appropriate techniques have been perfected (Strauss and Davis, 1990).

At birth

1. Diagnosis

Diagnosis at birth is usually immediate for babies born with cleft lip, but may be delayed by hours to weeks in cleft palate and by years in the case of submucous cleft palate (SMCP). To examine for cleft palate (CP) the midwife or junior doctor should obtain a clear view of the palate by inspection when the infant is crying or with a spatula and torch. Palpation alone is to be deprecated, and probably accounts for the delay in diagnosis of up to 10% of isolated CP (Gareth Davies, Chief Executive, National CLAPA, personal communication). A clinical pointer to SMCP may be the finding of a bifid uvula, although this is also found in 1% of normal babies. In others SMCP is indicated by the presence of a V-shaped notch at the junction of the hard and soft palate, usually identified through inspection and/or palpation. Moss et al. (1990) found slow feeding (>40 minutes) (85%) and nasal regurgitation of milk (50%) occurred in infants and young children with SMCP. It is the duty of consultant paediatricians to ensure that appropriate training of nursing and junior staff is in place to promote maximum rates of early detection. Frequently it is the midwife or most junior member of the medical team who makes the discovery. Delay in informing a parent in a misguided attempt to reduce suffering may lead to anger directed at medical services and sow the seeds of mistrust. The infant should never be whisked away, and the deformity should always be shown to the parents. As the baby is handed to the mother explicit reference to the defect should be made.

2. Initial assessment

If the diagnosis of cleft lip and/or palate is first made by a nurse or junior doctor, an urgent consultation with the middle grade or senior paediatrician is essential. Immediate problems to consider are airway obstruction, congenital abnormalities and feeding difficulties.

(i) Airway obstruction

This is a common presentation of the Pierre Robin sequence. It is associated with a small mandible (micrognathia), and classically a U-shaped cleft of hard and soft palate. The tongue is more posteriorly placed than usual, lacks the support of the genioglossi muscles, falls back and may occlude the airway if the infant is laid supine. Functional airway obstruction affecting both inspiration and expiration can be demonstrated (Moss et al., 1990). Other features include:

- Difficulty in intubation at birth.
- Intermittent obstruction relieved by turning into the prone position. An apnoea monitor may be recommended. A pulse oximeter or transcutaneous oxygen electrode is preferred as it detects the initial fall in oxygen. One that detects movement only may not alarm until after the termination of all respiratory effort, when the baby has finally failed to overcome the obstruction.
- In more severe cases, persistent soft tissue indrawing, cyanosis or apnoea. Complications of the Pierre Robin sequence include respiratory obstruction, hypoxia, hypercapnia, pulmonary oedema, cor pulmonale, vomiting, aspiration pneumonia and sudden death. Long-term effects might include failure to thrive and brain damage manifesting as learning or physical disability.

In the past infants were placed in a Burston frame (Campbell and Watson, 1980) for weeks or months, remaining in hospital because of the risk of hypoxia and aspiration. Opportunities for handling and stimulation of the infant were reduced. Insertion of a nasopharyngeal airway overcomes the obstruction, improves feeding, and reduces wasteful energy expenditure on increased effort of breathing, relieves associated congestive cardiac failure, and results in improved weight gain (Heaf et al., 1982). A Portex 3.0 or 3.5 mm endotracheal tube, cut to the correct length, is used. Careful positioning of the tube is required, just above the epiglottis. It is replaced every two weeks until there is no longer any obstruction; this is usually within four to twelve weeks. Home management is increasingly practised, especially if a Paediatric Home Care Nursing team is available. An alternative, less commonly used technique is tongue–lip adhesion (Cozzi et al., 1996). This can interfere with feeding and speech development (Masarei et al., 1999). Tracheostomy is rarely required. The development of Paediatric Home Care Nursing (PHCN) teams throughout the UK has reduced the hospitalization of many children with clefts. They usually work closely with ambulatory paediatricians (Meates, 1997), to provide anything from a five day service in office hours to continuous seven day 24 hour support. Oxygen saturation, oxygen dependency, changing of nasopharyngeal tubes for Pierre Robin sequence, gastrostomy care and feeding supervision initiated and established in the hospital is then supervised by the PHC nurse. Nurse specialists are often part of the team. For example, a respiratory nurse, in addition to the oxygen-related care, can assess and advise how best to give aerosolized asthma medication, via a nebulizer, face mask and spacer, or rotahaler for wheeze due to gastro-oesophageal reflux and aspiration, which is relatively common in multiply disabled children with facial clefts. The saving in hospital bed days and emotional trauma to child and family appear self-evident, although running costs of such teams are significant.

The Pierre Robin sequence is one of the named exceptions to the recommended supine posture in the 'Back to Sleep' campaign to reduce cot deaths (Recommendations of the Chief Medical Officer's Expert Group on the sleeping position of infants and cot death, Department of Health, 1993). In less severe cases a satisfactory compromise is to lay the infant on the side.

(ii) General examination

The baby should be examined systematically for other congenital abnormalities, particularly those requiring immediate attention such as congenital heart disease. Associated malformations of the heart and kidneys are commoner than in babies without clefts by a factor of ten or more. Features that can assist in identifying a syndrome are, for example, split-hand and syndactyly, and absence of eyelashes in the ectrodactyly–ectodermal dysplasia–cleft palate (EEC) syndrome (see Lees, Chapter 6). It is then possible to inform the parents of the clinical situation, to gently probe for information, and synthesize available data to decide on investigations and management strategies. A history should be taken, focusing particularly on drugs taken in the first trimester such as steroids, anticonvulsants, and diets low in folic acid. Periconceptional vitamin taking reduces the risk of clefting by a quarter (Shaw et al., 1995). The history may reveal a family history of clefting or associated abnormalities such as hearing difficulties and eye defects which are suggestive of Stickler syndrome, or the lip pits of van der Woude syndrome (see Lees, Chapter 6). Both are autosomal dominant conditions associated with cleft palate, and have a one in two chance of recurrence. Consanguinity should also be noted since this increases the risk of a wide range of congenital abnormalities.

(iii) Investigations to be arranged

Antenatal ultrasound may already have detected abnormalities, but this should not be taken for granted, and other tests may be indicated following the above assessments. Initial categorization is then possible into familial, syndromic or, by exclusion, isolated clefts (i.e. no affected relative).

(iv) Feeding

Limited data are available comparing the advantages and disadvantages of the many different feeding methods such as breast, bottle, cup and spoon, or supplemental tube feeds. Further work is required to put nutritional advice on a truly scientific basis. The paediatrician needs to work in close collaboration with the specialist nurse (see Bannister, Chapter 10).

A quarter of cleft infants have early feeding difficulties, with poor weight gain for the first two to three months of 145 g/week compared with an average of 200 g/week in non-cleft babies (Richards, 1994). Feeds are often prolonged, in part due to ulceration of the nasal mucosa. Infants with congenital heart disease or airway obstruction (e.g. in Pierre Robin sequence) often have increased metabolic needs.

Medical management decisions: neonatal period to two years

1. Admission to a Special Care Baby Unit

This is best avoided unless airway or congenital abnormalities require active help. Rooming-in with mother is to be encouraged even where feeding is a major problem.

2. Assessment for other congenital abnormalities

A careful clinical scrutiny is extended if dysmorphic features or more than one major anomaly are detected. Scanning (ultrasound, echo, X-ray, MRI/CT), genetic (chromosomes, DNA probes) and biochemical and haematological work-up are selectively applied.

3. Referral

Early referral to the CLP team is essential. A team member should visit within 24 hours of birth. Careful consideration is required before committing a child to a type of operation or treatments without the benefit of satisfactory audit or evidenced-based research. A powerful weapon in the search for evidence-based practice comes in the CSAG advice to Purchasers of CLP services within the National Health Service (CSAG, 1998). This states the requirement to produce a service specification requiring compulsory audits of treatment and outcome.

4. Breast milk

Breast milk fed to cleft infants may significantly reduce ear effusions and consequent hearing problems to 3% compared with 32% of children fed exclusively on formula (Paradise et al., 1994).

5. Feeding problems

1. The cause of inadequate intake needs to be established such as whether it is of a physical, airway, metabolic or neurological aetiology.
2. Breastfeeding difficulties are frequent due to an inability to generate negative suction or express sufficient for baby's needs. Bottles and teats need to be assessed, involving the specialist nurse (see Bannister, Chapter 10).
3. If calorie supplementation is needed the dietician should be involved.
4. A speech and language therapist experienced in dysphagia should be involved when there is significant oral-motor, pharyngeal or gastro-oesophageal dysfunction (Carroll and Reilly, 1996).
5. Sometimes it is necessary to involve a psychologist when there are behavioural problems.

Monitoring and counselling visits in the first year of life

1. Early weight gain

The paediatrician provides anticipatory support to minimize poor weight gain and parental anxiety. 'Catch up' after surgery, in weight and height, occurs on average by two years of age (Lee et al., 1996). Syndromic children grow poorly. In non-syndromic cleft lip and palate, those with isolated clefts of the palate grow the least well (Bowers et al., 1987).

2. Genetic assessment

The first step is to establish whether the cleft is isolated, familial, or if other abnormalities are present, syndromic (see Lees, Chapter 6). Major malformations are found in 40% of CP and 26% of CLP, and half have a recognized syndrome of which, to date, more than 400 have been described (Winter and Baraitser, 1998). Close attention should be paid to the apparently 'isolated cleft palate', both newly diagnosed and those attending for review. Two conditions are highlighted:

(a) Velocardiofacial (VCF) syndrome, often inherited from one parent, accounts for 10–20% of cleft palates.
(b) Stickler syndrome accounts for one third of those with the Pierre Robin sequence, which itself accounts for a half of cleft palates. The genetic implications of non-identification are of importance to the family as well as from the medico-legal perspective.

3. Stress

Children with a disability cause increased stress to families, leading to a greater frequency of parental break-up, mental breakdown and risk of child abuse.

4. Airway problems in infancy

Residual airway obstruction in the Pierre Robin sequence may continue to present as sleep-related obstructive episodes. Episodic hypoxia may elevate the pulmonary artery pressure to cause further oxygen desaturation and an increased danger of cot death. Sleep studies in which oxygen saturation, airway patency, sleep phase and body movement are synchronously recorded can identify the frequency, severity and duration of such episodes (Freed et al., 1988). Management decisions resulting from such studies include whether to continue prone posture, provide oxygen therapy, delay surgery, or anticipate the need for a nasopharyngeal airway postoperatively.

Preschool/school age monitoring

Growth measurement

Growth failure may be due to early nutritional problems. An additional cause in the Pierre Robin sequence may be lung aspiration or chronic hypoxia. Growth hormone deficiency is rare but may occur 40 times more commonly in isolated cleft palate than in non-cleft children (Rudman et al., 1978), and may also be associated with septo-optic dysplasia. A quarter of children under eight years of age with isolated cleft palate are below the fifth centile, that is a frequency five times greater than normal (Duncan et al., 1983). Children with unilateral CLP are two and a half times more likely to be below the tenth centile (Bowers et al., 1987; Dawkins, 1996a). Ideally cleft children should have their height measured annually. Where height is not routinely measured at clinics, cases of impaired growth may be missed until late on. Since parents of a cleft child are more likely to attend the CLP team than their community paediatrician or the family doctor for regular reappraisal, there is often a consequent failure of community surveillance. It is therefore of considerable importance for the team to monitor height attained and to communicate it to their colleagues. Growth monitoring should not be omitted in children with disabling conditions and dysmorphic syndromes. Appropriate growth charts are available for the following syndromes: Down's, Turner's, Noonan's, achondroplasia.

Developmental delay

Concern regarding the developmental progress of the child should initiate questioning and investigation to clarify whether delay is due to:

1. A valid association with clefting (hearing, speech).
2. Learning disability as part of a syndrome.
3. Multifactorial reasons such as hospitalizations, intercurrent illness, and/or reduced social opportunity.

When evidence of delay is found, the next step is to consider the involvement of community resources. This includes liaising with community paediatricians, who may arrange more specific assessments, such as speech and language therapy, physiotherapy, occupational therapy, a Portage stimulation programme (encouraging further developmental achievements by incremental steps) or a nursery placement with ordinary or special facilities, according to need.

The resources of the local authority social work department may be indicated to provide a family aid worker, social work input, help to apply for disability and invalid care allowances or appeals against their refusal, and in appropriate cases, the organizing of respite care, if requested, to give the family a rest from continued strain.

Educational resources include the school psychological service, with access to remedial help and the statutory authority to produce a Statement of Educational Needs (UK, 1981 Educational Act). These actions can be initiated by the paediatrician.

Psychological issues that are likely to manifest, and should be raised

The child's emerging awareness of being 'different', usually by the age of seven to eight years, may be exacerbated by teasing or bullying. A third of 12-year-olds with CLP admit to having been teased and a quarter are still worried by it (CSAG Report, 1998). The paediatrician has a responsibility along with other members of the CLP team to address the issues this raises (Dawkins, 1996a); (see Bradbury, Chapter 23).

Bullying is a form of child abuse, manifest as peer abuse. In the short term victims have lower self-esteem, feel less competent and have fewer close friends. Their schoolwork may be adversely affected. Self-harm and suicide may be more likely. Somatization with physical symptoms is common (Williams et al., 1996). As adults, they are more vulnerable to anxiety, depression and loneliness, and may be less likely to establish long-term relationships.

In cleft children and young adults, the awareness of 'difference', a manifest physical or articulatory disability, however mild, whether self-induced or expressed by others, becomes internalized. Boys with physical disability may be more vulnerable than girls (Dawkins, 1996a). Social relationships become impaired. In the long term the doubling in incidence of young adult suicides with CLP identified in Denmark (Herskind et al., 1993) is likely to have its roots in adverse childhood experience.

The warning signs include school refusal, and/or overdependency on adult company. Later, signs of depression (apathy, social withdrawal, anorexia) may emerge in adolescence. Girls tend to be more vulnerable, with the greater concern that they and their families have regarding facial appearance, and less 'acting out' with aggressive acts than boys.

Action

- Prophylaxis is the fostering of peer acceptance and good parent–child relationships. Social activities, Guides or Scouts, church groups, sports activities such as organized off street football, gymnastics or ballet foster self-confidence.
- Children can learn how to deal with everyday and confrontational situations from parental discussion, child guidance, or charities such as Changing Faces, which provides individual counselling and/or workshops. (Changing Faces, 1 & 2 Junction Mews, London W2 1PN, 020 7706 4232/4234).
- The Cleft Lip and Palate Team can provide support by supplying written information, being a contact point for parents, and giving individual consultations to the adolescent. At clinic reviews enquiries about headaches, abdominal pains, bed wetting, feeling sad and having sleeping difficulties may elicit symptoms that are associated with bullying (Dawkins, 1996b).
- Parent mediated action (Kish, personal communication)
  (a) Preschool. From three to four years old it is helpful to have a phrase ready to explain the deformity, e.g. 'my lip was sore and the doctor fixed it'. Parents should use appropriate language about a facial cleft and disfigurement, e.g. cleft lip ('hare' lip, although perhaps a pejorative expression, is still widely used and understood by the public and may be an alternative).
  (b) School age. It is important at this stage to reduce denial and encourage acceptance of disfigurement. Bullying should be acknowledged if it takes place, and parents should be informed that they cannot always solve all problems. Appropriate advice to deal with situations includes countering the bully by playing the fool, laughing back at tormentors, or, if able, being witty. It is advisable not to be

aggressive. It is sound advice to try and make friends with other children not involved in the bullying and inform the teacher or playground supervisor. Another helpful strategy is for parents to be encouraged to approach the school to promote classroom projects that enlist empathy and awareness, e.g. about hospitals, clinics and treatment.

It is vital that manifest bullying is tackled vigorously. Firstly, the child must be believed and reassured that by 'telling' he/she has acted correctly. Secondly, the parents should inform the school immediately. Thirdly, the school should act decisively. There are several useful resources for schools (Sharp and Smith, 1994; Department of Education and Employment's (1994) pack on bullying). A novel approach in which the pupils as a group support the victim and confront the bully with the consequences of their behaviour is outlined in a videotape entitled 'Bullying' (Available from Hopeline Videos, PO Box 515, London SW15 6LQ). In some cases, a referral to Child Guidance may be helpful for review of social function.

Adolescent issues for the paediatrician

Puberty and adult height

In isolated clefts puberty may be delayed by six months, and growth velocity in boys is slower. With the exception of isolated CP, which is associated with a slight reduction in final adult height, height achieved will be that predicted from mid-parental height in non-syndromic clefts (Bowers et al., 1988). Syndromic individuals are more likely to be of short stature, as for example in velocardiofacial syndrome, fetal alcohol syndrome and Stickler syndrome.

Psychological concerns

Teasing and bullying and the vulnerability of sexual relationships may show as depression, which is often not verbalized. It may be necessary to initiate afterschool social groups, assessment by the Department of Adolescent Psychiatry and/or contact with Changing Faces. A refusal of treatment may reflect reluctance to wear preoperative orthodontic appliances, fear of change, anticipation of pain, or be an assertion of independence. Sensitive handling, discussion of the issues and proceeding at the individual's pace all show respect for his/her viewpoint, and are likely to elicit cooperation in the fullness of time.

Genetics

The individual's type of cleft and family history will inform discussion about the likelihood of parenting similarly affected children. If the problem is complex, referral to a geneticist should be made. In isolated and familial cases of clefting the statistical risks tabulated in Chapter 6 apply.

Conclusion – a 'whole person' approach

The role of the paediatrician is to take a holistic view to the developing adult within the individual, addressing that person's medical, emotional and educational needs appropriate to their stage of development. Nowhere is this more challenging than among children with clefting.

References

Bowers EJ, Mayro RF, Whitaker LA, Pasquariello PS, LaRossa D, Randall R (1987) General body growth in children with clefts of the lip, palate, and craniofacial structure. Scandinavian Journal of Plastic and Reconstructive Surgery 21: 7–14.

Bowers EJ, Mayro RF, Whitaker LA, Pasquariello PS, LaRossa D, Randall R (1988) General body growth in children with cleft palate and related disorders: age differences. American Journal of Physical Anthropology 75: 503–515.

British Medical Journal (1995) Managing cleft lip and palate [letters] 311: 1431–1433.

Campbell ML, Watson ACH (1980) Management of the neonate. In: Edwards M, Watson ACH (eds) Advances in the Management of Cleft Palate. Edinburgh: Churchill Livingstone, pp. 123–133.

Carrol L, Reilly S (1996) The therapeutic approach to the child with feeding difficulty: II. Management and feeding. In Sullivan PB, Rosenbloom L, Bosma JF (eds) Feeding the Disabled Child. Clinics in Developmental Medicine No. 140. Cambridge: Cambridge University Press, 117–131.

Cozzi F, Bonanni M, Cozzi DA, Orfei P, Piacenti S (1996) Assessment of pulmonary mechanics and breathing patterns during posturally induced glossoptosis in infants. Archives of Disease in Childhood 74: 512–516.

CSAG Report – Cleft Lip and/or Palate. Clinical Standards Advisory Group (1998). London: HMSO.

Dawkins J (1996a) Bullying, physical disability and the paediatric patient. Developmental Medicine and Child Neurology 38: 603–612.

Dawkins J (1996b) Bullying in schools: doctors' responsibilities. British Medical Journal 310: 274–275.

Department of Education and Employment (1994) Bullying: Don't suffer in silence – an anti-bullying pack for schools. London: HMSO.

Department of Health (1993) Cot Death. PL/CNO (93) 3.

Drillien C, Ingram TTS, Wilkinson EM (1966) The Causes and Natural History of Cleft Palate. Edinburgh: Livingstone.

Duncan P, Shapiro L, Soley R, Turet S (1983) Linear growth patterns in patients with cleft lip or palate or both. American Journal of Diseases of Children 137: 159–163.

Freed G, Pearlman MA, Brown AS (1988) Polysomnographic indications for surgical intervention in Pierre Robin sequence: Acute airway management and follow-up studies after repair and take-down of tongue–lip adhesion. Cleft Palate Journal 25: 151.

Heaf DP, Helms P, Dinwiddie R, Matthew DJ (1982) Nasopharyngeal airways in Pierre Robin Syndrome. Journal of Pediatrics 100: 698–703.

Herskind AM, Christensen K, Juel K, Fogh-Anderson P (1993) Cleft lip: a risk factor for suicide. Paper given at seventh International Congress on Cleft Palate and Related Craniofacial Anomalies, Queensland, Australia.

Kaufman FL (1991) Managing the cleft lip and palate patient. Pediatric Clinics of North America 38: 1127–1147.

Lee J, Nunn J, Wright C (1996) Height and weight achieved in cleft lip and palate. Archives of Disease in Childhood 75: 327–329.

Masarei A, Sell D, Mitchell J, Habel A (1999) The Pierre Robin Sequence. RCSLT Bulletin 6–7.

Meates M (1997) Ambulatory paediatrics: making a difference. Archives of Disease in Childhood 76: 468–476.

Moss ALH, Jones K, Pigott RW (1990) Submucous cleft palate in the differential diagnosis of feeding difficulties. Archives of Disease in Childhood 65: 181–182.

Nicolaides K (1996) Guest Lecture at the Craniofacial Society of Great Britain Annual Meeting, Holloway, London.

Paradise JL, Elste BA, Tan L (1994) Evidence in infants with cleft palate that breast milk protects against otitis media. Pediatrics 94: 853–860.

Richards ME (1994) Weight comparisons of infants with complete cleft lip and palate. Pediatric Nursing 20: 191–196.

Rudman D, Davis T, Priest J, Patterson JH, Kutner MH, Heymsfield SB, Bethel RA (1978) Prevalence of growth hormone deficiency in children with cleft lip or palate. Journal of Pediatrics 93: 378–382.

Sharp S, Smith PK (1994) Tackling Bullying in your School: a Practical Handbook for Teachers. London: Routledge.

Shaw GM, Lammer EJ, Wasserman CR, O'Malley CD, Tolarova MM (1995) Risk of oropharyngeal clefts in children born to women using multivitamins containing folic acid periconceptionally. Lancet 346: 393–396.

Strauss RP, Davis JU (1990) Prenatal detection and fetal surgery of clefts and craniofacial abnormalities in humans: social and ethical issues. Cleft Palate Journal 27: 176.

Williams K, Chambers M, Logan S, Robinson D (1996) Association of common health symptoms with bullying in primary school children. British Medical Journal 313: 17–19.

Winter R, Baraitser M (1998) London Dysmorphology Database. Oxford: Oxford University Press.

CHAPTER 10

Early Feeding Management

P. BANNISTER

One of the first experiences in an infant's life is to be fed. Important connections between external stimuli and the development of cognitive patterns in the brain are set in motion as these experiences are encountered by the infant. It is at this time that the foundations are laid for both the physical and mental health in his/her adult life. For infants and their parents such experiences should produce feelings of contentment and security rather than tension, stress and fear (Anderson and Vidyasagar, 1979; Vandenberg, 1990). If too much emphasis is placed on feed volume, a parent may not pick up and respond to the social cues offered by the infant at this convivial time. The normal infant may respond in a variety of ways but often signals distress by becoming irritable and refusing to feed (Arvedson, 1993).

The immediate aims of feeding the infant with a cleft are the same as for any other baby and all aspects of infant feeding need to be considered when planning care. One of the most important challenges for professionals caring for the new family is the effective teaching of successful feeding.

Normal feeding

Full-term healthy babies are born with the natural ability to feed. To obtain milk from either the breast or the bottle they utilize a sucking reflex. For successful feeding the baby must be able to sustain effective sucking and coordinate respiration with the suck/swallow reflex. Because of the anatomical relationship of the soft palate to the epiglottis, the infant is able to breathe throughout the process of suckling with only a short period of apnoea during swallowing (Morris and Klein, 1987). Sucking activity is both an inborn (suckling) and conditioned (sucking) reflex dependent primarily on physiological maturation (Bosma, 1986). It is capable of being strengthened or changed in accordance with learning experience (Crump et al.,

1958; Anderson and Vidyasagar, 1979; Arvedson, 1993) and must be seen in the context of the whole development of the baby (Morris and Klein, 1987).

In bottle-feeding, the teat is placed in the baby's mouth following the rooting and/or gaping reflex initiated by the baby. The teat lies at the junction of the hard and soft palate which initially stimulates the sucking reflex (Woolridge, 1986). The tongue then moves forward under the teat and its lateral margins cup around the teat forming a central trough in which the teat lies. The tongue tip tilts upwards to assist in the withdrawal of milk. The lips close around the base of the teat, the mandible moves forward and the mouth becomes an airtight cavity. With each suck, negative intraoral pressure builds, the tongue compresses the teat towards the hard palate and milk is ejected into the mouth and deposited onto the tongue where it is propelled towards the pharynx. The swallow is triggered and milk passes into the oesophagus. During swallowing the major muscles in the soft palate pull the palate upwards and backwards much like a sling action. This closes off the nasopharynx from the oropharynx, thus preventing the nasal regurgitation of milk (Woolridge, 1986).

In breastfeeding the nipple and areola are drawn into the baby's mouth and stabilized into position by similar suction. As the baby gapes, the mother must present the nipple and breast tissue, to enable the baby to fix onto the breast. This is best achieved by holding the breast between the forefinger and middle finger and tilting the nipple up towards the baby's nose. As the mouth opens, the rim of the baby's lower lip is placed below the nipple and the breast is then folded into the baby's gaping mouth. This may be difficult at first, as it is easy to miss the gaping reflex. Once in the mouth it is important that the nipple lies adjacent to the tongue and lower jaw. The increase in negative intraoral pressure draws the nipple out to about three times its normal length (Woolridge, 1986). Milk is expressed from the breast with a simultaneous milking movement of the tongue and lower jaw and propelled backwards towards the pharynx for swallowing. The complete role of negative pressure remains unclear. During bottle-feeding its function is thought to assist the removal of milk from the bottle (Clarren et al., 1987), whereas in breastfeeding, the most likely function is to position and stabilize the nipple. Negative pressure, however, is not applied with the same intensity at every suck.

Studies have shown that newborn babies demonstrate two distinct patterns of sucking: nutritive and non-nutritive, and that both variants can be identified during the course of a feed (Brown, 1972; Smith and Erensberg, 1985). The principal difference is the effective delivery of milk into the mouth. Non-nutritive sucking is best observed when an infant is sucking on a dummy. It occurs in rapid short sharp bursts at a rate of two per second. Very little forward thrust of the mandible is observed. This type of suck is often demonstrated when a baby is first put onto the breast, prior to the stimulation of the hormonally controlled letdown reflex and the ejection of milk. Rhythmical non-nutritive sucking appears to be a necessary skill for oral feeding. Nutritive sucking, however, occurs at the slower rate of one per second and is observed once the milk has started to flow. As the feed progresses nutritive sucking is organized into a pattern of ten to fifteen bursts of sucking followed by a short pause and recommencing with two to three non-nutritive sucks.

Cleft lip/cleft lip and palate

Babies born with a cleft may present with a variety of feeding problems. The difficulties associated with cleft lip, and cleft lip and palate, can usually be resolved in the early neonatal period, whereas infants with isolated cleft palate, particularly in association with micrognathia, other medical problems or syndromes, may continue to experience difficulties for many months and require careful management. In this chapter both groups are considered separately.

Breastfeeding may be possible for some of these babies but it is difficult and requires commitment from the mother and informed support from the health professionals involved in their care (La Leche, 1992). A beneficial alternative is the use of expressed breast milk fed with a bottle. The general benefits of breast milk are well publicized. It is easily absorbed and thought less likely to cause localized inflammation of the nasal mucosa and associated middle ear problems (Paradise and Elster, 1984).

Many studies have identified a wide range of additional anomalies associated with oral clefting (see Lees, Chapter 6). Some of these additional problems are evident at birth but others only emerge as the developing infant matures. Often they are first indicated by an uncharacteristic dysfunctional feeding pattern. In a very small percentage of these infants oral feeding is an unachievable goal but in the majority of cases, with careful management, this can be achieved.

Problems associated with cleft lip or cleft lip and palate

Feeding difficulties related to full-term babies with isolated clefts of the lip and those involving lip and palate are generally primarily related to reduced sucking efficiency. Intraoral movements and tongue position are usually normal and the baby demonstrates an organized and functional breathe, suck/swallow coordination. For the infant with cleft lip only, and feeding difficulties, these are easily resolved by minor adjustments to the hole in the teat for the bottle-fed infant and more effective nipple placement in the breastfed infant (Danner, 1992). Where there is a cleft of the lip, alveolus and palate, whether unilateral or bilateral, a more pronounced sucking inefficiency is observed. Reduced efficiency of nutritive sucking can lead to lengthy feeding times, the ingestion of excessive amounts of air, and fatigue for both infant and parent if managed incorrectly. In the early neonatal period, it may be difficult for the baby to stabilize the nipple or teat in the mouth as the opposing palatal tissue surface for tongue compression is absent.

Problems associated with isolated cleft palate

Infants with these deformities may present with a different and often more complex feeding problem. In addition to the obvious anatomical anomalies of the palate, physiological alterations in the function of the oropharynx often contribute to these difficulties. It is perhaps useful to consider these babies on a continuum with those mildly affected at one end and those more severely affected at the other end. Minor feeding problems associated with the former are easily resolved with assisted feeding (see below); breast-feeding is an option but will usually require supplementation. However, for the more severely affected, particularly those with Pierre Robin sequence (see Watson, Chapter 1; Lees, Chapter 6; Habel, Chapter 9), micrognathia and glossoptosis place the infant at high risk of respiratory obstruction and aspiration (Shprintzen, 1988; Bath and Bull, 1997). These features may be part of a syndrome (see Lees, Chapter 6), which may contribute further to nutritional and feeding difficulties. Although glossoptosis may be evident at birth it may only emerge once feeding has commenced. The stability of the airway at rest must be established before teat feeding can be safely intro-duced. Babies with severe problems require naso-gastric tube feeding until breathing has been stabilised. Non-nutritive sucking will assist the continued development of sucking strength and pattern and enhance the growth in the cognitive link between sucking and the satiation of hunger. Once teat feeding has commenced, careful planning as to the frequency and length of time an infant is allowed to feed is important for the protection of the airway.

Management of feeding problems

Planning early care

As scanning technology improves antenatal diagnosis of clefting is now not infrequent (see Chitty and Griffin, Chapter 7). Comprehensive preparation for feeding, in terms of advice and supply of equipment, can therefore be undertaken. Following birth, the transfer to special care baby units is in the majority of cases inappropriate and only those babies who require medical intervention need to be separated from their mothers.

Early management

A feeding assessment should ideally be carried out by a feeding specialist within 24 hours of the birth. Arvedson (1993) considers three major factors of importance in the assessment and management of feeding: oromotor development, availability of nutritionally adequate food and the interaction between caregiver and infant. The infant must be awake and ready for a feed and, if possible, both parents should be present. The preferred methods of feeding are explored and integrated into the feeding plan. At this time the basic physiology of feeding is explained to the parents in simple but accurate language. It is often helpful to look at the normal feeding behaviours that the baby exhibits before moving on to the particular difficulties that may present. Both parents are given the opportunity to become involved with feeding and encouraged to feed the baby as often possible.

Multiple changes in carers creates inconsistencies that make learning difficult for the baby. In bottle-feeding it is important that the teat is placed well into the baby's mouth and is kept as still as possible whilst the baby suckles. Movement of the teat, a technique often used by health professionals to stimulate sucking, may cause ulceration of both the nasal septum and nasal turbinates. Ulceration of the latter can be extremely painful and cause a reluctance in the baby to teat feed. Parents need to be shown how to adjust the size of the hole in the teat, position the baby whilst feeding and be introduced to the concept of assisted feeding (see below) if appropriate. Where there are no perceived functional problems, the baby is fed comfortably cradled in the parent's arms with the head and upper body well supported, and the chin midway between flexion and extension (Macie and Arvedson, 1993). The feed should ideally be completed within 30–40 minutes with the minimal ingestion of air.

Where breastfeeding is the preferred choice, it is important that the baby is put to the breast as soon as possible after delivery. If necessary, supplementary feeds can be given via a spoon, cup or scoop bottle. Removal of the foremilk may become easier with time but the hindmilk may prove more difficult, necessitating supplementary feeds of expressed breast milk. A baby with cleft lip and palate may have to suckle at the breast for longer than normal before the effective delivery of milk. It has been suggested that the fitting of a feeding plate may help the infant stabilise the nipple. The use of a Supplementary Nursing System (SNS) or soft finger feeder has been found helpful in latching the baby onto the breast. If breastfeeding is unsuccessful and the baby requires supplementation, the use of expressed breast milk is a second option but requires a breast pump. Manual expression may be possible if taught properly.

Infants with airway and/or functional problems may require a combination of teat and nasogastric tube feeding. The baby should be encouraged to have frequent feeds but one or two teat feeds a day may be all that can be comfortably and safely tolerated. As the tongue moves forward under the teat, airway problems may appear to resolve. If the infant is overworked a deterioration in airway stability may be observed. The emphasis must be on feeding coordination rather than volume of feed consumed. Because of the potential for dysfunction in the oropharynx, care must be taken not to place too much milk in the mouth for swallowing. The use of an unadjusted teat is advisable with the introduction of assisted feeding (see below) as a coordinated suckling pattern emerges. The timing for this may vary from one week to two months of age. As bottle-feeding may take two to three months to establish, discharge home should be considered, with a feeding plan which includes a combination of tube and teat feeding during the day and tube feeding only at night. Once it has been established that the baby is able to organize an increased volume of milk, the teat may then be safely adjusted. Tiredness often results in the baby sleeping through feeds, making demand feeding difficult. A calorie supplement is often necessary to ensure adequate weight gain. Thickened feeds, or the use of Infant Gaviscon added to feeds, may be indicated when reflux is suspected. Feeding positions for these babies can vary but the normal cradling position is not recommended. The baby can be fed, either on its side facing the carer or in an upright position allowing any excess milk to dribble safely out of the mouth. These babies often cause a great deal of anxiety for parents as progress is often slow. Regular, informed community advice and counselling is vital for successful management.

In infants with Pierre Robin sequence the stability of the airway at rest must be established before teat feeding can be safely introduced. Babies with severe problems will require nasogastric tube feeding until breathing has been stabilized. Non-nutritive sucking will assist the continued development of sucking strength and pattern, and enhance the growth in the cognitive link between sucking and the satiation of hunger. Once teat feeding has commenced, careful planning as to the frequency and length of time an infant is allowed to feed is important for the maintenance of an adequate airway.

Where oral feeding is not possible, parents often require encouragement to become involved in activities which will enhance the possibility of normal feeding. These may include stroking of the face, cheeks and tongue where there appears to be no sucking reflex present, feeding small amounts of milk from cotton wool or gauze swabs where weak or dysfunctional skills require encouragement, or encouraging non-nutritive sucking with a dummy when the baby is being fed via a nasogastric tube. It is important for parents to have realistic expectations of feeding so that they are able to gain pleasure in the small advancements that their infant makes.

Feeding equipment is supplied to the parents and access to further teats and bottles and a breast pump must be arranged. Once mother and baby have gained sufficient confidence in the method of feeding, discharge home, with the support of preferably a specialist health visitor or community paediatric nurse, is possible. Liaison with the community health professionals will ensure that the continuation of the agreed plan is understood.

Assisted feeding

It can be very difficult for the baby with a cleft to remove milk successfully from a bottle. It can be made easier either by enlarging the existing hole in a latex teat, making an additional hole in the teat using a red hot intramuscular needle or combining the adjusted teat with a soft flexible bottle. The soft bottle is gently squeezed as the baby suckles, compensating for the oral stage difficulty. This process represents assisted feeding.

Assisted feeding enables the infant to gain adequate nutrition, within an acceptable time, whilst enhancing the continued development of nutritive sucking. It enables the carer of a bottle-fed infant to assist only when necessary. The need for such help will vary within a feed, from one feed to another and from one infant to another.

The frequency of squeezing will depend on many factors relating to the size of the cleft, the presence of other anomalies and the stage in the feed. At the beginning of a feed the baby may exhibit good nutritive sucking but this is usually short-lived as the baby begins to tire and efficiency at sucking is reduced. Effective feeding may require pressure to the bottle throughout the feed or pulse squeezing every two, three or five sucks. If the milk is delivered too fast the baby may communicate distress and nasal regurgitation of the milk may occur. Assisted feeding must be used with extreme caution in the presence of pharyngeal and/or oesophageal stage problems (Arvedson, 1993).

Feeding equipment

A clinical study into feeding methods (Shaw et al., 1999) recommended the use of standardized feeding equipment and this is now available through the mail order service provided by the Cleft Lip and Palate Association, a UK national voluntary parent's support group (see Davies, Chapter 24). In this study, 95% of parents expressed a desire to use feeding equipment that was as close to normal appearance as possible. The type and shape of teat, size of hole and viscosity of the liquid have been shown to influence the feeding behaviour of neonates (Adram et al., 1968).

- The most widely used teat was the Nuk, size 2, orthodontic shaped latex teat, which can be successfully combined with a soft plastic bottle. This sized teat is tolerated by neonates with a birth weight above 2.5 kg. The shape of the Nuk teat attempts to simulate the mother's nipple as it functions during the feeding process. This action enhances the continuing development of the mandible, which is important for all babies but particularly important for those babies presenting with micrognathia (Herrman, 1988).

- The Nuk cleft palate teat works on the same principle but is not aesthetically acceptable to many parents. Its size precludes its use with smaller babies.

- The Haberman feeding system is another form of assisted feeding but it does not attempt to simulate the breastfeeding action of the mandible. Because of its adjustable flow system, modification of the teat is unnecessary (Haberman, 1988). The prohibitive cost of the initial equipment and the renewal of teats means it is unavailable to low income families.

- The Rosti scoop bottle is particularly useful in conjunction with breastfeeding but can be used effectively for feeding babies who do not have either the energy or muscular ability to sustain sucking. Sucking satisfaction may be reduced so that the baby may require increased non-nutritive sucking.

- A variety of soft flexible bottles are available for use in assisted feeding. The Mead Johnson bottle is particularly useful for parents with problems with their hands, such as arthritis or carpal tunnel syndrome, as it is more pliable than the Chicco equivalent. Most parents, however, prefer the more regular shape of the Chicco bottle.

- The Lamb's teat is long and cumbersome. Milk is deposited so far back in the oral cavity that many infants will experience difficulty in maintaining a coordinated suck/swallow pattern.

- A soft latex or silicone nipple shield is sometimes helpful for babies who are unable to acquire the skills necessary for successful nipple placement for breastfeeding.

- The Supplementary Nursing System (SNS, Medela) is a useful method of giving the infant expressed breast milk whilst encouraging suckling at the breast. Success with its use is more likely once the immediate neonatal period is past.

- A finger feeder used in conjunction with a syringe can be effective in encouraging a breastfeeding infant to latch on to the breast. It is less cumbersome than the SNS system but requires the assistance of another person. A video on its use is available (Herzog-Isler, 1994).

Some examples of feeding equipment are shown in Figure 10.1.

Feeding plates as obturators

Although once extensively used these are now considered unhelpful and unnecessary in bottle-feeding. If correctly made and fitted they seem to have a limited use as a breastfeeding aid (Herzog-Isler, 1994). They are

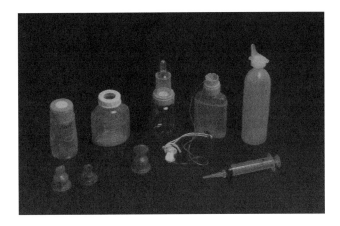

Figure 10.1. Back row, from left: Chicco, Mead Johnson, Haberman, Supplementary Nursing Feeding System (SNS), Rosti bottle. Front row, from left: Nuk size 2, Nuk Cleft Palate, Finger Feeder.

sometimes used to stabilize the tongue in infants with large isolated clefts of the palate.

Oral hygiene

For the first eight weeks, two to three teaspoons of cooled boiled water given after formula feeds only, from a spoon or teat, will keep the oral and nasal cavities clean. From about two to three months of age this may be discontinued because of a maturational increase in saliva production. The regular application of an edible lubricant to the areas around the cleft lip and premaxilla will help to prevent the development of soreness. It is not advisable to use cotton wool buds to clean the inside of the mouth and nose but their use may be helpful to remove debris around the alar rim.

Weaning

It is now generally recommended that infants should not be given solid foods before the age of four months and that a mixed diet should be offered by six months of age (Coma Report, 1994). At about four months developmental age, neurological maturation and increased intraoral spaces enable the infant to begin to use a posterior stripping action of the tongue (Schechter, 1990) recognized as a pre-chewing skill. The acquisition of these skills allows the infant to learn to control pureed foods as weaning commences. Immaturity results in much of the food being pushed out of the baby's mouth or, where there is a cleft palate, nasal regurgitation. For the first few weeks it is helpful to rest the spoon in the baby's mouth whilst he removes the food at his own pace. Babies are usually able to compensate for these early difficulties and develop a functional eating pattern before closure of the cleft palate. The transition to mashed and lumpy foods generally occurs at a similar age to that of any other infant and it is important not to miss these sensitive periods. Confidence is often gained by encouraging parents to offer tastes of mashed and family foods at meal times.

References

Adram GM, Kemp FH, Lind J (1968) A cineradiographic study of infant bottle feeding. British Journal of Radiology 31: 11–22.

Anderson GC, Vidyasagar D (1979) The development of sucking in premature infants from 1–7 days. Birth Defects 15(7): 45–171.

Arvedson JC (1993) Feeding with craniofacial anomalies. In: Arvedson JC, Brodsky L (eds) Pediatric Swallowing and Feeding. Assessment and Management. London: Whurr, pp. 417–437.

Bath AP, Bull PD (1997) Management of upper airway obstruction in Pierre Robin Sequence. Journal of Laryngology and Otology 111: 1155–1157.

Bosma JA (1986) Development of feeding. Clinical Nutrition 5: 210–218.

Brown J (1972) Instrumental control of sucking response in newborns. Journal of Experimental Child Psychology 14: 66–88.

Clarren SK, Anderson B, Wolf LS (1987) Feeding infants with cleft lip, cleft lip and palate or cleft palate. Cleft Palate Journal 24: 244–249.

Cleft Lip and Palate Association. Feeding Bottles and Teats Catalogue. 3rd Floor, 235–237 Finchley Road, London NW7 6LD.

Coma Report (1994) Weaning and the weaning diet. Report on Health and Social Subjects 45. London: HMSO.

Crump PE, Gore PM, Horton CP (1958) The sucking behaviour in premature infants. Human Biology 30: 128–141.

Danner SC (1992) Breast feeding the infant with a cleft defect. NAACOG 3(4): 634–639.

Haberman M (1988) A mother of invention. Nursing Times 84(2): 52–53.

Herrman DB (1988) Jaw development from infancy to early childhood. 2730 Zeven, Germany.

Herzog-Isler C (1994) Video showing Breastfed Infants with Cleft lip and Palate. C. Herzog, Pilatusstrasse 4, CH-6033 Buchrain, Switzerland.

La Leche (1992) Nursing a baby with a cleft lip or cleft palate. La Leche League Book, Leaflet no 122, 160 Blenheim Street, Hull, HU5 3PN.

Macie D, Arvedson J (1993) Tone and positioning. In: Arvedson J, Brodsky L (eds) Pediatric Swallowing and Feeding. Assessment and Management. London: Whurr, p. 209.

Morris ES, Klein DM (1987) Pre-Feeding Skills: A comprehensive source for feeding Development. Therapy Skill Builders, Arizona.

Paradise JL, Elster B (1984) Evidence that breast milk protects against otitis media with infants with cleft palate. Pediatric Research 18: 283.

Schechter GL (1990) Physiology of the mouth, pharynx and oesophagus. In: Bluestone CD (ed.) Pediatric Otolarynglogy, 2nd edn. Philadelphia: WB Saunders, p. 816.

Shaw WC, Bannister RP, Roberts CT (1999) Assisted feeding is more reliable for infants with clefts – a randomized trial. Cleft Palate–Craniofacial Journal 36(3): 262–268.

Shprintzen R (1988) Pierre Robin, micrognathia and airway obstruction: The dependency of treatment on accurate diagnosis. International Anesthesiology Clinic 26: 64–71.

Smith WC, Erensberg J (1985) Physiology of sucking in normal term infants. Radiology 156: 379–381.

Vandenberg KA (1990) Nippling management of the sick neonate in NICU. The Disorganized Feeder. Neonatal Network 9(1): 9–16.

Woolridge MW (1986) The anatomy of infant sucking. Midwifery 2(4): 164–171.

CHAPTER 11

Presurgical Orthopaedics

I.S. HATHORN

Introduction

The principal aim of presurgical orthopaedic treatment for babies with cleft lip and palate is to realign the bony elements of the cleft to provide a more normal base for surgery. Historically, McNeil was associated with significant development of presurgical orthopaedics in the United Kingdom (McNeil 1950, 1956). The reasoning behind early attempts at presurgical orthopaedics was to reduce the distance between the cleft elements to help make surgical correction easier and reduce postsurgical breakdown. This work was not, however, the first in the field. A recent review paper on presurgical orthopaedics by Winters and Hurwitz (1995) referred to facial binding, which was used by Hoffman in the seventeenth century to narrow the cleft in order to prevent postsurgical breakdown. A similar technique was used by Desault in the eighteenth century to retract the premaxilla before surgical repair of the bilateral cleft lip. In the nineteenth century, Hullihen stressed the importance of presurgical preparation of clefts using an adhesive tape binding. This technique resulted in the approximation of the ends of the alveolar cleft in four to six weeks, and required that the binding should be used when the infant was very young. Von Esmarch in the late nineteenth century used a bonnet and strapping which very closely resembles that used by McNeil. Unlike modern presurgical orthopaedics, Von Esmarch's aim was to stabilize the premaxilla after surgical retraction. A different approach to this external pressure applied to the cleft maxilla, was that published by Brophy (1927) in the early part of the 20th century. He described the use of silver wire passed through both ends of the cleft alveolus, which was then progressively tightened in order to approximate the ends of the alveolus before lip repair.

Burston (1958) developed the work done by McNeil, popularizing presurgical orthopaedics in the United Kingdom and internationally. His treatment was focused on the realignment of the maxillary alveolar processes, which was thought to encourage more normal facial growth and dental arch development. By carrying out this realignment he also expected to produce a reduction in the cleft gap, which would lead to more successful surgery. It was also believed that the appliances used would help with feeding, hence the reference often used to the presurgical appliances as 'feeding plates'.

During the development of the Burston and McNeil techniques, presurgical orthopaedics were seen as accomplishing non-surgical closure of palatal defects by stimulating the 'growth impulse' by mechanical means and reducing the need for orthodontic treatment. These claims were clearly extravagant and were not supported by evidence from properly conducted studies. In the latter part of this chapter the evidence for and against the use of presurgical orthopaedics will be considered.

Presurgical orthopaedic techniques

There are a number of variations in the technique of presurgical orthopaedics. Robertson (1983) described various methods of preparing a cleft child presurgically, along similar lines to those described by McNeil and Burston. Robertson used active or passive acrylic appliances and external strapping, depending on the presenting clinical problem, to reposition the alveolar segments and encourage shelf growth. Active appliances were constructed by making a plaster model of a baby's cleft palate, sectioning the model by dividing the alveolar segments and moving them in a planned way to restore a more normal maxillary arch form. The cleft area was plastered out (filled with plaster so that a gap would be left between it and the appliance) to prevent ulceration and to leave a clear space for shelf growth. An acrylic appliance was then constructed on the new model. This appliance, once placed in the baby's mouth, was stabilized by means of external fixation. The appliance would move the bony segments by moulding them in the planned direction.

Passive appliances were constructed on a plaster model without moving the alveolar segments, but by plastering out the cleft area, the space created under the acrylic appliance would allow lateral shelf growth. Extraoral strapping, elasticated adhesive plasters or other elastic materials were used to apply pressure to the displaced segments to help reposition them in a more normal relationship within the face. Generally in the United Kingdom, presurgical treatment continued from soon after birth until primary lip surgery at approximately three months old.

Before describing examples of presurgical treatment using the techniques outlined above, it is worth reviewing the normal baby's facial relationships. The normal baby has a symmetrical frontal appearance with the nares of equal size. The mandible is set back compared to the maxilla, with the result that the upper gum pad lies ahead of the lower by up to 3 mm (Robertson, 1983). In planning presurgical techniques, the aim is to restore the cleft face to as near normal as possible. If we consider the cleft problems in turn:

1. Clefts of lip and alveolus

There is usually relatively little facial and alveolar distortion in this group of patients. External strapping can, however, be used to redirect any errant distortions of the lip and alveolus.

2. Unilateral clefts of lip and palate

This is the group where most of the presurgical treatment has been directed. The individual variation is considerable. As a consequence, at one end of the spectrum, with little distortion, a passive appliance can be fitted to keep the tongue out of the cleft gap and encourage lateral shelf growth. At the other extreme, where there is significant distortion, a combination of intraoral appliances and extraoral strapping might be required.

3. Bilateral clefts of lip and palate

The main presenting distortion is the prominent premaxilla which in the bilateral cleft child is brought about by vigorous growth of the nasal septum. Extraoral strapping can be used to restrain further forward growth of the premaxilla and to allow the posterior segments to advance. Presurgical appliances can be used as required either to stabilize the existing arch form or to expand the posterior segments in preparation for retraction of the premaxilla.

4. Clefts of hard and soft palate

Passive presurgical plates have been fitted to wide and extensive clefts of the hard and soft palate in order to exclude the tongue from the cleft and to encourage lateral shelf growth. In the Pierre Robin sequence, which is the combination of hard and soft palate cleft with a retrusive mandible and respiratory distress (see Habel, Chapter 9), it has been felt that a passive plate combined with nursing directed at keeping the tongue forwards would have a beneficial effect on the baby's maxillary shelf growth laterally and on anterior mandibular growth.

Other workers such as Hotz (1990), have used passive orthopaedic appliances with continuous adjustment to guide growth over a prolonged period. This approach delays lip closure until six months and soft palate closure until 18 months with final hard palate closure at six years. The technique does not use any form of external strapping on the basis that it may retard maxillary growth. All presurgical preparation is focused on allowing as much unrestricted growth to occur as possible before primary surgery is carried out.

Brogan (1986) described a technique that combines elements of both of the above. There is a period using external strapping to align the major segment with a loose fitting intraoral appliance to maintain maxillary arch form. Extraoral appliances are discontinued when the segments are restored to their 'normal' position, prior to repair of the defect. A second intraoral appliance is fitted to guide growth by selective trimming. This passive appliance is worn until primary lip and nose correction takes place at three to four months.

Di Biase (Di Biase and Hunter, 1983; Ball and Di Biase, 1995) has designed an orthopaedic appliance that combines the facility for manipulation of the segments on a continuous basis and the ability with trimming to allow favourable lateral shelf growth. This appliance is used from birth until primary lip closure at approximately three months. It is then worn for a further three months until final palate closure takes place. The Di Biase appliance is shown in Figure 11.1. The palatal view shows the expandable spring which allows selective adjustment. There is also a split in the acrylic with overlapping edges, which can be seen more clearly in the posterior view of the appliance. This also shows the clearance of the plate from the palatal shelves which allows shelf growth, unhindered by the tongue. The changes in shelf growth under such an appliance are also illustrated (Figure 11.1c).

Mylin et al. (1968) have used active pin-retained appliances to manipulate the segments using screws. However, serious concern has been expressed as to the potential damage to the dentition and to the probable large forces generated on the bony structures by the screws, when they are activated.

Results of presurgical orthopaedics

As well as the realignment of the bony elements of the alveolar cleft to provide a more normal base for surgery, presurgical orthopaedics can result in an improved angulation of the palatal shelves as they drop into a more horizontal position, contributing to a narrowing of the cleft gap (Robertson, 1971; Fish, 1972; Hochban and Austerman, 1989) These changes are achieved by the presurgical appliance keeping the tongue out of the cleft gap and allowing growth to take place unhindered.

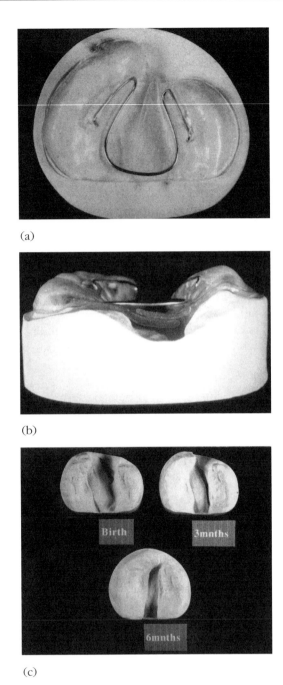

(a)

(b)

(c)

Figure 11.1. The presurgical orthopaedic appliance. (a) Palatal view; (b) posterior view; (c) changes in palatal shelf growth with use of appliance. (By kind permission of Mr D. Di Biase.)

McNeil (1984) considered that not only was presurgical treatment creating more normal arch form, but that the process also stimulated tissue growth. However, Huddart and Crabb (1977) demonstrated that there was in fact no extra tissue growth. It is generally recognized, therefore, that presurgical treatment is directed at realignment of the maxillary bony elements, also encouraging lateral palatal shelf growth when possible. McComb (1990) states that the first step in correction of the cleft lip nose is preparation of a symmetric bony platform by means of presurgical treatment.

Presurgical appliances were also considered to help with feeding. In a study by Shaw et al. (1999) a randomized feeding trial took place with one group using 'feeding plates'. It was found that the plates were not necessary in establishing successful feeding and they were abandoned early in the trial. Many centres around the world which produce excellent long-term results do not use so-called 'feeding plates' and their babies thrive in preparation for surgery with careful and experienced nursing support (see Bannister, Chapter 10).

It is thought that the intensive contact between the family and the clinicians carrying out the presurgical treatment gives emotional support during the period of adjustment to the child's deformity (Huddart, 1990). This has not been properly tested, although in the Shaw feeding trial the clearest outcome of the study was the recognition that the health visitor outreach programme was a significant advance in care, giving unique opportunities for family counselling and support. This was an unanticipated finding from the study.

The effect of presurgical orthopaedics on dental alignment has been considered a logical consequence of the improved alveolar symmetry (O'Donnell et al., 1974). Subsequent studies have not shown significantly improved occlusal results after presurgical treatment (Mars et al., 1992; Hathorn et al., 1996). On the contrary, the study model analysis actually showed worse occlusal outcomes for the units which used presurgical orthopaedics when compared with those units which did not use any form of presurgical orthopaedics. Although good occlusal results have been shown in the primary dentition (Huddart, 1972) longer-term studies have not confirmed this in the permanent dentition. It is now generally accepted that presurgical treatment does not confer any special benefits on the alignment of the permanent dentition (Ross, 1970). Any dental malocclusions prevented by presurgical orthopaedic treatment could be resolved easily in the later routine orthodontic management (Pruzansky, 1964).

Complete unilateral and bilateral clefts present with many variations of distortion of the cleft elements. The disturbed functional matrix surrounding the cleft allows rotation of the segments and the base of the nose is often severely disturbed. McCance et al. (1993) in their Sri Lankan study have shown that without surgery or any other form of treatment, the unoperated maxilla grows relatively normally. The influence with the greatest potential for disturbing growth in the treatment of cleft lip and palate is the nature of the surgery. In the Eurocleft study (Mars et al., 1992) the two best centres had not used presurgical orthopaedics and demonstrated significantly better results than the two centres where presurgical orthopaedics had been practised. Ross (1970) in his multicentre study showed that there was no significant advantage derived from presurgical orthopaedics in the long-term outcome of cleft treatment and that the most significant effect on treatment outcome was the surgeon.

More recently, Ross and MacNamera (1994) found no differences in facial aesthetics in forty patients with bilateral clefts of lip and palate, all treated by the same surgeon, half of whom had had presurgical orthopaedics and half of whom had not. On the other hand, Sommerlad's surgical outcomes as measured by the Goslon Yardstick have shown better occlusal results than those of the best centres in the Eurocleft study (Chate et al., 1997), in using Di Biase's technique of presurgical orthopaedics.

Presurgical orthopaedics is also a very costly procedure, taking up considerable time and resources of the professionals involved. It is simply not possible in many parts of the world to transport the mother and baby to distant clinics for the extensive treatment required for presurgical support. Also the management of the appliances necessary for the orthopaedic movements can be a considerable extra burden to a stressed parent.

There is still a need for careful long-term studies to evaluate fully the benefits of presurgical work. The preliminary work of Kujpers-Jagtman and Prahl-Anderson (1997), in a randomized controlled trial of presurgical orthopaedics versus no presurgical treatment, may go a long way to resolving many of the key issues. The preliminary finding of this trial is that there is no significant benefit from presurgical orthopaedics.

It may be that if the correct atraumatic surgery were carried out, the relatively subtle and time-consuming presurgical orthopaedics would result in a minor long-term contribution to the overall outcome. It is, however, difficult to see more than a minor effect on the final outcome when so many more profound effects such as the surgical technique, timing and the skill of the surgeon come into play. At the present time it seems doubtful that presurgical oral orthopaedics is a cost-effective addition to the management of clefts.

References

Ball JV, Di Biase D (1995) Transverse maxillary arch changes with the use of preoperative orthopaedics in unilateral cleft palate infants. Cleft Palate–Craniofacial Journal 32: 483–488.

Brogan WF (1986) Cleft lip and palate. The state of the art. Annals of the Royal College of Dental Surgeons 9: 172–184.

Brophy TW (1927) Cleft lip and cleft palate. Journal of the American Dental Association 14: 1108–1115.

Burston WR (1958) The early orthodontic treatment of cleft palate conditions. Transactions of the BSSO. Dental Practitioner 9: 41–56.

Chate RAC, De Biase DD, Ball JV, Mars M, Sommerlad BC (1997) A comparison of the dental occlusions from a United Kingdom sample of complete unilateral cleft lip and palate patients, with those from the Eurocleft Study. Transactions, 8th International Congress on Cleft Palate and Related Craniofacial/Anomalies 371: 276.

Di Biase DD, Hunter SB (1983) A method of presurgical oral orthopaedics. British Journal of Orthodontics 10(1): 25–31.

Fish J (1972) Growth of the palatal shelves of post-alveolar cleft palate infants. Effects of stimulation appliances. British Dental Journal 132: 492.

Hathorn IS, Roberts-Harry DP, Mars MM (1996) The Goslon Yardstick applied to a consecutive series of unilateral clefts of the lip and palate patients, treated at Frenchay Hospital. Cleft Palate–Craniofacial Journal 33(6): 494–496.

Hochban W, Austerman KH (1989) Presurgical orthopaedic treatment using hard plates. Journal of Craniomaxillofacial Surgery 17(suppl. 1): 2–4.

Hotz M (1990) Infant orthopedics and later monitoring for unilateral cleft lip and palate patients in Zurich. In: Bardach J, Morris HL (eds) Multidisciplinary Management of Cleft Lip and Palate. Philadelphia: WB Saunders, pp. 578–585.

Huddart AG (1972) A comparative study of treatment and occlusion in unilateral cleft subjects. Transactions of the European Orthodontic Society 48: 167–176.

Huddart AG (1990) Presurgical orthopaedic treatment of cleft lip and palate. In: Bardach J, Morris HL (eds) Multidisciplinary Management of Cleft Lip and Palate. Philadelphia: WB Saunders, pp. 574–578.

Huddart AG, Crabb JJ (1977) The effect of presurgical treatment on palatal tissue area in unilateral cleft lip and palate subjects. British Journal of Orthodontics 4(4): 181–185.

Kujpers-Jagtman AM, Prahl-Anderson B (1997) Value of presurgical orthopaedics: an inter-centre randomised clinical trial. Presentation to 8th International Congress on Cleft Palate and related Craniofacial Anomalies, Singapore.

Mars M, Asher-McDade C, Brattstrom V, Dahl E, McWilliam J, Molsted K, Plint D, Prahl-Anderson B, Semb G, Shaw W (1992) A six centre international study of treatment outcome in patients with clefts of lip and palate: Part 3. Dental Arch Relationships. Cleft Palate–Craniofacial Journal 29: 405–408.

McCance A, Roberts-Harry DP, Mars MM, Sherriff M, Houston WJB (1993) Sri Lankan Cleft Lip and Palate Study model analysis. Cleft Palate–Craniofacial Journal 30: 227–230.

McComb H (1990) Primary unilateral and bilateral cleft lip nose reconstruction. In: Bardach J, Morris HL (eds) Multidisciplinary Management of Cleft Lip and Palate. Philadelphia: WB Saunders, pp. 197–203.

McNeil CK (1950) Orthodontic procedures in the treatment of congenital cleft palate. Dental Record 70(5): 126–132.

McNeil CK (1956) Congenital oral deformities. British Dental Journal 101: 191–196.

McNeil CK (1984) Oral and Facial Deformity. London: Pitman, pp. 81–89.

Mylin WK, Hagerty RF and Hess DA (1968) The pin-retained prosthesis in cleft palate orthopaedics. Cleft Palate–Craniofacial Journal 5: 219–223.

O'Donnell JP, Kirscher JP, Shiere FR (1974) An analysis of presurgical orthopaedics in the treatment of unilateral cleft lip and palate. Cleft Palate–Craniofacial Journal 11: 374–393.

Pruzansky S (1964) Presurgical orthopedics and bone grafting for infants with cleft lip and palate: A dissent. Cleft Palate–Craniofacial Journal 1: 164–187.

Robertson NRE (1971) Recent trends in the treatment of cleft lip and palate. Transactions of the BSSO. Dental Practitioner 21: 326–338.

Robertson NRE (1983) Oral orthopaedics and orthodontics for cleft lip and palate. London: Pitman, pp. 33–74.

Ross RB (1970) The clinical implications of facial growth in cleft lip and palate. Cleft Palate–Craniofacial Journal 7: 37–47.

Ross RB, MacNamera MC (1994) Effect of presurgical infant orthopaedics on facial aesthetics in complete bilateral cleft lip and palate. Cleft Palate–Craniofacial Journal 31: 68–73.

Shaw WC, Bannister P, Roberts CT (1999) Assisted feeding is more reliable for infants with clefts – a randomised trial. Cleft Palate–Craniofacial Journal 36: 262–268.

Winters JC, Hurwitz DJ (1995) Presurgical orthopedics in the surgical management of unilateral cleft lip palate. Plastic and Reconstructive Surgery 95: 755–764.

CHAPTER 12

Primary Surgery

A.C.H. WATSON

Introduction

Children with an untreated cleft lip have a dreadful deformity. If they have a cleft of the palate they cannot speak normally, are likely to suffer from earache and deafness, have the embarrassment of food and drink coming down the nose, the prospect of impaired dental and facial development and suffer major psychosocial consequences. The aim of treatment is to make these children anatomically and functionally as near normal as possible, and the basis of treatment is the surgical closure of the cleft (Figure 12.1).

The pioneers of cleft surgery aimed no further than getting the cleft closed and, were the deformity simply a cleft in otherwise normal tissues, this would have been adequate. In reality, the problem is much more complicated. Not only is there a cleft but there is also to a greater or lesser extent a deficiency of tissue in the line of the cleft. Intrauterine growth of the involved tissues, in which the normal constraints and attachments have been disturbed, gives rise to distortions and displacements of these structures from their normal positions, which add to the difficulties of successful treatment. The amount by which postnatal growth is affected if the cleft is untreated, and the extent to which different methods of surgical treatment interfere with facial growth, are matters of argument about which research has not yet been able to provide all the answers (see Mars, Chapter 4). Only very recently has agreement been reached in the UK on how to assess and record speech in cleft children (Harding et al., 1997, Sell et al., 1994, 1999) and there is still no generally accepted way of scoring facial appearance. Add to these uncertainties the variable influence of other factors such as the techniques and timing of surgery, the skill of the surgeon, deafness, intelligence, home environment and orthodontic management, and it is not

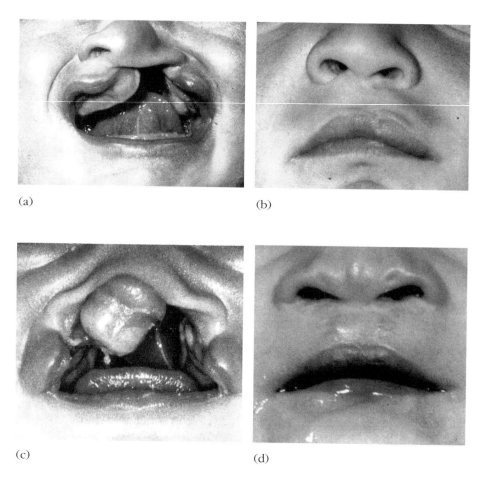

Figure 12.1. Examples of infants with complete clefts of lip and palate. (a) Unilateral cleft, preoperative view. (b) Postoperative view. (c) Bilateral cleft, preoperative view. (d) Postoperative view.

surprising that there is still no consistent evidence to suggest that any one operative procedure gives better results than others.

At present the accepted main outcome measures are speech and facial growth.

Factors related to poor speech

The recent CSAG report (1998) indicated an incidence of poorly intelligible speech, in five-year-old children with clefts, ranging from 0 to 36% across the UK. There are several factors which are likely to result in poor speech, over which the nature of the treatment will have little or no influence. For example, children of low intelligence and those whose parents are uninterested in their progress tend to speak poorly (Drillien et al., 1966). The choice of surgical regime is unlikely to influence these children to speak more normally.

Deaf children with cleft palates speak less well than those with good hearing. Secretory otitis media is very commonly associated with cleft palate and can lead to intermittent hearing loss (see Lennox, Chapter 15). Closure of the cleft may sometimes reduce its incidence, but there is no evidence that one type of operation is any better than another in this respect, and every published series includes a proportion of children whose poor speech is associated with deafness. Whatever surgical regime is chosen, a close watch must be kept on the patient's hearing and active steps taken to deal with middle ear disease.

Patients with complete clefts of the secondary palate have been shown by Glover (1961) and others to run a high risk of poor speech. Many of these clefts are associated with a greater tissue deficiency than any other type, but Berkowitz (1996) has stressed that there is a great variation in the conformation and degree of underdevelopment in all types of cleft. Many clefts are part of syndromes that are themselves associated with poor speech (see Lees, Chapter 6). These factors will influence the results of surgery quite independently of the choice and timing of operation and may actually be more important in determining the final result.

The inevitable incidence of children with low intelligence, poor homes, deafness and severe tissue deficiency in any cleft palate population will ensure that no single operation will allow all patients to achieve normal speech.

If we now attempt to set down those variations in operative treatment that are known to contribute to poor speech results, we face problems. Almost the only fact which is generally accepted is that the later the palate is closed, the worse the speech (Sell, 1992). Early closure of the soft palate with delayed repair of the hard palate – a protocol that was believed to allow satisfactory speech development while ensuring good maxillary growth – has become less popular since it has been shown that speech results are, in fact, relatively poor (Bardach et al., 1984; Witzel et al., 1984). Children with cleft palates have abnormal babbling before speech develops (see Russell and Harding, Chapter 14) and as a result many surgeons are now closing the palate at six months or younger (Kaplan, 1981; Randall et al., 1983; Malek and Psaume, 1983). Some close the soft palate at three months and the hard palate at a second stage, but still at 18 months or less. These arguments will be considered further in the coming pages.

Factors relating to poor growth of the maxilla

The growth of the maxilla of the cleft palate patient is influenced by several factors which are quite independent of surgical treatment. One is the variable primary deficiency of tissue adjacent to the cleft; another is the growth potential of the maxilla, which is deficient in some syndromic clefts (see Lees, Chapter 6). However, studies of adults with unoperated clefts show that most have the potential for normal facial growth (see Mars, Chapter 4).

All operations designed to close the cleft involve the early union of the two halves of the lip and the soft palate which create the normal muscular union between the two elements of the maxilla, and the muscular pull causes these elements to be drawn together. If there is a great deficiency of tissue, the resulting narrowing of the cleft will produce an abnormal medial displacement of the lateral element (or elements) of the maxilla and 'alveolar collapse' without the operation interfering with growth in any way. As a result, there is no surgical regime that can guarantee to prevent some degree of collapse, but its effects can be overcome by later orthodontic treatment.

Closure of the cleft in the alveolus and hard palate involves, in one way or another, mobilizing tissue from the maxilla on each side of the cleft and displacing it across the cleft to be sutured to tissue from the other side. With most techniques this produces raw areas laterally, which are usually left to epithelialize. Operations to close the soft palate have often involved quite extensive dissection of soft tissues lateral to it. The scarring produced by all these manoeuvres has been blamed for many of the deformities seen in patients who have had their clefts repaired (Dixon, 1966; Kremenack et al., 1970; see Mars, Chapter 4), and techniques have been developed to minimize the growth disturbance from these causes (Malek and Psaume, 1983; Delaire and Precious, 1985; DeMay et al., 1992; Murison and Pigott, 1992; Thatte et al., 1992, 1997; Sommerlad et al., 1997).

The arguments for the different protocols of surgical treatment will be developed in the following pages, the most commonly used techniques described and an attempt made to place them in perspective.

The choice of a treatment protocol

There are two basic areas of disagreement: the timing of surgery and the operative technique. They will be considered in turn.

Timing of surgery

Lip and primary palate

There is a school of thought which states that a cleft lip should be closed in the neonatal period so that the parents do not have to suffer the distress of looking after a baby stigmatized in this way (Desai, 1979). Surgery in the neonate is more risky than in the older baby; in particular, the cardiovascular and respiratory systems are immature and clefts can be associated with other congenital abnormalities, especially cardiac ones (see Lees, Chapter 6). It is therefore essential, if neonatal surgery is to be considered, that it is carried out in a centre with expert paediatric anaesthesia and intensive care facilities, and that a thorough preoperative assessment is performed by a paediatrician (see Habel, Chapter 9). What evidence there is suggests that the results of neonatal cleft lip repair are no better than later repair and that the psychological impact on the parents is no different (Slade et al., 1999).

The majority of surgeons prefer to wait until the child is older – usually between three and six months – before operating as, with reduced risks of anaesthesia, they feel that they can spend more time and get a better result when the lip and nose are more developed. In addition, many believe that it is better for the parents to spend some weeks coming to terms with their child's deformity, as this will prepare them to accept the various problems which may arise during childhood and which will require treatment (see Bradbury and Bannister, Chapter 8).

In those centres which favour presurgical oral orthopaedics (see Hathorn, Chapter 11) the timing of surgery to the lip and alveolus is dependent on the time it takes the orthodontist to move the segments of the alveolar arch into proper alignment. This can usually be done by about three or four months.

Many surgeons obtain soft tissue closure of the alveolar and anterior palatal cleft at the same time as they close the lip. There is no doubt that this area is easier to close at this stage when the cleft is wide open, and access may be very difficult after lip closure when the pull of the united muscles has drawn the two halves of the maxilla together so that they abut each other. Nevertheless, some leave this area untouched at the primary operation as they believe such surgery interferes with growth; they close it at the time of alveolar bone grafting in later childhood (see Mars, Chapters 4 and 20).

Secondary palate

It has become clear that the child has a better chance of speaking normally if the cleft is closed early (Veau, 1931; Kaplan, 1981; Dorf and Curtin, 1982; Randall et al., 1983). Most surgeons therefore aim to close the whole palate by 18 months, and many do so at six months.

Unfortunately, surgery to the bony cleft of the alveolus and palate has been shown to interfere with maxillary growth (see Mars Chapter 4) and this has made some people believe that no surgery should be performed on bony structures until maxillary growth is almost completed.

Gillies and Fry (1921) developed an operation in which they closed only the soft palate and left the hard palate open, to be filled in by an obturator, and in this way avoided maxillary collapse. They subsequently abandoned this practice, which condemned the patient to wearing the obturator for the rest of his life, but suggested it would be best to delay hard palate surgery until the age of four or five years, when 80% of transverse maxillary growth has taken place. Hotz et al. (1978) advocated this approach. Some, like the Schweckendiecks (father and son), even waited until the child was 12 to 14 years old, when maxillary growth is virtually completed. Schweckendieck (1978) published a series of over 250 cases treated in this way, with a 25-year follow-up of patients, none of whom apparently had any maxillary deformity. However, an independent review of Schweckendieck's cases (Bardach et al., 1984) showed that their speech results were significantly poorer than those of children with early hard palate closure, and this was supported by other reports (Cosman and Falk, 1980; Jackson et al., 1983; Witzel et al., 1984). Since then, this type of regime has lost much of its popularity. However, there are those who use a two-stage approach but close the hard palate at 18 months or even earlier, for example Malek and Psaume (1983), Lohmander-Agerskov et al. (1995).

Recently published evidence (CSAG, 1998; Sommerlad et al., 1997) indicates that good facial growth and good speech can both be achieved following closure of hard and soft palate, in a single stage before one year of age, providing dissection and raw areas are kept to a minimum.

Operative techniques

Cleft lip

The history of cleft lip repair is of a steady improvement in the cosmetic result, as surgeons have gradually come to appreciate the true nature of the defect. The recognition that, in the unilateral cleft, most of the cupid's bow and philtrum are already present and should be preserved, and the development of operations in which almost none of the precious tissue is thrown away, have resulted in lips that look far more natural. The nasal deformity which always coexists with the cleft lip is now more effectively dealt with than ever before (McComb and Coghlan, 1996).

Although a repaired cleft lip may look excellent at rest, it will not move symmetrically unless the muscles within it are properly realigned; the deformity will become apparent when the child smiles or pouts. The muscle of the cleft lip runs parallel to the free margins of the cleft and is abnormally attached to the edge of the piriform fossa and alar base (see Sommerlad, Chapter 3). (In the bilateral cleft the muscle in each lateral element of the lip runs in this way, and there is no muscle in the prolabium – see Figure 12.2.) In this respect the lip resembles the cleft soft palate, and the importance of muscle mobilization is the same. Reconstitution of the muscle sphincter around the mouth not only allows the lip to function more naturally. If there is a complete cleft of the lip, alveolus and palate then the muscle pull across the repaired lip draws the two halves of the maxilla together anteriorly and narrows the alveolar cleft and the anterior part of the cleft palate.

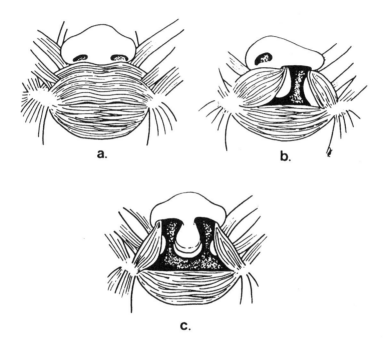

Figure 12.2. The configuration of the orbicularis oris muscle. (a) Normal. (b) Unilateral cleft lip. The orbicularis oris muscle runs parallel to the edges of the cleft and inserts into the margins of the piriform fossa. (c) Bilateral cleft lip. There is no muscle in the prolabium.

In many infants born with a complete cleft of lip and palate the two parts of the maxilla are displaced laterally, making the cleft very wide and surgical closure very difficult. In the complete bilateral cleft the prolabium and premaxilla are suspended from the tip of the nose and the lateral elements may be collapsed far behind them (Figure 12.3). The definitive closure of the lip can be made easier, and therefore possibly better, by narrowing the cleft preoperatively. This narrowing can be achieved by the fitting of a series of presurgical orthopaedic splints by the orthodontist (see Hathorn,

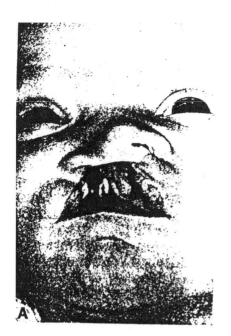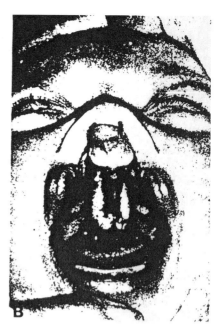

Figure 12.3. Displacements of the elements of the alveolar arch in complete clefts. (a) Unilateral cleft. Note the wide gap between the two parts of the alveolus. (b) Bilateral cleft. Note how the prolabium and premaxilla are suspended from the tip of the nose and lateral elements of the maxilla lie far behind them.

Chapter 11), by adhesive strapping across the cleft, or by a simple preliminary operation known as a lip adhesion carried out in the first few weeks of life. Such a procedure was popularized by Randall (1965) and modified by Millard (1976) so that it does not interfere with tissues that will be needed in the definitive lip closure (Figure 12.4). The muscles are exposed in the opposing margins of the upper half of the cleft. They are sutured together across the cleft after minimal undermining, so converting the complete cleft into what is, in effect, an incomplete cleft. Presurgical orthopaedics should produce a similar effect in a more controlled but time-consuming way, and moreover can expand a collapsed lateral segment, which an adhesion cannot do. When the time comes for the definitive operation the available tissue does not have to be stretched across a wide gap, and the surgeon can concentrate on using it to the best advantage in constructing the features of the normal lip and nose.

Unilateral cleft lip

The principles of unilateral cleft lip repair are illustrated using Millard's widely used rotation advancement operation, which he first described in

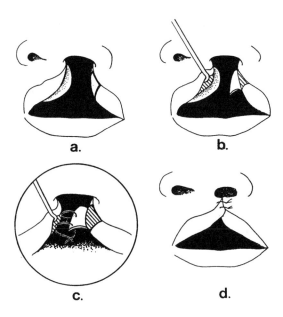

Figure 12.4. The lip adhesion operation (after Millard). (a) Incisions marked. The medial element of the lip is elevated from the maxilla enough to allow it to advance laterally to meet the lateral element. (b) A mucosal flap is raised from the lateral element. (c) The lateral flap is sutured to the posterior edge of the raw area on the medial lip. (d) The muscles are sutured separately and finally mucosa is stitched to skin.

1955 (Millard, 1957) and expounded in great detail in his book *Cleft Craft* (1976). Other techniques have their advocates (e.g. Tennison, 1952; Randall, 1959; Delaire, 1978) and all can give good results in the right hands. The rotation advancement procedure is relatively simple to plan and does not involve complicated markings and measurements, but this means that experience and an artistic eye are needed to get the best results (Figure 12.5). It is a 'cut as you go' method, so that at no point in the operation has an irrevocable step been taken, and adjustments can be made up to the very end of the procedure. It allows as much correction of the nasal deformity as the surgeon feels is wise to carry out at the primary operation. Any tightness is high up under the nose in the normal position, and the free margin of the lip remains pleasingly full. The two-thirds of the cupid's bow and philtrum, which are already present, are preserved and rotated into their normal positions, fixed there by the advancement flap from the lateral side, which moves across the downwardly rotated medial flap. In doing so, this advancement flap draws the splayed out alar base into its correct position. Even the little 'C' flap can be slid upwards to lengthen the deficient cleft side of the columella. Most important of all, the operation can be carried out in

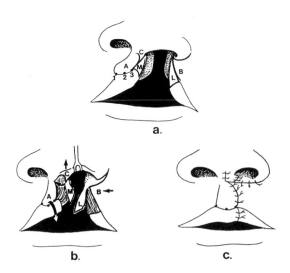

Figure 12.5. Millard's rotation advancement operation for unilateral cleft lip. (a) The peak of the cupid's bow on the non-cleft side (2) can be identified and marked. Point 3 lies an equal distance from point 2, and represents the peak of the cupid's bow on the cleft side. The first incision passes from point 3 parallel to the cleft and then curves under the base of the columella and must not go further than the philtral ridge on the non-cleft side. It cuts through the whole thickness of the lip and if necessary can be extended by a back cut. The incision at point 3 is completed by cutting through the free margin at right angles to the edge of the cleft. This frees flap A (the rotation flap). Flaps C and M are freed by an incision along the mucocutaneous junction continued along the membranous septum. On the lateral lip element flap B (the advancement flap) and flap L are created by the incisions shown. The length of the incision along the mucocutaneous junction should equal the length of the incision delineating flap A and can be adjusted later in the operation if necessary. (b) Flap A rotates downwards to bring the cupid's bow into the horizontal position. If rotation is inadequate it can be increased by a back cut as indicated in (a) above. Flap B advances into the triangular defect left in the upper part of the lip. Muscle is freed from its attachment to the piriform margin and rotated downwards towards the horizontal position. Flap C advances upwards to lengthen the cleft side of the columella. Flaps M and L can be used in various ways, to construct the nasal floor, provide extra lining for the nostril or close the alveolar cleft. A small 'white roll' flap is raised from the lateral element at the mucocutaneous junction to fit into an incision on the medial element and break up the line of the scar at this point. (c) The flaps are sutured into position. Closure is in layers, particular attention being paid to suturing the muscle in its correct alignment. The contour of the free margin can be adjusted by excision of excess mucosa and transposition of mucosal flaps to augment deficiencies.

such a way that no tissue whatever need be discarded. Every piece of tissue seems to fall so naturally into its proper place that it feels intuitively that the operation must be 'right'. Yet it has its limitations. In complete clefts the free margin of the cleft side of the lip can be too short (from cupid's bow to the angle of the mouth) if the lateral element of the lip is small. It can sometimes be difficult to achieve sufficient rotation of the medial flap without making an excessively large back cut, and, if so, many surgeons increase its length by adding a small Z-plasty above the cupid's bow.

When the rotation flap is cut, the skin is detached from the underlying muscle for a few millimetres but the philtral dimple and ridge on the non-cleft side are preserved. As the flap is rotated downwards it brings the medial orbicularis muscle into its proper position. On the lateral side, however, the skin of the advancement flap must be dissected free from the muscle, which is abnormally attached to the alar base. The bulk of the orbicularis is freed from this attachment and transposed downwards to be sutured to the medial muscle and create the orbicularis sphincter. Some tissue is left attached to the alar base to be sutured to the area of the anterior nasal spine and base of the septum to aid rotation of the alar base and centralization of the septum.

Primary nasal correction

The deformity of the cleft lip nose is as noticeable as that of the lip itself (Figures 12.3 and 12.6). In the unrepaired unilateral cleft the base of the ala and lateral crus of the alar cartilage are displaced laterally and posteriorly, and the anterior nasal spine with its attached septum, medial crura and columella are displaced to the non-cleft side. The stretched alar cartilage is splayed and rotates inferiorly, lengthening the cleft side of the nose. If specific measures are not taken to correct this deformity it will remain obvious and ugly. Fears that attempts to correct it at the primary operation would interfere with growth have proved unfounded and several methods are in use. That of McComb (1975) is the best documented, for he has published a consecutive series of his first ten cases as they have grown, with good results at 18 years old (McComb and Coghlan, 1996). He widely undermines the skin over the cleft half of the nose without making any internal incisions, and elevates the cleft alar dome with through-and-through mattress sutures before closing the nostril floor. These initial sutures may have to be repositioned at the end of the procedure (Figure 12.7). Anderl (1985) carries out a similar procedure but is more radical. In addition to the skin undermining and alar lifting, he central-izes the septum and elevates the alar base by creating a subperiosteal pocket which he fills with Surgicel, and has shown that this is replaced by bone. Matsuo et al. (1989) have demonstrated good results without a surgical attack on the nose by using silicone stents preoperatively.

Bilateral cleft lip

The bilateral cleft lip is a much more severe deformity than the unilateral. The absence of muscle in the prolabium, the lack of any vestige of a cupid's

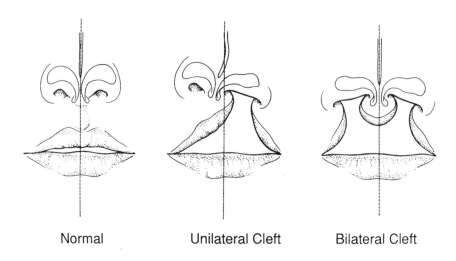

Figure 12.6. Distortion of the alar cartilages and septum in cleft lip.

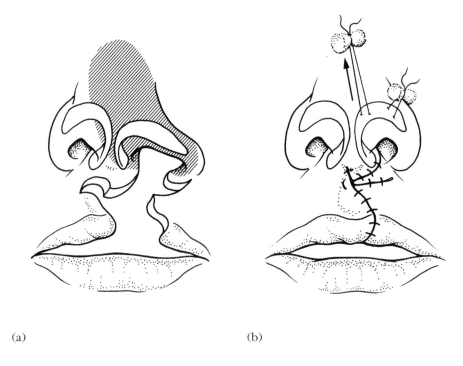

(a)   (b)

Figure 12.7. McComb unilateral nasal correction. (a) Alar deformity with area of undermining shaded. (b) Alar cartilage held in elevated position with suspension sutures.

bow or philtrum, the missing columella, and the fact that the deficiency of tissue is in general greater, make the challenge of surgical repair much more difficult.

When the bilateral cleft is complete, the projection of the prolabium and premaxilla and recession of the lateral elements behind them add to the surgeon's problems. Lip adhesions or strapping can help by tilting the premaxilla backwards, and skilled presurgical orthopaedics can add expansion of the lateral elements, so allowing the premaxilla to fit between them. Correct alignment of the alveolar arch brings the lip elements closer together. The practice of surgically repositioning the protruding premaxilla has fallen into disrepute because of the disastrous effect it can have on growth.

Closure of the lip can be carried out in one stage or in two. There is a choice of techniques, and no one technique has pre-eminence at the present time (McComb, 1975, 1986; Manchester, 1965; Millard, 1959, 1971, 1976; Mulliken, 1985; Veau, 1938). An important point to remember when making a choice is that the prolabium, even if it seems very small, stretches greatly after it is united to the rest of the lip, so that no technique should be chosen which introduces skin from the lateral elements below the prolabium. This results in a lip which is too tight and too long. The vermilion of the prolabium is of a different quality from that of the rest of the lip, and should be hidden, or it remains as an obvious blemish.

It is possible to close one side of a bilateral cleft lip at a time (Millard, 1959). This is perhaps most appropriate in incomplete, asymmetrical clefts.

Millard (1971) (Figure 12.8) closes the lip in one stage, leaving a prolabial element which looks much more like a philtrum than the other methods, and brings muscle across behind the prolabium. At the second stage the 'banked' forked flap is used to lengthen the columella (Figure 12.9). It produces excellent early results, but if the bony elements are very displaced, muscle union may be tenuous, and it may be better delayed.

McComb (1975, 1986) lengthens the columella before operating on the lip, using forked flaps from the prolabium. Six weeks later he repairs the lip and nasal tip using a technique similar to his unilateral nasal tip repair.

Alveolar cleft

At the time of closure of the cleft lip it is usually possible to close the cleft in the alveolus without difficulty, together with a greater or lesser part of the hard palate. Such a closure can be carried out in one layer, by elevating the septal mucoperichondrium and suturing it to the mucosa of the side wall of the nose (Figure 12.10). This is usually enough to achieve closure, but the raw undersurface will contract and drag the edges of the cleft together. This may not necessarily be a bad thing if the alveolar segments are properly oriented, but if they are not it may contribute to the collapse of the alveolar

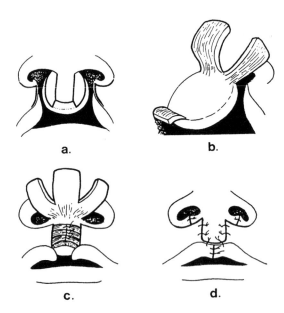

Figure 12.8. Millard's method of bilateral cleft lip repair: first stage. (a) The incisions marked out. The prolabium is divided into three flaps, based superiorly. The central flap is shaped to resemble a philtrum and the lateral ones are to be banked to lengthen the columella at the second stage. The vermilion of the prolabium, based on its attachment to the premaxilla, is separated from the philtral flap. The flaps on the lateral elements resemble the advancement flap in the rotation advancement procedure, and incisions along the mucocutaneous junctions are the same length as the philtral flap. (b) The prolabial flaps have been raised. The prolabial vermilion is shown turned down, but will be turned up to line the raw area on the front of the premaxilla and help form a buccal sulcus. (c) The mucosa and muscle of the lateral elements have been advanced in front of the premaxilla and sutured together. Vermilion flaps are turned down. (d) The philtral flap has been laid back over the approximated muscles and sutured to the skin of the lateral elements. The vermilion flaps have been approximated with a slight excess to form a midline tubercle in the free margin. The two lateral prolabial flaps are being banked in the floor of the nose, where they form little mounds. Alternatively, they can be inserted between alar base and lateral tip element, where they do not obstruct the airway.

arch. The Oslo regime (Semb et al., 1990) has been shown to produce very good results. It involves a single layer closure of the nasal floor using a vomer flap, not only through the alveolus but also of as much of the hard palate as possible, at the time of the lip repair.

Veau (1931) described a flap of palatal mucoperiosteum, based posteriorly, which he swung across the cleft to reinforce the nasal closure behind the alveolus, but it cannot reach forward into the critical area of the alveolar cleft (Figure 12.11). A two-layer closure in this area can be obtained by

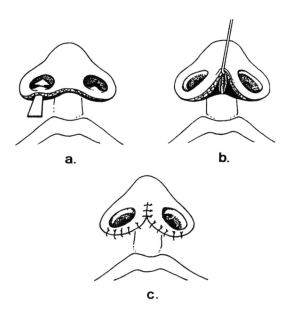

Figure 12.9. Second stage of Millard's bilateral cleft lip repair: columellar lengthening. (a) The banked flaps and nostril sills are separated from the lip and from the floor of the nose posteriorly by parallel incisions so that they remain attached medially to the columella and laterally to the alar bases. The columella is also freed from the lip and from the septum. (b) The bipedicled flaps so formed are rotated medially into the columella and sutured together. The columella is lengthened and the tip of the nose raised. (c) Incisions sutured. If the flaps are banked below the nostril floors they can be freed so that they retain only a medial attachment to the columella and are advanced as before to lengthen the columella.

bringing a flap of lip mucosa as described by Muir (1966) or Burian (1978), but these are not often used now that secondary bone grafting has become popular, as teeth will not grow through buccal or labial mucosa.

Primary bone grafting of the alveolar cleft has been shown to be disastrous in terms of maxillary growth and has been virtually abandoned. In most centres bone grafting is carried out according to the Oslo protocol at the time of eruption of the permanent canines (Åbyholm et al., 1981) (see Mars, Chapter 20).

The alveolar cleft may deliberately be left unrepaired at the time of primary surgery, to avoid interfering with bony structures, and closed at the time of alveolar bone grafting. The alveolar fistula is often non-functional as the margins lie in apposition, but it can sometimes be a great nuisance, allowing particles of food and drink to escape into the nose and having a significant effect on speech. This may make earlier closure necessary.

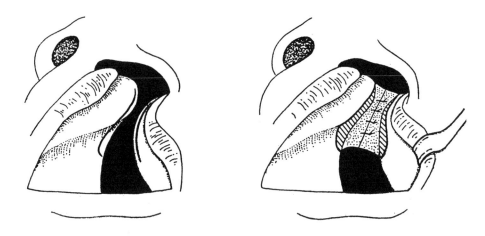

Figure 12.10. Single layer closure of cleft alveolus and nasal floor. Incisions are made at junction of oral and nasal mucosa on each side of the cleft. Nasal mucosal flaps are then elevated from septum (cartilage anteriorly and vomer posteriorly) and lateral wall of nose and sutured together.

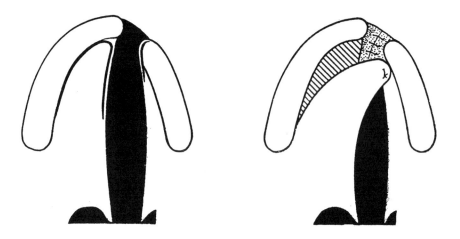

Figure 12.11. Veau mucoperiosteal flap for closure of oral aspect of anterior palate cleft. Shown in association with nasal mucosal closure of alveolar cleft. Incisions are made and the mucoperiosteal flap elevated and transposed across cleft.

Hard palate closure as part of a one-stage procedure

The von Langenbeck operation

Von Langenbeck (1861) was the first surgeon to devise a reliable method of closing the cleft hard palate, and his operation is still widely practised, with modifications, to this day (Figure 12.12). The mucous membrane of the hard palate is densely adherent to the underlying periosteum and in this proce-dure the two are stripped off the bone as a single strong and thick layer. The edges of the cleft are incised and the soft tissues of the two halves of the palate – that is, mucoperiosteum anteriorly and soft palate posteriorly – are slid towards each other and stitched together in the midline. To allow this to happen, release incisions have to be made on each side and these run just inside the alveolar process from the region of the canine anteriorly, curving round the maxillary tuberosity, to end just behind the region of the ptery-goid hamulus. The mucoperiosteum is then elevated from the bone as a bipedicled flap, attached anteriorly and posteriorly, and dissection is carried out through the posterior ends of the release incisions to relax the soft palate. After this dissection has been completed, the mucoperiosteal flaps of the hard palate and the two halves of the soft palate can be approximated in the midline. The dissection involves freeing the aponeurotic and muscular attachments of the soft palate from the back of the hard palate, and under-mining the nasal mucosa as far as possible from the upper surface of the hard palate. The mucoperiosteal flaps remain tethered by their vascular pedicles, the greater palatine vessels, as they emerge from the greater palatine foramina, but these may be lengthened by teasing them out of the foramina. The modern von Langenbeck operation nearly always involves closure of the nasal mucosa with the help of a flap (or flaps if bilateral) raised from the vomer.

The medial displacement of the palatal tissue in the von Langenbeck procedure leaves raw areas on each side. Over the hard palate bare bone is exposed. Epithelialization takes place quickly and healing is usually complete within two weeks, but scar tissue is inevitably formed, which can restrict palatal growth and pull medially the teeth to which it is related (Dixon, 1966; Kremenak et al., 1970 see Mars, Chapter 4).

The main criticism levelled against the von Langenbeck operation was that the procedure, as originally described, did not free the muscles from the back of the hard palate and so allow the creation of a muscle sling. The palate was short, and it was very common for patients who had been operated upon by the method to have hypernasal speech. Veau, who was a pioneer in the careful recording and reporting of the speech of his patients, reported that none of them spoke normally after a von Langenbeck opera-

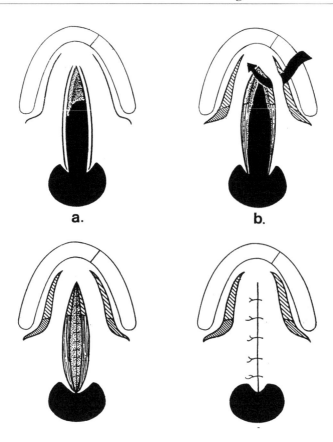

Figure 12.12. The von Langenbeck operation for closure of the secondary palate. (a) The margins of the cleft have been pared and the release incisions have been made medial to the alveolar processes curving behind the maxillary tuberosities. (b) Mucoperiosteum stripped from the oral surface of the hard palate. The arrow on the right of the diagram indicates how the mucoperiosteum is raised as a bipedicled flap. The nasal mucosa on the upper surface of the hard palate and, if necessary, the septum is mobilized far enough to allow it to meet across the cleft. (c) Appearance after suturing the nasal layer. (d) Closure of the cleft completed. Raw areas are left on each side, exposing the bare bone of the hard palate anteriorly.

tion. He developed a 'push-back' operation to lengthen the palate, and obtained very much better speech results (Veau, 1931). Unfortunately these push-back procedures, subsequently adapted by Wardill (1937) and Kilner (1937), leave larger raw areas than the von Langenbeck operation and inter-fere more severely with maxillary growth. Most centres have abandoned them and other more elaborate attempts to lengthen the palate. However, Thatte reports good early results after closing the raw areas with a primary tongue flap (Thatte et al., 1992, 1997).

Closure of the hard palate without release incisions

If the hard palate cleft is narrow it may be possible to close it without making release incisions (Sommerlad et al., 1997). The absence of raw areas might be expected to reduce the effect of scarring on maxillary development. However, closure of the cleft can only be achieved by allowing the mucoperiosteal flaps to fall away from the bony palate so that there may be a considerable dead space between the nasal and oral layers (Figure 12.13). If this is thought to be a problem, a single release incision may be sufficient to allow the mucoperiosteum to slide medially when the tongue presses upwards, so relieving the tension. Reid and Watson (1988) suggested that scoring the periosteum while leaving the mucosa intact would allow the flap to stretch and give a tension-free closure.

Murison and Pigott (1992) recommend incisions medial to the greater palatine neurovascular bundles which, they suggest, leave scars that do not interfere with growth. Delaire and Precious (1985) use these where necessary with delayed hard palate closure.

Soft palate

A cleft of the soft palate may be part of a more extensive cleft or be an isolated deformity. A submucous cleft may never cause problems (McWilliams in 1991 reported that 44% of 130 patients did not require

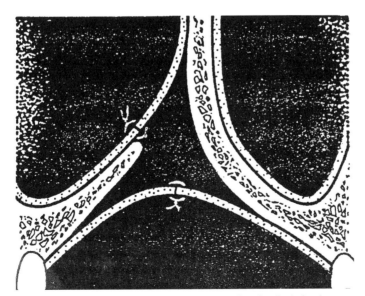

Figure 12.13. Coronal section through septum and palatal cleft, demonstrating that closure of the cleft without lateral relaxing incisions can only be achieved by allowing the mucoperiosteal flaps to fall away from the bone, leaving a large dead space.

surgery) and such a cleft, if diagnosed in infancy, should not be repaired unless there are serious feeding problems or middle ear disease. However, most submucous clefts are missed in infancy and are not identified unless the child develops speech problems. If surgery is needed, then the same principles apply as for other clefts.

Intravelar veloplasty

This term was coined by Kriens (1970) and describes a radical dissection of the muscles of the soft palate, freeing them from the back of the hard palate and from the oral and nasal mucosa and transposing them medially. This allows the construction of the normal levator sling in the posterior part of the soft palate. The technique was, in fact, previously described by Braithwaite and Maurice in 1968 in relation to the push-back operation. It can be used in conjunction with the von Langenbeck repair of the hard palate or with delayed hard palate closure. Sommerlad et al. (1994) have shown that it results in lengthening and improved function of the soft palate when carried out as a secondary procedure for velopharyngeal insuffi-ciency, but they and many others also use it for the primary repair (see Sommerlad, Chapter 3).

Fracture of the hamulus

During the dissection of the muscles the pterygoid hamulus is exposed and may be fractured to relax the tensor palati muscle, which passes round it, and make it easier to close the soft palate. This manoeuvre was first described by Billroth in 1889 and is carried out as part of many operations. It is frowned upon by some, e.g. Kriens (1970), on the grounds that it inter-feres with the normal function of the tensor palati, but Thomson and Harwood Nash (1972) showed by X-ray studies that the hamulus returns to its normal position after a few months.

It is not usually necessary to fracture the hamulus if a thorough mobiliza-tion of the muscles and aponeurosis medial to it is carried out, but if the cleft is very wide and closure is difficult it can probably be done without risk to the tensor palati.

Furlow's double opposing Z-plasty

Furlow described this technique in 1986 and it has been championed by Randall (Randall et al., 1986). It is an ingenious operation which allows radical realignment of the levator muscles and formation of the muscle sling and, at the same time, lengthens the soft palate. Two Z-plasty flaps are raised from the oral mucosa of the soft palate, the one based posteriorly incorpo-rating the muscles which are detached from the back of the soft palate and from the nasal mucosa. These flaps are held out of the way and an opposite

Z-plasty is raised from the nasal side, again incorporating the muscles with the posteriorly based flap. When these Z-plasties are transposed, the muscles are overlapped in the posterior half of the palate (Figure 12.14).

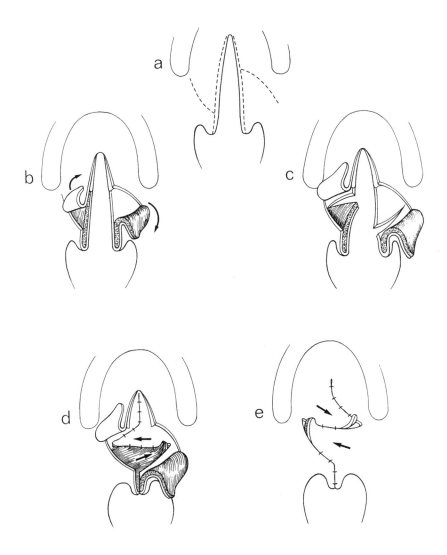

Figure 12.14. Furlow double reversing Z-plasty repair of soft palate. (a) Oral flaps marked. (b) Oral flaps raised. Note muscle in posteriorly based flap on right. (c) Nasal flaps raised. Again, note muscle in posteriorly based flap on left. (d) Nasal flaps transposed. (e) Oral flaps transposed.

In practice, this is a straightforward operation in a narrow cleft, but there can be problems when the cleft is wide. A Z-plasty produces lengthening in one direction at the expense of shortening in the other, and in the wide cleft there is no tissue to spare to allow this. Furlow described his oral Z-plasty incisions extending to overlie the hamulus, but in the author's experience such large flaps cannot be transposed in a wide cleft. However, smaller mucosal flaps, as described by Randall, can be raised and transposed and the muscle can be dissected widely as in an intravelar veloplasty. Sometimes release incisions may be required around the maxillary tuberosity in conti-nuity with von Langenbeck incisions in the hard palate, but frequently no release incisions are required, or an incision on only one side.

Primary pharyngeal flap

Schoenborn in 1876 was the first to use the posterior pharyngeal flap as a primary procedure after he had become dissatisfied with the speech results of the von Langenbeck operation. Its use was advocated by Burian (1978) in Prague, and was used by his successor, Fara, and by Stark in New York (Stark and de Haan, 1960) among others. (The details of the various types of pharyngeal flap are found in Chapter 17.) However, they are now rarely used as part of the primary operation unless the palate is extremely deficient as they can obstruct the nasal airway.

Primary closure of the soft palate with delayed closure of the hard palate

If hard palate closure is to be delayed, the soft palate can be closed using an intravelar veloplasty (Figure 12.15). The muscles can be covered by using flaps from the posteromedial hard palate or vomer, but this clearly involves losing some of the theoretical advantage of the procedure. The Furlow double reversing Z-plasty operation can also be adapted for use with delayed hard palate closure.

After the soft palate has healed a large hard palate defect is left in front of it. The tension of the muscle sling in the soft palate draws the halves of the maxilla together and narrows this fistula to such an extent that, when the time comes to close it, it may be possible to do so without making any lateral relaxing incisions, but simply by undermining the mucoperiosteum from the free edges of the palate. It is perhaps this conservative dissection, rather than the age at which it is done, which allows good maxillary development.

The Malek regime

Malek and Psaume (1983) reported a very large series of clefts in which the soft palate was closed first, at three months, and the hard palate, alveolus

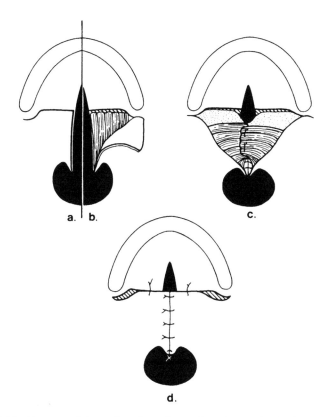

Figure 12.15. Closure of the soft palate alone after the method of Widmaier. (a) Flap outlined, reaching no further than the posterior edge of the hard palate. (b) Flap elevated to expose muscle which is mobilized in the usual way. (c) After mobilization of the soft palate, the muscle has been transposed and it and the nasal mucosa have been sutured. (d) Closure completed. The raw areas lie behind the hard palate.

and lip were closed at a second operation at six months. They stated that the early closure of the soft palate brings the tongue forward and down into a normal position where it opposes the tendency of the lesser maxillary segment to collapse after lip repair. Soft palate repair also causes narrowing of the posterior hard palate cleft and it is easier to close the hard palate when the lip is still unrepaired. He originally used a single layer closure of the hard palate, but had a high fistula rate and now uses a small vomerine flap and oral mucoperiosteal flaps with minimal elevation. Ross (1995) reviewed his results in terms of mid-face growth of complete unilateral clefts at 10 years and found them 'excellent'. De Mey has reported good results using a similar technique in a single stage (De Mey et al., 1992). Perhaps the most important point to note is that, in this procedure, excellent maxillary growth is reported even after hard palate surgery has been completed by six months.

The Delaire regime

Delaire and Precious (1985) close lip and soft palate at seven months, and state that the vomerine mucosa must not be touched when repairing the hard palate. They believe that the scarring produced by vomer flaps inhibits vertical growth of the maxilla and advocate closing the hard palate with a single layer of oral mucoperiosteum when this can be done with minimal elevation – at any age from 18 months to six or seven years. Delaire (1978) also holds strong opinions on how the lip and nose should be repaired. Unfortunately, neither he nor his disciples have yet published any long-term results in a way in which they can be compared with those using different approaches and, until this is done, Delaire's theories remain unproven. It is hoped that this unsatisfactory situation can be remedied quickly so that this method of management can be properly assessed.

Conclusion

At the present time it is not possible to say with certainty which are the best operations for closing a cleft lip or cleft palate, or when they should be done, and there is a great need for multicentre randomized controlled trials to clarify the issues (see Shaw and Semb, Chapter 25). One dilemma surgeons have faced is that some operations appear to offer a better chance of good speech at the possible sacrifice of facial growth, while others may give the patient a more normal appearance in adult life but run a higher risk of giving poor speech. Evidence is beginning to emerge, however, that it may be possible to achieve excellent results in both speech and growth.

References

Åbyholm F, Bergland O, Semb G (1981) Secondary bone grafting of alveolar clefts. Scandinavian Journal of Plastic and Reconstructive Surgery 15: 127.

Anderl H (1985) Simultaneous repair of lip and nose in the unilateral cleft (A long-term report). In: Jackson IT, Sommerlad B (eds) Recent Advances in Plastic Surgery (3). Edinburgh: Churchill Livingstone.

Bardach J, Morris HL, Olin WH et al. (1984) Late results of primary veloplasty: the Marburg project. Plastic and Reconstructive Surgery 73: 207–215.

Berkowitz S (1996) Cleft Lip and Palate. Perspectives in Management, Vol. 1. San Diego: Singular Publishing Group, p. 358.

Billroth T (1889) Ueher uranoplastik. Wien, Klinische Wochenschrift 2: 241.

Braithwaite F, Maurice D (1968) The importance of the levator palati muscle in cleft palate closure. British Journal of Plastic Surgery 21: 60.

Burian F (1978) The Plastic Surgery Atlas 1. New York: Macmillan.

Cosman BA, Falk AS (1980) Delayed hard palate repair and speech deficiencies: a cautionary report. Cleft Palate Journal 17: 27.

CSAG: Clinical Standards Advisory Group Report (1998) Cleft Lip and/or Palate. London: HMSO.

De Mey A, Lacotte B, Malevez C, Mansbach AL, Lejour M (1992) Traitement des fentes labiopalatines: resultats à long terme. Annales de Chirurgie Plastique et Esthetique 37: 174–178. deformity.

Delaire J (1978) Theoretical principles and technique of functional closure of the lip and nasal aperture. Journal of Maxillo-Facial Surgery 6: 109–116.

Delaire J, Precious D (1985) Avoidance of use of vomerine mucosa in primary surgical management of velopalatine clefts. Oral Surgery, Oral Medicine, and Oral Pathology 60: 589–597.

Desai S (1979) Primary cleft lip repair in newborn babies. Transactions of the 7th International Congress of Plastic and Reconstructive Surgery, Rio de Janeiro.

Dixon DA (1966) Abnormalities of the teeth and supporting structures in children with clefts of the lip and palate. In: Drillien CM, Ingram TTS, Wilkinson EM. The Causes and Natural History of Cleft Palate. Edinburgh: Livingstone.

Dorf DS, Curtin JW (1982) Early cleft palate repair and speech outcome. Plastic and Reconstructive Surgery 70: 74–79.

Drillien CM, Ingram TTS, Wilkinson EM (1966) The Causes and Natural History of Cleft Palate. Edinburgh: Livingstone.

Furlow LT (1986) Cleft palate repair by double opposing Z-plasty. Plastic and Reconstructive Surgery 78: 724–736.

Gillies HD, Fry K (1921) A new principle in the surgical treatment of congenital cleft palate and its mechanical counterpart. British Medical Journal i: 335.

Glover DM (1961) A long range evaluation of cleft palate repair. Plastic and Reconstructive Surgery 27: 19.

Harding A, Harland K, Razzell RE (1997) Cleft Audit Protocol for Speech (CAPS). Available from K Harland, Speech/Language Therapy Department, St Andrew's Centre for Plastic Surgery, Broomfield Hospital, Chelmsford, Essex.

Hotz MM, Gnoinski WM, Nussbaumer H et al. (1978) Early maxillary orthopaedics in cleft lip and palate cases: Guidelines for surgery. Cleft Palate Journal 15: 405.

Jackson IT, McLennan G, Scheker LR et al. (1983) Primary veloplasty or primary palato-plasty: some preliminary findings. Plastic and Reconstructive Surgery 72: 153–157.

Kaplan EN (1981) Cleft palate repair at three months. Annals of Plastic Surgery 7: 179–190.

Kilner TP (1937) Cleft lip and palate repair technique. In: Maingot R (ed.) Postgraduate Surgery, Vol. 3. London: Medical Publishers.

Kremenak CR, Huffman WC, Olin WH (1970) Maxillary growth inhibition by mucope-riosteal denudation of palatal shelf bone in non-cleft beagles. Cleft Palate Journal 7: 817–825.

Kriens OB (1970) Fundamental findings for an intravelar veloplasty. Cleft Palate Journal 7: 27.

Langenbeck B von (1861) Die Uranoplastik mittels ablösung des mukös-periostalen Gaumen überzuges. Archiv für klinische Chirurgie 2: 205.

Lohmander-Agerskov A, Soderpalm E, Fried H, Lilja J (1995) A longitudinal study of speech in 15 children with cleft lip and palate treated by late repair of the hard palate. Scandinavian Journal of Plastic and Reconstructive Surgery and Hand Surgery 29: 21–31.

Malek R, Psaume J (1983) Nouvelle conception de la chronologie et de la technique chirurgicale du traitement des fentres labio-palatines. Annales de Chirurgie Plastique 28: 237.

Manchester WM (1965) The repair of bilateral cleft lip and palate. British Journal of Surgery 52: 878.

Matsuo K, Hirose T, Otagiri T, Norose N (1989) Repair of cleft lip with non-surgical correction of nasal deformity in the early neonatal period. Plastic and Reconstructive Surgery 83: 25.

McComb H (1975) Primary repair of the bilateral cleft lip nose. British Journal of Plastic Surgery 28: 262.

McComb H (1986) Primary repair of the bilateral cleft lip nose: A 10-year review. Plastic and Reconstructive Surgery 77: 701–713.

McComb HK, Coghlan BA (1996) Primary repair of the unilateral cleft lip nose: completion of a longitudinal study. Cleft Palate–Craniofacial Journal 33: 23–31.

McWilliams BJ (1991) Submucous clefts of the palate: How likely are they to be symptomatic? Cleft Palate–Craniofacial Journal 28: 247–251.

Millard DR Jr (1957) A primary camouflage of the unilateral harelook. In: Transactions of the First International Congress of Plastic Surgeons. Baltimore: Williams & Wilkins.

Millard DR Jr (1959) Adaptation of the rotation-advancement principle in bilateral cleft lip. In: Wallace AB (ed.) Transactions of the International Society of Plastic Surgeons. 2nd Congress. Edinburgh: Livingstone.

Millard DR Jr (1971) Closure of bilateral cleft lip and elongation of columella by two operations in infancy. Plastic and Reconstructive Surgery 47: 324.

Millard DR Jr (1976) Cleft Craft: the Evolution of its Surgery, Vol. 1, Boston: Little Brown.

Muir IFK (1966) Repair of the cleft alveolus. British Journal of Plastic Surgery 29: 30.

Mulliken JB (1985) Principles and techniques of bilateral cleft lip repair. Plastic and Reconstructive Surgery 75: 447.

Murison MSC, Pigott RW (1992) Medial Langenbeck: experience of a modified Von Langenbeck repair of the cleft palate: A preliminary report. British Journal of Plastic Surgery 45: 454–459.

Randall P (1959) A triangular flap operation for the primary repair of unilateral clefts of the lip. Plastic and Reconstructive Surgery 23: 331.

Randall P (1965) A lip adhesion operation in cleft lip surgery. Plastic and Reconstructive Surgery 35: 371–376.

Randall P, La Rossa DD, Fakhrase SM et al. (1983) Cleft palate closure at 3–7 months of age: a preliminary report. Plastic and Reconstructive Surgery 71: 624–628.

Randall P, La Rossa DD, Solomon M et al. (1986) Experience with the Furlow double reversing Z-plasty for cleft palate repair. Plastic and Reconstructive Surgery 77: 569–574.

Reid CD, Watson JD (1988) Preliminary report of a new method of cleft palate repair. British Journal of Plastic Surgery 41: 234–238.

Ross RB (1995) Growth of the facial skeleton following the Malek repair for unilateral cleft lip and palate. Cleft Palate–Craniofacial Journal 32: 194-198.

Schoenborn D (1876) Ueber eine neue methode der staphylorrhaphie. Archiv für klinische Chirurgie 19: 527.

Schweckendieck W (1978) Primary veloplasty: long term results without maxillary deformity. Cleft Palate Journal 15: 268.

Sell D (1992) Speech in Sri Lankan cleft palate subjects with delayed palatoplasty. Unpublished PhD, De Montfort University.

Sell D, Harding A, Grunwell P (1994) GOS.SP.ASS. A screening assessment of cleft palate speech. European Journal of Disorders of Communication 29: 1–15.

Sell D, Harding A, Grunwell P (1999) Revised GOS.SP.ASS (98): Speech assessment for children with cleft palate and/or velopharyngeal dysfunction. International Journal of Disorders of Communication 34(1): 7–33.

Semb G, Borchgrevink H, Saelher I L, Ramsted T (1990) Multidisciplinary management of cleft lip and palate in Oslo, Norway. In Bardach J, Morris H L (eds) Multidisciplinary Management of Cleft Palate. Philadelphia: WB Saunders, pp. 27–37.

Slade P, Emerson DJM, Freedlander E (1999) A longitudinal comparison of the psychological impact on mothers of neonatal and 3 month repair of cleft lip. British Journal of Plastic Surgery 52: 1–5.

Sommerlad BC, Henley M, Birch M, Harland K, Moremen N, Boorman JG (1994) Cleft palate re-repair – a clinical and radiographic study of 32 consecutive cases. British Journal of Plastic Surgery 47: 406–410.

Sommerlad BC, Hay NHJ, Moss JP (1997). Transactions of the 8th International Congress on Cleft Palate and Related Craniofacial/Anomalies. Singapore.

Stark RB, De Haan CR (1960) The addition of a pharyngeal flap to primary palatoplasty. Plastic and Reconstructive Surgery 26: 378.

Tennison CW (1952) The repair of the unilateral cleft lip by the stencil method. Plastic and Reconstructive Surgery 9: 115.

Thatte RL, Govilkar P, Patel J (1992) The tongue flap in the primary treatment of cleft palate: a report of 19 cases. British Journal of Plastic Surgery 45: 150.

Thatte RL, Sahasrabuddhe P, Shirsat S (1997) 25 consecutive cleft palates treated primarily with tongue flaps – results at 5 years of age. Transactions VIIIth International Congress on Cleft Palate and Related Cranio-facial Anomalies, Singapore, p. 505.

Thomson HG, Harwood-Nash D (1972) The fate of the infractured hamulus. Plastic and Reconstructive Surgery 50: 354.

Veau V (1926–27) Proceedings of the Royal Society of Medicine 10:(3) Sec Surg 127.

Veau V (1931) Division palatine. Paris: Masson.

Veau V (1938) Bec de lievre. Paris: Masson, p. 184.

Wardill WEM (1937) Technique of operation for cleft palate. British Journal of Surgery 25: 97.

Witzel MA, Salyer KE, Ross RB (1984) Delayed hard palate closure: the philosophy revisited. Cleft Lip and Palate Journal 21: 263–269.

CHAPTER 13

Pre- and Postoperative Nursing Care

V. MARTIN

The best possible outcome from cleft lip and palate surgery can only be achieved with appropriate nursing care. It is important to identify minimum standards of care for cleft children whilst accommodating variations in practice in different units. No single treatment or regime has been identified as the optimum.

The setting

The Patient's Charter: Services for Children (Department of Health, 1996), which sets the standards for the care of children in hospital, states that infants should be nursed in a paediatric setting 'under the supervision of a consultant paediatrician or paediatric specialist and have a qualified children's nurse responsible for their nursing care'. This applies equally to children with a cleft lip and/or palate.

When in hospital, parents and other family members need 'complete ease of access to the child'. It is important to recognize that children are members of a family unit, the support of which is essential to their well-being (Department of Health, 1991). Facilities for parents are required to allow family life to continue with the least possible disruption.

Parents should be well prepared for every aspect of their child's hospital stay. Verbal preparation should be supported by the provision of information leaflets dealing with all aspects of preparation, treatment and aftercare (Action for Sick Children, 1996). Familiarity with the available facilities and equipment is best achieved by a visit to the ward area before the child's admission. Parents should be encouraged to bring the child's own clothes to wear in hospital, to have a selection of favourite toys and food, and to undertake familiar tasks in as close a routine to the home one as possible.

184

Preoperative preparation

Safety

The majority of units screen infants for group A beta-haemolytic strepto-coccal infection prior to admission by sending nose and throat swabs for culture and sensitivity, as suggested by Armstrong et al. (1993). The virulent potential of this organism may on occasions require surgery to be deferred.

Infants undergoing surgery for a cleft lip only may be admitted to the ward on the day of surgery, provided a preoperative assessment indicates that they are fit and healthy and that growth and development are within the normal range. Before surgery, best practice dictates that photographic records of the cleft be obtained for hospital records, showing antero-poste-rior, inferior and lateral views. These are needed to provide a baseline for follow-up and audit purposes.

Infants requiring a more thorough assessment and those undergoing surgery for a cleft palate may require admission the day before surgery. Prior to a cleft palate repair, the child's assessment should include obtaining a full blood count and grouping and cross matching. The operating surgeon should confirm that informed consent has been obtained. Arm splints have been widely used to prevent interference with the repair of both lip and palate but they have been shown to be of no apparent benefit, particularly if the palate repair is undertaken at the earlier age of six months rather than 14 to 18 months (Jigjinni et al., 1993). However, some surgeons may request them.

The nurse should record an accurate weight of the infant for the calcula-tion of anaesthetic and postoperative drug dosage. Baseline observations of temperature, pulse, respiration and blood pressure and a urine test should be documented and a urine test obtained.

Infants may have food and formula milk up to five hours, and breast milk, water or weak juice up to two hours prior to surgery (Phillips et al., 1994). They can be bathed and should be dressed warmly in easily remov-able garments. Local anaesthetic cream should be applied over suitable venous access sites unless contraindicated (Twycross et al., 1998).

Emotional support

Parents should be encouraged to be present during the induction of anaes-thesia and during postoperative recovery (Department of Health, 1996). This allows them to give their child the love and support they need. This is a traumatic time for parents and they require good preparation and support from nursing staff.

Postoperative care

Breathing

It is important to assess hourly the rate and quality of the infant's respirations following a primary repair to the lip or palate. It is helpful to have the additional safeguard of an apnoea monitor and also to monitor the infant's oxygen saturation levels. It is usual for the saturation rate of an infant of two months to be between 97 and 100% (Stebbens et al., 1991). The child should be laid on one side to allow blood and secretions to drain naturally from the mouth and nose. Suction should be used with caution as the nose and palate are vulnerable to damage following the operation.

It is also very important to be aware that infants of less than six months of age are obligate nasal breathers (Advanced Life Support Group, 1997). An infant used to a large airway has to cope with a smaller one following the repair. Initial signs of an infant having airway difficulties are 'sucking in' of the lower lip on inspiration and sternal, intercostal or subcostal recession. It is essential that these early signs of distress are acted upon promptly as an infant's condition can deteriorate rapidly. The anaesthetist should be alerted immediately if there are any concerns about the child's airway. Postoperative airway obstruction can result from oedema, the presence of blood or exudate in the respiratory tract or certain drugs. Some children may benefit from a nasal airway, particularly following a complete bilateral cleft lip repair.

Another safety measure used in some units to guard the infant's airway is a tongue stitch (Millard, 1980). An oral airway would irritate the palatal suture line, so a tongue stitch is inserted into the posterior aspect of the tongue. This can be used to pull the tongue forward and open up the oral airway in an emergency. It is removed as soon as the child is fully alert.

Eating and drinking

Following cleft surgery, infants usually return from theatre with a maintenance intravenous infusion of half strength Hartmann's solution or 4% dextrose with 0.18% saline. In infants up to 10 kg this will be infused at 100 ml per kg body weight per 24 hours. Unless the lip is very bruised, infants who have had surgery for a cleft lip will often drink from the breast or a bottle soon after return from theatre. Most units offer infants their normal feed postoperatively as soon as they appear hungry. The infusion can be discontinued once the regular feeding regime has been restored.

Cleft palate surgery is more invasive, and infants are much more reluctant to drink. Although some surgeons prefer infants to be fed with a spoon or cup after cleft palate surgery, most allow them to drink from their bottle using a short orthodontic teat. It is easier for infants to drink if they are pain free. Plenty of time should be allowed to reassure and persuade the child to begin drinking again. This is not a task that should be left to the mother, as initially she will find it distressing. Patience and plenty of praise is needed. A nasogastric tube passed at the time of surgery can settle the infant who is reluctant to drink as it can be used to 'top up' after feeds. In the majority of units, a soft diet is commenced after 24 to 48 hours (Cuthbert, 1994). This is continued for a month to six weeks following surgery.

Comfort

Following a simple repair to a cleft lip, paracetamol and regular feeds usually settle infants comfortably. An occasional dose of codeine phosphate or a non-steroidal anti-inflammatory drug (NSAID) may be needed, especially if the lip is very bruised.

Following repair of a cleft palate, infants are very uncomfortable. A standard protocol has been developed for drugs used in paediatric pain management, of opioids, codeine phosphate, NSAID and paracetamol. If a combination of these is used, a much greater pain relief effect will be produced than by using any on their own. Similarly, an NSAID and parac-etamol together produce a greater pain relief effect than either individually (Twycross et al., 1998). Yaster and Maxwell (1993) indicated that doctors were still hesitant to prescribe opioids for children of less than a year old. They stressed that, if opioids are needed, they should be given, but regular observation recordings and oxygen saturation monitoring is vital (Yaster and Maxwell, 1993; Royal College of Paediatrics and Child Health, 1997). Protocols of pain relief should be developed with the anaesthetists and audited regularly.

Safety

Lip care

Care of the suture line is important. The presence of food and debris can cause infection. The formation of scabs should be discouraged, as the removal of scabs with the sutures will remove any new cells that have formed on the scar line (Miller, 1994). Regular cleaning with warm normal saline and an application of an antibiotic cream or soft paraffin helps to protect the area. Care can be negotiated with parents, and, if they agree, they can be taught to care for their child's suture line. They will tend to do this diligently. It is important to use a gentle rolling action with a cotton bud for cleaning. Sutures are removed on the fifth day, usually under sedation (Cuthbert, 1994). This is a skilled procedure, as great care is needed around the columella and lip margin, which are very delicate.

Palate care

Regular fluids are necessary to keep the mouth moist and clean, attempting to create an environment that promotes healing (Miller, 1994). Sterile water should be given following milk, food and medicine to keep the suture line clean. Prophylactic antibiotics and analgesic suspensions must be administered using sterile spoons and/or oral syringes. The use of dummies is either discouraged from birth or they are removed for a period of five weeks postoperatively (Cuthbert, 1994).

Some infants develop sore areas at the angles of the mouth because they are stretched at the time of surgery. These can be soothed by regularly applying sterile soft paraffin, thus attempting to create the ideal environment to accelerate wound healing (Miller, 1994). Soft paraffin is also soothing to dry lips.

All children are discharged from hospital when they are eating and drinking normally and parents are confident about caring for them at home.

Children with syndromes

The pre- and postoperative care of children with a syndrome who are undergoing cleft surgery is similar to that of any other child with a cleft. They will, however, require a more detailed assessment preoperatively and the evaluation of care needs to be negotiated even more thoroughly with parents. This acknowledges the experience of parents in the care of their child and helps to define the role of nurse and parent in hospital.

Parents of children with hypoplastic mandibles have usually been warned that intubation may be difficult. Similarly, children with Pierre Robin sequence may already have had surgery delayed to allow sufficient jaw development to ensure surgical access and preservation of the airway. (Nottingham City Hospital, 1994).

A higher proportion of children with syndromes admitted for cleft surgery may have a tracheostomy than children admitted for other surgical procedures. Parents become very competent in caring for their child's tracheostomy, but still need support while in a hospital environment. There are general principles of care of which staff should be aware. The environment in hospital is drier than that of the home. This means that there is a potential for crusts to form inside the tracheostomy tube, which could be fatal (Serra et al., 1986). The administration of regular humidity is essential. This can be given by the use of a 'Swedish nose', a device that clips to the end of the tube, by the regular instillation of saline before suction, and by the use of a humidifier. Suction should be given not only to remove secretions, but also to evaluate the patency of the tube. A spare tube the same size as the child's should always be ready with tapes attached, in the event of an emergency. Staff responsible for a child with a tracheostomy should have been instructed in the procedure for changing the tube and have practised a tube change, so that their first experience is not in an emergency situation.

Discharge advice

Cleft lip

Parents are encouraged to leave scabs, that form on the child's lip following suture removal, to drop off naturally.

A few weeks after surgery when the lip has healed totally, parents are encouraged to keep the scar line supple by massaging it twice daily with a non-perfumed oil-based cream, for example E45 or Nivea. This helps to break down the irregular pattern formation of collagen fibres in scar tissue (Gollup, 1997; Bosworth, 1997). This is continued until the scar is white and mature and may take a year or more.

Parents are also told to protect the scar from the sun by using a total sun block regularly, both in the morning and at lunchtime.

Cleft palate

Parents are asked, when they return home, to keep their child away from children or adults with coughs and colds as these children appear more vulnerable to infection in the immediate postoperative period.

Parents should be given advice on nourishing foods to give their child and when to return to a normal diet. Pulses are discouraged in their diet at first, as the skins can stick to the suture line. Fruit yoghurts with pips are also discouraged. Parents are asked to continue rinsing their child's mouth with water after food for at least two weeks.

In units using arm splints, children may have to continue wearing them at home for a few weeks, especially when they are not being supervised, and at night (Berkowitz, 1994).

References

Action for Sick Children (1996) Health services for children and young people, a guide for commissioners and providers: Principles for commissioning and providing service: Action for Sick Children Publication, p. 5.

Advanced Life Support Group (1997) Advanced Paediatric Life Support: The Practical Approach. London: British Medical Journal Publishing Group, pp. 9 and 66.

Armstrong AJ, Finch RG, Bailie FB (1993) Serious group A streptococcal infections complicating cryotherapy to lip haemangiomas. Clinical and Experimental Dermatology 18: 537–539.

Berkowitz S (1994) The Cleft Palate Story. Chicago: Quintessence Publishing Company, p. 79.

Bosworth C (1997) Burns Trauma Nursing Procedures. London: Whurr, p. 229.

Cuthbert AM (1994) Cleft lip and palate survey: an examination of 16 hospitals' protocols for cleft lip and palate surgery. Unpublished, Royal Victoria Hospital, Newcastle, September–December.

Department of Health (1991) Welfare of children and young people in hospital (Guidance Document). London: HMSO, p. 16.

Department of Health (1996) The Patient's Charter: Services for Children and Young People, and My rights and what I can expect. DoH, p. 7.

Gollup R (1997) Burns aftercare and scar management. In: Bosworth C (ed.) Burns Trauma. London: Baillière Tindall, p. 165.

Jigjinni V, Kangesu T, Sommerlad BC (1993) Do babies require arm splints after cleft palate repair? British Journal of Plastic Surgery 46: 681–685.

Millard DR (1980) Cleft Craft: The Evolution of its Surgery, Vol. III: Alveolar and Palatal Deformities. Boston: Little Brown and Company, p. 154.

Miller M (1994) The ideal healing environment. Nursing Times 90: 62–68.

Nottingham City Hospital (1994) Parent information booklet, Hello, my name is Jade, Nottingham City Hospital NHS Trust, p. 3.10.

Phillips S, Daborn AK, Hatch DJ (1994) Pre-operative fasting for paediatric anaesthesia. British Journal of Anaesthesia 73: 529–536.

Royal College of Paediatrics and Child Health (1997) Prevention and control of pain in children: a manual for health care professionals. London: British Medical Journal Publishing Group, pp. 55 and 124.

Serra AM, Bailey CM, Jackson P (1986) Ear, Nose and Throat Nursing. Oxford: Blackwell Scientific Publications, p. 230.

Stebbens VA, Poets CF, Alexander JR, Arrowsmith WA, Southall DP (1991) Oxygen saturations and breathing patterns in infancy: 1. Full term infants in the second month of life. Archives of Disease in Childhood 66: 569–573.

Twycross A, Moriarty A, Betts T (1998) Paediatric Pain Management – A Multi-disciplinary Approach. Oxford: Radcliffe Medical Press, pp. 128–129.

Yaster M., Maxwell LG (1993) Opiate agonists and antagonists. In: Schecter NL, Berde CB, Yaster M (eds) Pain in Infants, Children and Adolescents. Baltimore: Williams & Wilkins, pp. 145–171.

CHAPTER 14

Speech Development and Early Intervention

V.J. RUSSELL AND A. HARDING

Introduction

It is now recognized that the speech and language therapist has an active role in the early management of infants born with clefts of the lip and palate (LeBlanc, 1996; McWilliams et al., 1990). The therapist provides support and information regarding communication development for parents and monitors the child's progress with the aim of facilitating normal development, preventing problems and providing appropriate early intervention for problems which are identified. Although the majority of children with clefts will achieve normal speech patterns with little or no speech and language therapy involvement, 'at least 20% of nonsyndromic cleft palate individuals and individuals with syndrome-related cleft palates' (LeBlanc, 1996) may have significant speech difficulties (Golding-Kushner, 1995, LeBlanc, 1996; McWilliams et al., 1990). It is important, therefore, to identify the latter group as soon as possible so that appropriate intervention can be implemented. It has been established that potential problems can be identified in the pre-speech stage of development and preventative work undertaken to promote more normal patterns of development (Golding-Kushner, 1995; Russell and Grunwell, 1993).

In addition, early speech and language therapy involvement contributes to research and good practice by providing an opportunity to monitor and keep records of all infants' patterns of phonetic development. These data can be utilized in retrospective studies investigating possible relationships between cleft types (Albery and Grunwell, 1993), surgical timing/technique, speech therapy and other factors in relation to those children who develop normal speech and those who experience difficulties (CSAG, 1998).

This chapter discusses the possible influences of the structural defect on the speech development of cleft palate children. Speech and language therapy involvement from birth is outlined and examples provided of early intervention strategies.

Influences of the cleft palate on communication development

The presence of a cleft may influence the earliest stages of communication development because of physical factors which may also disrupt parent/child interaction and social development. These factors, in isolation and in combination, can contribute to delayed and deviant speech and language development.

One of the initial consequences of the cleft, except in the case of a very minor defect, is early feeding difficulties (see Bannister, Chapter 10). These infants are more prone to wind and can take longer to feed, which creates anxiety and distress for both mother and child. Both abnormal feeding patterns and the physical defect itself can affect oral motor and oro-sensory development. Bzoch (1979) suggests that abnormal neuromotor patterns may develop because both decoding and encoding skills are learned while 'the vast majority of infants with clefts have an abnormal (speech) mechanism'. Both the abnormal physical structures and neuromotor patterns may result in delayed or deviant pre-speech development.

A further effect of feeding difficulties is the disruption of normal mother–child interaction. This relationship is inevitably vulnerable when a baby is born with a facial deformity (see Bradbury, Chapter 23). While having to cope with feeding problems some mothers grieve over the lost opportunity to breastfeed. This sorrow, combined with the fatigue of frequent, lengthy feeds may limit the mother's motivation to communicate with her baby. As Neiman and Savage (1997) comment in their study of the development of children with clefts from birth to three years of age, the feeding context helps to shape early communicative sequences. The authors suggest that feeding difficulties and associated environmental adjustments may account for 'early cognitive lags (in the cleft lip and palate group) and language lags (in the cleft palate group)' (Neiman and Savage, 1997). Some mothers, however, seem to fear that their baby might feel rejected and actively compensate for their own reactions by consciously interacting intensively with their cleft palate infant. This can result in more advanced communicative abilities rather than delayed development.

In addition to the effect of the feeding situation on parent–child interaction, it is also possible that the presence of a physical defect will affect the parents' attitude to the child and thus their response to and initiation of communication. As Edwards (1980) points out, 'it has been shown that parents of a child with a congenital handicap tend to regard them as being different long after they have in fact moved towards normality'. This means that parents may underrate their child's potential. Attempts by the child to communicate may not be recognized as words by the parents because of the effects of the cleft on articulation development (Harding, 1993; Russell, 1991). Additional stress may also be placed on the parent–child relationship and early communicative interaction by hospitalization, surgery and outpatient clinic appointments.

Another physical consequence of a cleft palate is the frequent occurrence of otitis media due to Eustachian tube malfunction (Heller, 1979; Lencione, 1980; Maw, 1986; McWilliams et al., 1990; see Lennox, Chapter 15). This results in a conductive hearing loss which may fluctuate and can seriously affect auditory skills and communication development (Bamford and Saunders, 1990). A recent study by Broen et al. (1996) provides evidence that the majority of cleft palate children have reduced hearing levels unless ventilation tubes have been inserted. Although the exact nature of the relationship between otitis media and speech development remains unclear, those children who suffer early and frequent episodes of otitis media seem to be at greater risk for speech and language problems (Bamford and Saunders, 1990, Hall and Hill, 1986). Russell and Grunwell (1993) demonstrate how the presence of fluctuating hearing loss associated with otitis media, combined with other factors, might have contributed to the greater severity of the atypical and delayed patterns of speech development in three of their subjects.

There is general agreement that the language skills of cleft palate children tend to be delayed, particularly in the development of expressive language (Bzoch, 1989; Chapman and Hardin, 1990; McWilliams et al., 1990; Neiman and Savage, 1997; Scherer and D'Antonio, 1995). There is, however, considerable variation in the aspects of language investigated and the variables taken into account. The causes of any delay, for example, may be more closely related to associated hearing loss, linguistic environment and other psychosocial factors than to direct effects of the physical defect itself. There is, therefore, a need for close monitoring of the language development of cleft palate children commencing in the prelinguistic period of development and continuing into later childhood.

Early vocalizations – pre-speech phonetic development

Recent research has described atypical pre-speech development in cleft palate children (Harding and Grunwell, 1993; Russell and Grunwell, 1993) and there is, therefore, a need to consider this development from birth. The range of consonant-like sounds available to any infant is dependent on several other aspects of development. Articulatory development can be thought of as a product of the ongoing synergy between: growth of the skeletal structures, the maxilla and the mandible; increasing neuromuscular control of the moving parts of the speech mechanism, the lips, tongue, velopharyngeal sphincter and the respiratory system; cognitive development; social interaction skills, and the individual's motivation to communicate. All these aspects contribute to the changing 'shape' of early vocalizations. If any aspect of development is disturbed, then the pattern of progress might be affected. Given the variability between individuals in ages and stages of development, it is remarkable that the majority of 'normal' children follow similar developmental patterns (Kent, 1992; Trost-Cardamone, 1990). The influences of a cleft, as described above, therefore, highlight the potential for these children to exhibit delayed and atypical speech sound development.

In the first few months of life there is little difference between cleft and non-cleft infants. Neonates with cleft palate produce much the same nasalized vowel-like cries and cooing noises as non-cleft infants. This is due to the fact that all infants have limited control of the velopharyngeal sphincter and immature movements of the articulatory muscles (Trost-Cardamone, 1990). As a result, the vocal tone is hypernasal with glottal and pharyngeal articulations, but during the first four to six months of life non-cleft infants develop a range of consonant-like sounds (contoids) in the oral cavity. Infants with unrepaired cleft palates are not able to progress to these oral consonants because they cannot establish the intraoral pressure (achieved by closure of the velopharyngeal isthmus so that the airstream is directed orally) to produce contoids such as /b d g/ for example (Wyatt et al., 1996). These are the first consonants requiring intraoral pressure to appear in the babble of children who do not have clefts. Repair of palate clefts at about the age of six months may be timely in facilitating normal babble development.

There is evidence, however, of atypical development in the pre-speech vocalizations of children with cleft palate both preoperatively and postoperatively (Dorf and Curtin, 1982; Henningsson, 1989; Mousset and Trichet, 1985; O'Gara and Logemann, 1988; Russell and Grunwell, 1993). Preoperative vocalizations are characterized by a lack of labial and lingual and a corresponding dominance of glottal and pharyngeal articulations. This marked difference from normal babble is undoubtedly physically based and results from the structural inadequacy of the intraoral mechanism. Postoperatively the improved mechanism facilitates progress towards more normal patterns. There is an increase in labial and lingual articulations as infants discover the potential of their changed intraoral structure, although there is still a delay in comparison with normal development (Russell and Grunwell, 1993). Some studies indicate a tendency for children who receive earlier repair to develop more normal articulations sooner than those children who have later operations (Dorf and Curtin, 1982; Henningsson, 1989, Mousset and Trichet, 1985; O'Gara and Logemann, 1988) and empirical evidence supports this view. Trost-Cardamone (1990) suggests that the speech pathologist should monitor early babble development so that palate repair can be 'timed to precede and facilitate' the stage at which babbling becomes more speech-like.

Early speech development

In studies of normal children it has been clearly established that there is a link between the phonetic repertoire of babbling and the basic sound system of a child's language, whatever that language might be (Locke, 1983; Oller et al., 1975). Studies have shown that this relationship is also evident in the cleft palate population and, therefore, that the early speech patterns of children with cleft palate are related to their babbling patterns (Estrem and Broen, 1989; Russell and Grunwell, 1993).

Estrem and Broen (1989) compared first words used by non-cleft and cleft groups of children. The cleft palate group used more words beginning with nasals [m n ŋ], approximants [w l j] and vowels and fewer words beginning with pressure consonants. In addition, the children with cleft palate produced more words starting with velar and glottal consonants, but targeted fewer alveolar consonants than the normal group. Estrem and Broen (1989) comment that: 'Deviant production patterns, characteristic of the speech of children with cleft palate appeared very early in the speech of some children'. Chapman (1991) also identified that cleft palate children tended to produce more words containing nasal consonants. Hence words like 'more, mummy, mine, no' might emerge early but those such as 'bye bye, ball, daddy' are less likely to be attempted or are not understood by parents.

In the study reported by Russell and Grunwell (1993) patterns that were evident in the children's pre-speech vocalizations were also evident in their early speech. For one subject this was a range of predominantly back of tongue, pharyngeal and glottal fricatives, and for four subjects, pre-speech front of tongue articulations were still evident as palatal fricatives in speech. Pre-speech patterns showing a lack of plosives and a predominance of nasal articulations were subsequently evidenced as the same restricted range of consonants. Interestingly, the single subject whose pre-speech phonetic inventory was developmentally normal went on to show a near normal pattern of development in early speech.

Evidence of the link between the phonetic repertoire of babbling and the basic sound system of a child's language in the cleft palate population highlights the need for speech and language therapists to monitor babbling development and to implement intervention if there are indications of delay or deviance. It is recommended that all children who have cleft palate should receive routine screening of speech and language development at 18 months. In the study reported by Russell and Grunwell (1993) it was at this age that children most 'at risk' for delayed and deviant speech development could be identified. An absence of plosives indicates that there may be a delay in plosive consonant acquisition in the child's future speech development.

Phonetic and phonological development

Articulatory constraints

In the non-cleft child, early vocalizations are produced in the pharynx and glottis but by six months tongue and velopharyngeal function have developed such that babble and first words contain more anterior labial and alveolar contacts [m b] and [d]. In addition, control of the velopharyngeal sphincter facilitates the development of pressure consonants [p b t d] which are acquired during the next six months. The acquisition of the consonants used in speech is a lengthy process and takes place in a series of stages or levels (Grunwell, 1987a). At the time of starting to speak, all children have access to a limited range of consonants [m p b w t d n] which extends with increasing articulatory skill, neuromotor development and practice. Cleft palate articulatory simplifications are to some extent superimposed on non-cleft immaturities. However, they can be directly associated with specific structural deficiencies imposing articulatory constraints.

Conditions which impose articulatory constraints are velopharyngeal insufficiency (VPI), residual clefts or fistulae, nasal obstruction and dental and occlusal anomalies. VPI is characterized by hypernasal resonance, nasalized weak pressure consonants and/or nasal emission accompanying pressure consonant production (Wyatt et al., 1996). In severe VPI oral consonants may be realized as nasals, for example /b/ as [m], but this could also be a result of abnormal learned neuromotor patterns (Bzoch, 1989). VPI is also associated with a persistence of non-oral articulations such as pharyngeal and glottal realizations (Sell et al., 1994, 1999; see Grunwell and Sell, Chapter 5 and Sell and Grunwell, Chapter 16) for explanation of these characteristics.

A fistula may perpetuate a preference for back articulation, for example velar /k,g/, because pressure can be built up more easily behind the fistula. Backing may affect any of the alveolar and post-alveolar consonant targets and is the reverse of the normal developmental pattern of fronting (Grunwell, 1987a). Fistulae are particularly likely to affect the quality of grooved alveolar fricative consonants [s ʃ] because of difficulty establishing central airflow between the tongue tip and the hard palate without loss of air through the fistula.

Whilst cleft palate is most commonly associated with VPI and excessive nasal resonance, nasal obstruction can precipitate hyponasal resonance in developing cleft palate speech. In severe hyponasality the nasal consonants sound like plosives, for example 'Mummy' sounds like 'bubby'. Causes of nasal obstruction resulting in hyponasality are described by Whetmore (1992). Nasal obstruction usually precipitates mouth breathing, snoring, slow eating and disturbed sleep patterns. Mouth breathing or open mouth posture warrants attention because normal facial growth is dependent on nose breathing and sustained lip closure (Moss, 1969; Oblak and Kozelj, 1984). Where habitual open mouth posture is the result of upper lip immobility, and no obstruction exists, strategies can be devised to encourage sustained lip closure. Lip closure cannot, however, be targeted when the open mouth posture results from nasal obstruction, when medical intervention may be required (see Lennox, Chapter 15).

Dental and occlusal anomalies may also influence speech production, resulting particularly in palatalization and lateralization of alveolar consonant targets (Albery and Grunwell, 1993; Albery and Russell, 1990). However, palatalization and lateralization may also result from atypical phonetic development (Russell and Grunwell, 1993).

The effect of the cleft palate condition on phonetic development may result in a different order of consonant acquisition from that which occurs in a non-cleft child (Harding, 1993; O'Gara and Logemann; 1988; Russell and Grunwell, 1993). In particular, velar plosives may occur before alveolar plosives, as discussed above, and voiceless prior to voiced consonants. This has implications for clinical management and the selection of therapy targets, which will be discussed below. In addition, the early speech of cleft palate children may contain a vocabulary which reflects a limited repertoire of consonants. Chapman (1991) made the point that since a nasal consonant colours the neighbouring vowels, a prevalence of nasals would increase the overall nasal resonance throughout speech.

Given the potential constraints on developing speech it is somewhat surprising that many children born with a sizeable cleft develop normal speech patterns without any apparent effect from the cleft. For many children this will be the result of the surgeon's expertise but sometimes excellent speech patterns have been achieved despite structural impairment. Fletcher (1985) studied an adult patient who produced a perfect /s/ despite an unrepaired palate. He concluded that individuals with cleft palate may develop adaptive strategies. Furthermore, he proposed that clinicians should study these strategies, which might be taught to less adaptive individuals.

Studies of early speech reveal that there is considerable variability in the speech patterns of younger children with cleft palate. However, in an extensive review McWilliams et al. (1990), although confirming the high risk of disordered articulation for children with cleft palate, highlighted also the occurrence of improvement with age, especially in the production of plosives and fricatives. In addition, they point out the variability between individual children with cleft palate in the nature and extent of their speech sound errors and conclude that this is a heterogeneous population in this respect. Riski and DeLong (1984), in a longitudinal study that investigated the articulation development of 108 children from 3;0 to 8;0 years of age, also conclude that children with cleft palate are a heterogeneous group.

Phonological development

From about one year of age, all infants gradually organize the few consonants available to them into speech which is immature but can be understood by their immediate family. As described above, this early speech is subject to simplifications. Such simplifications affect whole groups of consonants; for example, all words that begin with /t, s, ʃ, ʤ/ are realized with a [d] as the initial consonant. These simplifications resolve gradually following a predictable developmental pattern until a mature phonological system is achieved by the age of seven years (Grunwell, 1987a). It has been established that the speech development of cleft palate children also reveals systematic patterns (Harding and Grunwell, 1996; Ingram, 1976, 1989). As Grunwell (1987a) comments: '...a child with a repaired cleft is developing a phonological system as well as coping with and compensating for the effects of the organic malformation'.

Cleft palate speech development is a combination of normal simplification processes and cleft type strategies. Whole groups of consonants may be affected by cleft palate articulatory constraints in addition to normal immature patterns (Harding and Grunwell, 1996). If, for example, a child with a cleft palate backs /d/ to [g] and 'door' is pronounced as 'gore', it follows that all the consonants grouped with /d/ in normal development will also be backed. Therefore, 'do, two, zoo, shoe, chew, Jew' will all be produced as 'goo'. Later, when fricatives begin to emerge, a persistent backing process will result in the backing of the alveolar fricatives /s/ and /z/ to velar [xɣ]. Existing processes in a child's phonological system are sufficiently strong that realizations of a new target, such as /s/, which might be produced accurately in sound play, would always conform to the existing phonological rules, whether cleft related or developmental. This effect of an articulatory constraint on the phonological system is described as a phonological consequence of an articulatory disorder (Grundy and

Harding, 1995). Normal immaturities usually resolve spontaneously, but cleft type processes are likely to stabilize and require therapeutic intervention.

There is, therefore, a need to employ phonological techniques of analysis to cleft palate speech in order to determine the extent and nature of any deviance or delay and to determine whether these result primarily from phonetic or phonological bases (Crystal, 1989). Broen et al. (1986) illustrate how phonological analysis helped to identify children at the age of two and a half years who required secondary surgery for velopharyngeal insufficiency. Lynch et al. (1983) studied the developing phonological systems of two cleft palate children. One of their subjects evidenced speech cleft type characteristics associated with structural inadequacy whereas the other showed evidence of developmental delay. Both these subjects, and those in the non-surgical group studied by Broen et al., differed from non-cleft subjects with regard to consonant development. Russell and Grunwell (1993) report considerable individual variation but also common tendencies in the developing phonological systems of eight subjects. Characteristics of cleft palate speech were detected in the data of all their subjects at some stage but the number and types of characteristics varied. The results of this study indicated that more normal phonetic development leads to normal phonological development but delay in phonetic development causes further delay in the establishment of a child's phonological system.

Children with cleft palate may follow exactly the same progression as those with no cleft but they may initially evidence 'cleft type' patterns which resolve and match normal development by approximately four years (Russell, 1991; Harding, 1993). If, however, their early idiosyncrasies show no sign of resolving spontaneously then they require early therapeutic intervention to facilitate modification of their speech production. In addition, later surgical intervention may also be required.

Speech and language therapy management and intervention

Birth to palate repair

The most significant part of the speech and language therapist's role prior to palate repair is to provide parents with support and information concerning communication development. This includes an explanation of the function of the palate (with the aid of diagrams), the possible effects of the cleft on speech development and an outline of the therapist's preventative and therapeutic roles. In addition, the therapist will encourage normal patterns of parent–child interaction in 'an environment that will facilitate normal speech and language development' (LeBlanc, 1996). As Russell (1989) describes, it is important to emphasize that many cleft palate children will achieve normal communication skills with little or no help, but others may need greater involvement from the speech and language therapist. Specialist clinicians, therefore, observe and monitor all infants with cleft palate in order to support the parents and to ensure that the child receives any help required at the appropriate time. Prior to palate repair, mothers are encouraged to engage in vocal play and vocal stimulation with their infants in order to establish early patterns of turn taking and vocal response.

Palate repair to eighteen months

In most instances the palate will have been repaired within the first year of life. However, even when surgery has not taken place, for example in some cases of submucous cleft palate or if the child's health prevents it, the following procedures remain applicable.

During this period general communication development will be observed. Discussion with the parents will particularly focus on the development of babble patterns. It is important to obtain evidence that the child's postoperative vocalizations progress towards more anterior patterns as described above. Evidence of progress includes an increase in labial and lingual articulations, e.g. [p m l] and the development of oral plosives [p b t d k g]. If oral pressure consonants fail to develop, it is not possible to determine at the pre-speech stage whether this is due to velopharyngeal insufficiency (VPI) or other factors. However, it is important to identify this atypical pattern as soon as possible in order to initiate appropriate management.

Early intervention for children who are not using plosives, especially the voiceless plosives [p t k], is recommended by Russell and Grunwell (1993) and Mousset and Trichet (1985). As suggested in Albery and Russell (1994), early intervention should be implemented when there is evidence of the following:

- An absence of plosive articulations such that the child is only using nasals, vowels, approximants and possibly glottal articulations [m n l w j h ʔ].
- A predominant pattern of non-oral glottal and pharyngeal articulations [ʔ ħ ʕ].
- A lack of labial and front of tongue plosives. The child may be using velars but no other plosives, which can lead to a backing pattern as the phonological system develops.
- Any other evidence of deviant or delayed communication development, for example, language delay.

Early intervention would usually take the form of an indirect approach where the parents are given target consonants to model in participative babble (Albery and Russell, 1994). The more children see, hear and feel particular sounds which are repeatedly modelled in specific ways, the more likely they are to produce similar sounds themselves (Stoel-Gammon, 1992). Through this approach, the acquisition of new sounds may be completely effortless for the child. Parents should also be advised to interpret babbled utterances as potentially meaningful in order to encourage vocal output.

Early intervention and home programmes for cleft palate children are described by Albery and Russell (1994) and Golding-Kushner (1995). Parents are trained to facilitate and reinforce appropriate patterns in babble and first words. Albery and Russell (1994) stress the importance of taking advantage of what the child is doing naturally to encourage appropriate development. Specialist programmes are not required for most infants with cleft palate, but for those developing an atypical phonetic repertoire they can be very effective in eliciting more normal production, thereby preventing a need for later therapy (Golding-Kushner, 1995). To be effective home programmes require close contact between the parents and the speech and language therapist. Some parents need frequent demonstration of modelling techniques before they are confident to apply them. In addition, audio or, in particular, videotapes of modelled activities are effective in helping parents carry out the programme. They extend the therapeutic experience to the home. Children can re-absorb the clinician's model and parents can be reminded of the precise modelling techniques.

Eighteen months to three years

Even if there has been no previous concern about communication development, all children who have had cleft palate should be routinely assessed at the age of 18 to 20 months. This is to ensure that the child is making satisfactory progress along normal lines and also for the collection of records which can be used for audit and research purposes. Information about babble patterns and speech development is an essential contribution to the ongoing debate about the timing and type of surgical repair. An audit of 50 consecutive assessments of children with cleft palate at 18 months found that 'at risk' children can be accurately identified on 98% of occasions by a specialist speech and language therapist (Bowden et al., 1997).

Assessment

At the 18 month assessment all aspects of communication development should be screened and any areas of concern, including verbal comprehension and expressive language, investigated in greater detail (Russell, 1989;

Albery and Russell, 1990). In addition, it is important for the speech and language therapist to have information about the child's hearing status, developmental milestones and other data related to the nature of the cleft and the medical history. Information about play, language and speech skills is obtained using selected age-appropriate toys.

At subsequent assessments, when children are producing more language, a systematic phonological screening assessment such as PACS TOYS (Grunwell and Harding, 1995) can be particularly useful. It elicits specific target words whilst also offering opportunities to probe verbal comprehension and to transcribe samples of spontaneous speech.

Consonant production

The child's phonetic repertoire is assessed through transcription of babble and parent report. Consonant production may initially be recorded using a phonetic inventory (Grunwell and Harding, 1995) or the phonetic diagram (Sell et al., 1994). Figure 14.1 shows the phonetic diagram of a child at 18 months. This subject is using the nasals /m/ /n/ and /ŋ/ but only the velar plosive /k/ and glottal stop. It is evident from this atypical and restricted inventory that therapy is required. Harland (personal communication) recommends circling consonants heard during the assessment session and using a dotted line for those reported by the parents but not heard by the clinician. A colour coding system is described by Sell et al. (1994).

An absence of oral pressure consonants may be followed by an increase in cleft type characteristics as the consonant system develops. For example, newly acquired plosives might be accompanied by nasal emission so that

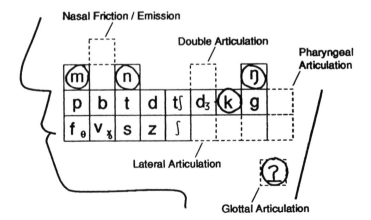

Figure 14.1. Phonetic diagram showing a child's phonetic repertoire at 18 months.

'pea' originally realized as 'me' becomes [p̃i]. Similarly, transition from the normal stopping process to the production of fricative consonants may result in speech cleft type characteristics such as velar or uvular fricatives or non-oral pharyngeal or nasal fricatives. For example, 'four' is firstly realized as 'pour', which is developmentally normal, but as the child starts to use nasal fricatives to realize the [f] consonant it becomes [m̥̃]. Expansion of the phonological system may, therefore, give the impression of deteriorating speech and/or increasing VPI. This also highlights the importance of continuing to monitor progress until speech development is complete because each maturational stage may result in a cleft related error.

Intervention

Intervention strategies include a combination of the indirect approach used for younger children and more direct articulation therapy. For younger children, still largely in the pre-speech stage of development, therapy is indirect with change being facilitated by the parents modelling and feeding back. In addition, games using manipulated vocabulary (Grundy and Harding, 1995; Hahn, 1989) in which specific target words are repeatedly used is effective. The aim of these approaches is to use a structured repetitive input model to destabilize existing atypical articulatory patterns. Harding and Bryan (1998) suggest that the specific aims of therapy during this critical period are to develop each child's attentiveness to the structure of language and their ability to reflect subconsciously on the articulatory processes involved.

New motor programmes are encouraged with the following aims:

- To encourage the child to experiment with his/her articulators so that new consonants may be produced.
- To encourage the child to use new consonants in different word positions.
- To increase the child's awareness of differences between speech sounds and to improve listening and discrimination skills.
- To produce consonants with correct articulatory placement (and if possible the appropriate manner of articulation, for example plosive or fricative).

Activities designed to achieve these aims are described in Albery and Russell (1994), who recommend associating consonants and vowels with specific pictures and using these for discrimination and production games. It may be helpful to use a specific system such as The Nuffield Dyspraxia Programme (1985, 1992). Even very young children respond to this type of approach provided it is presented as a game. Nose-holding in sound play may reveal new articulatory possibilities which subsequently might be achieved without nose-holding (Harding and Grunwell, 1998; Golding-Kushner, 1995). As soon as consonants have been produced in play, then a more direct approach can be adopted which encourages repeated productions of newly achieved target consonants.

Three to four and a half years

From about the age of three years and sometimes earlier, intervention should be based on a comprehensive phonetic and phonological assessment. Data are obtained using PACS TOYS (Grunwell and Harding, 1995) or PACS Pictures (Grunwell, 1987b), and GOS.SP.ASS (Sell et al., 1994, 1999). Elicitation of the sentences for the latter is facilitated by the use of the Picture Stimuli (Sell et al., 1996). Analysis of the data obtained from the speech assessment enables the clinician to use 'principled decision making' (Grunwell, 1992) when designing therapy programmes for children with cleft palate This will ensure that the most effective therapy approach is implemented, i.e. articulatory, phonological or a combined articulatory and phonological approach (Grunwell and Dive, 1988; Grundy and Harding, 1995).

Articulation therapy

Target consonants can be selected using the rationale outlined by Harding and Grunwell (1998) and/or the criteria for phoneme selection described by Hoch et al. (1986). Following assessment those consonants that are most easily elicited in isolation are selected. It is generally accepted that voiceless targets will be easier to elicit than voiced targets (Harding and Grunwell, 1998). In addition, it may be appropriate to target fricatives before plosives and sometimes, especially when there is a fistula or alveolar defect, back prior to front articulatory placements. It is apparent, therefore, that it is common to follow an idiosyncratic sequence of consonant acquisition when working with cleft palate children. It is recommended that a number of different targets are selected, although it is occasionally necessary to work on only one consonant in therapy.

Techniques for eliciting specific consonants are described by Albery and Russell (1994). Consonants that are produced correctly in terms of place or manner of articulation may be used to help the child to attempt particular targets. For example, similar consonants provide phonetic and tactile cues. Auditory, visual, verbal and manual cues can also be used and the clinician will ascertain which type or combination of cues is most effective for the individual child (Golding-Kushner, 1995). Nose-holding may be effective in helping the child to experience oral versus nasal airflow, particularly if reduced intraoral pressure precipitates passive processes (Harding and Grunwell, 1998). Golding-Kushner (1995) describes using a sustained /h/ in order to inhibit glottal realizations whilst facilitating production of aspirated voiceless consonants. Overaspiration of the target sound followed by an elongated vowel can facilitate new articulatory achievements. Gentle blowing with subsequent production of a voiceless bilabial fricative can be an effective precursor to achieving /f/. When working with cleft palate children it is important to remember that 'it is possible for different individuals to make different articulatory gestures to produce a sound which is perceptually the same' (Grundy and Harding, 1995). The therapist is, therefore, encouraging the child to experiment with his lips and tongue in order to achieve an acceptable auditory match with the adult target rather than precise articulatory movements.

It is evident from the above that articulation therapy is a direct approach and part of a structured programme based on a comprehensive assessment. It is important for activities to be motivating whatever the age and ability of the client and specific individual reward systems may be required (Russell and Sell, 1998). It is often helpful to agree and discuss therapy aims with both the child and parent. Once a new articulatory target has been achieved and is being consistently used in non-word activities, phonological therapy approaches using meaningful words (Grunwell and Dive, 1988; Grundy and Harding, 1995) are used to establish it in different word positions and facilitate generalization. Phonological therapy activities include:

- Consonant recognition and discrimination, in isolation and in different word positions.
- Sorting words according to contrasting consonants, e.g. [t] versus [k].
- Producing the correct word from a minimal pair (words which differ by one consonant, e.g. tea – key, bat – back, paw – four). Using the word to convey the correct meaning in sentences and stories.

Velopharyngeal insufficiency

When velopharyngeal insufficiency is suspected, speech analysis provides important information for the differential diagnosis. It is essential to determine whether hypernasality and/or nasal emission occur consistently throughout speech (Sell et al., 1994, 1999). These features may be present on individual or groups of consonants only (phoneme specific) or because the child is only using nasal consonants. Analysis of speech data also establishes whether the child's speech is affected by active and/or passive processes (Harding and Grunwell, 1998). Any active processes will require therapy whereas passive processes are more likely to need surgical intervention. Suspected velopharyngeal insufficiency cannot be fully investigated during early speech development because young children are unable to cooperate with procedures such as nasendoscopy. It is important, however, to commence therapy in order to facilitate normal articulatory patterns (LeBlanc, 1996; Russell, 1997).

Frequency of therapy

It is clear from the literature and clinical experience that cleft palate children respond best to focused, intensive and frequent therapy sessions (Golding-Kushner, 1995; Hoch et al., 1986; LeBlanc, 1996). In many situations there may have to be a compromise with regard to the frequency of therapy sessions but progress may still be made provided the therapy is appropriate and there is consistent daily follow-up. This can be achieved with weekly (or occasionally less frequent) therapy sessions if the parent undertakes to continue the therapy programme at home. In some instances this will consist of structured parental input with minimal conscious effort from the child. It may be necessary to involve significant other people in the home and/or school environment. In addition, video and audio tapes, as described above, are valuable aids. The therapist, therefore, needs to invest time in devising the programme, preparing therapy materials and training the parent and others appropriately. This is, however, time well spent in comparison to the time wasted and frustration caused by inadequate weekly therapy. As Golding-Kushner (1995) points out, if articulation errors do not start to resolve within three to six months, it is usually the fault of the therapy and not the patient. In some cases a therapy programme designed by a specialist therapist and implemented by a community therapist has proved to be effective.

Summary

This chapter has described the pre-speech and speech development of cleft palate children. It has illustrated the need for early involvement from the speech and language therapist and the importance of providing intervention as soon as potential problems are identified. A description of speech and language therapy management from birth onwards is provided. Examples are given of specific treatment strategies with reference to other texts.

References

Albery E, Grunwell P (1993) Consonant articulation in different types of cleft lip and palate. In: Grunwell P (ed.) Analysing Cleft Palate Speech. London: Whurr, pp. 83–111.

Albery E, Russell J (1990) Cleft palate and orofacial abnormalities. In: Grunwell P (ed.) Developmental Speech Disorders. London: Whurr, pp. 63–82.

Albery E, Russell J (1994) Cleft Palate Sourcebook. Oxford: Winslow.

Bamford J, Saunders E (1990) Hearing Impairment, Auditory Perception and Language Disability, 2nd edn. London: Whurr.

Bowden M, Harland K, Sommerlad B (1997) How early should speech and language skills be assessed? An audit of 50 consecutive assessments undertaken at 18 months of age. Paper presented at The Craniofacial Society of Great Britain annual scientific conference, Writtle, Essex.

Broen PA, Felsenfeld S, Kittleson-Bacon CK (1986) Predicting from the phonological patterns observed in children with cleft palate. Paper presented at the Symposium on Research in Child Language Disorders, Madison, Wisconsin.

Broen PA, Moller KT, Carlstrom J, Doyle SS, Devers M, Keenan KM (1996) Comparison of the hearing histories of children with and without cleft palate. Cleft Palate–Craniofacial Journal 33: 127–133.

Bzoch KR (1979) Communicative Disorders Related to Cleft Lip and Palate, 2nd edn. Boston, MA: Little Brown.

Bzoch KR (1989) Communicative Disorders Related to Cleft Lip and Palate, 3rd edn. Boston, MA: College Hill Press.

Chapman KL (1991) Vocalizations of toddlers with cleft lip and palate. Cleft Palate–Craniofacial Journal 28: 172–178.

Chapman KL, Hardin MA (1990) Communicative competence in children with cleft lip and palate. In: Bardach J, Morris HL (eds) Multidisciplinary Management of Cleft Lip and Palate. Philadelphia: WB Saunders, pp. 721–726.

CSAG Report – Clinical Standards Advisory Group (1998) Cleft lip and/or palate. London: HMSO.

Crystal D (1989) Clinical Linguistics. London: Whurr.

Dorf DA, Curtin JW (1982) Early cleft palate repair and speech outcome. Journal of Plastic and Reconstructive Surgery 12: 74–79.

Edwards M (1980) Speech and language disability. In: Advances in the Management of Cleft Lip and Palate. Edinburgh: Churchill Livingstone.

Estrem T, Broen PA (1989) Early speech production of children with cleft palate. Journal of Speech and Hearing Research 32: 12–24.

Fletcher SG (1985) Speech production and oral motor skills in an adult with an unrepaired palatal cleft. Journal of Speech and Hearing Disorders 50: 254–261.

Golding-Kushner KJ (1995) Treatment of articulation and resonance disorders associated with cleft palate and VPI. In: Shprintzen R (ed.) Cleft Palate Speech Management: A Multidisciplinary Approach. St Louis: CV Mosby, pp. 327–335.

Grundy K, Harding A (1995) Disorders of speech production. In: Grundy K (ed.) Linguistics in Clinical Practice, 2nd edn. London: Taylor & Francis, pp. 329–357.

Grunwell P (1987a) Clinical Phonology, 2nd edn. London: Croom Helm.

Grunwell P (1987b) PACS Pictures: Language Elicitation Materials. Windsor: NFER-Nelson.

Grunwell P (1992) Principled decision-making in the remediation of children with phonological disability. In: Fletcher P, Hall D (eds) Specific Speech and Language Disorders in Children. London: Whurr.

Grunwell P, Dive D (1988) Treating 'cleft palate speech': combining phonological techniques with traditional articulation therapy. Child Language Teaching and Therapy 4: 193–210.

Grunwell P, Harding A (1995) PACS TOYS: a Screening Assessment of Phonological Development. Windsor: NFER-Nelson.

Hahn E (1989) Directed home training programme for infants with cleft lip and palate. In: Bzoch KR (ed.) Communicative Disorders Related to Cleft Lip and Palate, 2nd edn. Boston, MA: Little Brown.

Hall D, Hill P (1986) When does secretory otitis media affect language development? Archives of Disease in Childhood 61: 42–47.

Harding A (1993) Speech development related to timing of cleft palate repair. Unpublished PhD Thesis, De Montfort University.

Harding A, Bryan A (1998) Facilitating phonological awareness through input-modelling. Paper presented at Royal College of Speech and Language Therapists conference, Liverpool.

Harding A, Grunwell P (1993) Relationship between speech and timing of hard palate repair. In: Grunwell P (ed.) Analysing Cleft Palate Speech. London: Whurr, pp. 48–82.

Harding A, Grunwell P (1996) Characteristics of cleft palate speech. European Journal of Disorders of Communication 31: 331–357.

Harding A, Grunwell P (1998) Active versus passive cleft-type speech characteristics. International Journal of Disorders of Communication and Language 33: 329–352.

Heller J (1979) Hearing loss in patients with cleft palate. In: Bzoch KR (ed.) Communicative Disorders Related to Cleft Lip and Palate. Boston, MA: Little Brown.

Henningsson G (1989) Cleft palate babbling related to time of palate repair. In: Kriens O (ed.) What is a Cleft Lip and Palate? Proceedings of an Advanced Workshop, Bremen, 1987. New York: Thieme.

Hoch L, Golding-Kushner K, Siegel-Sadewitz VL, Shprintzen RJ (1986) Speech therapy. In: McWilliams BJ (ed.) Seminars in Speech and Language: Current Methods of Assessing and Treating Children with Cleft Palates. New York: Thieme.

Ingram D (1976) Phonological Disability in Children. London: Edward Arnold.

Ingram D (1989) Phonological Disability in Children, 2nd edn. London: Whurr.

Kent RD (1992) The biology of phonological development. In: Ferguson CA, Menn L, Stoel-Gammon C (eds) Phonological Development, Models, Research, Implications. Maryland: York Press.

Leblanc EM (1996) Fundamental principles in the speech management of cleft lip and palate. In: Berkowitz S (ed.) An Introduction to Craniofacial Anomalies, Vol. II. Cleft Lip and Palate: Perspectives in Management. San Diego: Singular Publishing.

Lencione RM (1980) Associated conditions. In: Edwards M, Watson A (eds) Advances in the Management of Cleft Palate. Edinburgh: Churchill Livingstone.

Locke JL (1983) Phonological Acquisition and Change. New York: Academic Press.

Lynch JL, Fox DR, Brookshire BL (1983) Phonological proficiency of two cleft palate toddlers with school-age follow-up. Journal of Speech and Hearing Disorders 48: 274–285.

Maw AR (1986) Ear disease. In: Albery EH, Hathorn I, Pigott R. Cleft Lip and Palate: A Team Approach. Bristol: Wright & Sons.

McWilliams BJ, Morris HL, Shelton RL (1990) Cleft Palate Speech, 2nd edn. Philadelphia: BC Decker.

Moss ML (1969) The primary role of functional matrices in facial growth. American Journal of Orthodontics 55: 566–577.

Mousset MR, Trichet C (1985) Babbling and phonetic acquisitions after early complete surgical repair of cleft lip and palate. Paper presented at the Fifth International Congress on Cleft Palate and Related Craniofacial Anomalies, Monte Carlo.

Neiman GS, Savage HE (1997) Development of infants and toddlers from birth to three years of age. Cleft Palate–Craniofacial Journal 34: 218–225.

Nuffield Dyspraxia Programme (1985, revised 1992) Nuffield Hearing and Speech Centre, Royal National Throat Nose and Ear Hospital, London.

Oblak P, Kozelj V (1984) Basic principles in the treatment of cleft at the University Clinic for Maxillofacial Surgery in Lubljana and their evolution in 30 years. In: Hotz M, Gnoinski WM, Perko MA, Nussbaumer H, Hof E (eds) Early Treatment of Cleft Lip and Palate. Proceedings of the Third International Symposium. Zurich: Hans Huber.

O'Gara MM, Logemann JA (1988) Phonetic analysis of the development of babies with cleft palate. Cleft Palate Journal 25: 122–134.

Oller DK, Wieman LA, Doyle W, Ross C (1975) Infant babbling and speech. Journal of Child Language 3: 1–11.

Riski JE, Delong E (1984) Articulation development in children with cleft lip/palate. Cleft Palate Journal 21: 57–64.

Russell VJ (1989) Early Intervention. In: Stengelhofen J (ed.) Cleft Palate: The Nature and Remediation of Communication Problems. Edinburgh: Churchill Livingstone.

Russell VJ (1991) Speech development in children with cleft lip and palate. Unpublished PhD thesis, Leicester Polytechnic.

Russell J (1997) The timing of consonant articulation therapy in relation to velopharyngeal surgery. Paper presented at The Craniofacial Society of Great Britain annual scientific conference, Writtle, Essex.

Russell J, Grunwell P (1993) Speech development in children with cleft lip and palate. In: Grunwell P (ed.) Analysing Cleft Palate Speech. London: Whurr, pp. 19–47.

Russell J, Sell D (1998) The GOS–CLAPA therapy project. Paper presented at The Craniofacial Society of Great Britain annual scientific conference, Oxford.

Scherer NJ, D'Antonio LL (1995) Parent questionnaire for screening early language development in children with cleft palate. Cleft Palate–Craniofacial Journal 32: 7–13.

Sell D, Harding A, Grunwell P (1994) A screening assessment of cleft palate speech (Great Ormond Street Speech Assessment). European Journal of Disorders of Communication 29: 1–15.

Sell D, Harding A, Grunwell P, Razzell R, Harland K (1996) Picture stimuli for revised GOS.SP.ASS. C.A.P.S. Sentences. Thameside Community Healthcare NHS Trust.

Sell D, Harding A, Grunwell P (1999) GOS.SP.ASS.'98: An assessment for speech disorders associated with cleft palate and/or velopharyngeal dysfunction (revised). European Journal of Disorders of Communication 34: 17–33.

Stoel-Gammon C (1992) Prelinguistic vocal development. In: Ferguson CA, Menn L, Stoel-Gammon C (eds) Phonological Development, Models, Research, Implications. Maryland: York Press.

Trost-Cardamone JE (1990) Speech: anatomy, physiology and pathology. In: Kernahan DA, Rosenstein SN (eds) Cleft Lip and Palate: A System of Management. Baltimore, MD: Williams & Wilkins, pp. 91–103.

Whetmore RF (1992) Importance of maintaining normal nasal function in the cleft palate patient. Cleft Palate–Craniofacial Journal 21: 263–269.

Wyatt R, Sell D, Russell J, Harding A, Harland K, Albery E (1996) Cleft palate speech dissected: a review of current knowledge and analysis. British Journal of Plastic Surgery 49: 143–149.

CHAPTER 15

Hearing and ENT Management

P. LENNOX

Introduction

The association between cleft palate and ear disease is well established and was first recognized over 100 years ago in a report of a seven-year-old child with discharge from the ear and hearing impairment which resolved after closure of the cleft palate (Alt, 1878). This chapter will look at the structure and function of the Eustachian tube and middle ear and how they are altered by the presence of a cleft palate. It will then describe the common pathological conditions affecting the middle ear and review their management.

Anatomy and physiology

The middle ear is a gas-filled cavity which is bounded laterally by the tympanic membrane and medially by the inner ear. Within it are a number of structures including the ossicular chain, the horizontal portion of the facial nerve, and anteriorly the opening of the Eustachian tube (Figure 15.1). It is in continuity with the mastoid air cell system posteriorly via the attic and aditus.

At the point where the Eustachian tube opens into the middle ear it is a bony canal. Passing medially and inferiorly this narrows down to an isthmus, which has an internal diameter of about 1 mm and a length of about 2 mm. The medial portion is formed by a plate of cartilage forming the roof and posteromedial wall and is completed by a mucosal and muscle sheet. This muscle consists of the tensor palati muscle, which arises from the scaphoid fossa and greater wing of the spheroid bone and the cartilaginous roof of the Eustachian tube. It converges into a short tendon which passes medially around the hook of the hamulus and spreads out within the soft palate. The levator palati muscle contains some fibres that originate from the inferior surface of the cartilaginous Eustachian tube.

The gas in the middle ear is derived from air which enters it from the nasopharynx through the Eustachian tube. Two of its constituents, namely carbon dioxide and oxygen, constantly diffuse across the mucosal barrier down a pressure gradient into the venous blood draining the middle ear. There is therefore a constant tendency for middle ear pressure to be negative unless a periodic supply of air is available through the Eustachian tube. The medial collapsible segment of the Eustachian tube can be considered as a bellows. This is opened when the tensor palati contracts on swallowing or yawning, allowing air to flow down a pressure gradient from the nasopharynx into the newly created volume of the Eustachian tube. Passage of air through the isthmus may well require more than passive diffusion as the pressure difference between the middle ear and the nasopharynx may be no more than 1-2 mm water. It may occur as the collapsible portion of the tube returns to its normal state assisted by the levator palati muscle. As well as ventilating the middle ear the Eustachian tube is also responsible for clearing inflammatory exudate from the middle ear via a mucociliary clearance system.

Effect of a cleft palate on the Eustachian tube

Failure of the Eustachian tube to ventilate the middle ear adequately and clear mucus results in a middle ear effusion. Eustachian tube dysfunction and middle ear effusions are almost universal in infants with cleft palate (Paradise et al., 1969). Histopathological studies of temporal bones of children with cleft palate have identified a number of anatomical abnormalities of the Eustachian tube. The tube is shorter than in age-matched children under the age of six years (Siegel at al., 1988). Abnormal insertion of the tensor palati muscle into the tubal cartilage has been demonstrated (Matsune et al., 1991a). The lateral lamina of the cartilage is deficient and the lumen is poorly developed (Matsune et al., 1991b). None of these studies have shown any evidence of anatomical obstruction of the tube, suggesting that the Eustachian tube dysfunction associated with cleft palate is functional. This is supported by radiographic and manometric Eustachian tube function tests. It is possible to measure middle ear pressure with a ventilation tube *in situ*. The opening and closing pressure of the Eustachian tube can then be measured as middle ear pressure is raised or lowered, and the effect of swallowing noted. Infants with cleft palates have variable degrees of difficulty equilibrating increased middle ear pressure and are unable to correct negative pressure by swallowing (Doyle et al., 1980). It is also possible to measure the effect of swallowing on the resistance of the Eustachian tube. The resistance of the tube increases with swallowing, suggesting a tubal constriction rather than dilation (Doyle et al., 1980).

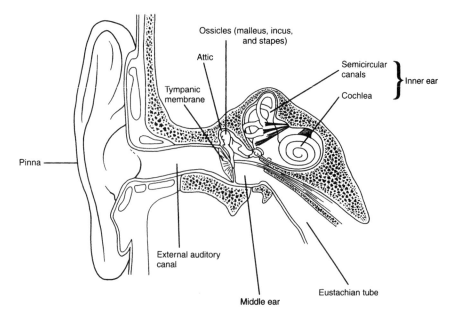

Figure 15.1. Coronal section through a right ear.

Contrast studies have shown that liquid media will flow from the middle ear into the nasopharynx, but not in the opposite direction, also implying a functional rather than a mechanical obstruction of the tube (Bluestone et al., 1972a).

Otitis media with effusion

Otitis media with effusion (OME) has a number of synonyms. Commonly known as glue ear, it is also referred to as middle ear effusion, chronic secretory otitis media or non-suppurative otitis media. It can be defined as a prolonged effusion in the middle ear space which is either serous or mucoid, but not frankly purulent. This needs to be distinguished from an acute effusion, which commonly develops after an upper respiratory tract infection and resolves spontaneously within three months.

The incidence of OME in young children with cleft palate is high. Prospective trials in which myringotomy has been undertaken routinely at the same time as cleft repair demonstrate an incidence of 92% in children between two and 20 months old (Grant et al., 1988; Robinson et al., 1992). This compares with a prevalence of 20% at age two years in children without a cleft palate (Zielhuis et al., 1990). Eustachian tube function improves in older children with cleft palates and from the age of six years there is likely to be resolution of the OME (Moller, 1981). The presence of fluid in the middle ear results in a conductive hearing loss. The hearing impairment is variable and unpredictable. It may be as little as 10 dB (decibels) or as much as 40 dB, in which case the child will be missing quiet conversation and may experience difficulty with consonant discrimination. The hearing loss may not be noticed but may present instead as speech and language difficulties, behavioural or educational problems.

Acute otitis media

Acute otitis media is an episode of inflammation of the middle ear associated with pain, fever, hearing loss and sometimes discharge. The latter follows perforation of the tense bulging tympanic membrane with release of pus (acute suppurative otitis media). This usually heals with resolution of the infection. Over 50% of children with cleft palate have recurrent episodes of acute suppurative otitis media (Van Cauwenberge et al., 1998).

Tympanic membrane abnormalities

Both otitis media with effusion and acute otitis media can predispose to damage to the tympanic membrane and chronic ear disease. A ruptured tympanic membrane may not heal, resulting in a persisting perforation. Even when it does heal it may be atrophic with loss of its fibrous middle layer or with formation of scar tissue (tympanosclerosis). A floppy atrophic tympanic membrane may become retracted into the middle ear, particularly if there is negative middle ear pressure secondary to persisting Eustachian tube dysfunction. Pockets can form which, if deep enough, may accumulate keratin (cholesteatoma).

Perforations

The tympanic membrane can be divided into the pars flaccida and pars tensa (Figure 15.2). It is usually part of the central pars tensa that ruptures during an episode of acute otitis media with subsequent healing. However, if healing fails to occur due to persistent infection, poor blood supply or necrosis, the perforation may persist. This central perforation can vary in size but the fibrous annulus remains intact (Figure 15.3). Although this may result in recurrent episodes of infection with discharge of pus through the perforation (active chronic suppurative otitis media), it is regarded as safe as it is not associated with the accumulation of keratin (see below). A perforation in the pars flaccida, however, is associated with cholesteatoma and is therefore regarded as being unsafe. The degree of hearing loss resulting from the presence of a perforation depends on the size and site of the defect. For example, a small anterior inferior central perforation may produce no more than a 10 dB hearing loss whereas a subtotal perforation may result in a 40 dB hearing loss, or more, if there is associated damage to the ossicular chain.

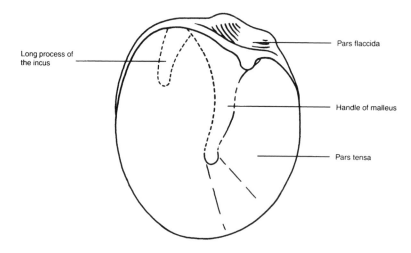

Figure 15.2. Diagram of a right tympanic membrane.

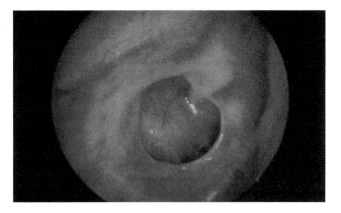

Figure 15.3. A central perforation in the right ear with a rim of normal tympanic membrane surrounding the defect. (Reproduced with permission of Professor A. Wright, University College London.)

Cholesteatoma

Cholesteatoma is the presence of skin (keratin) in the middle ear cleft. It appears as a cyst-like structure containing pale keratinous debris. The most useful classification relates to its anatomical site. Pars flaccida cholesteatoma, or attic cholesteatoma (Figure 15.4), results from a perforation or retraction

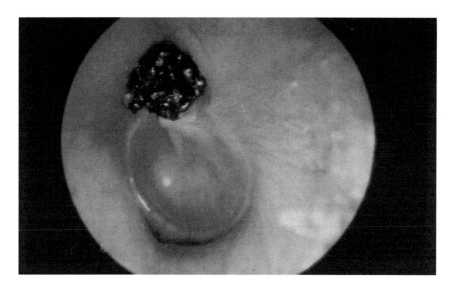

Figure 15.4. Attic cholesteatoma in the left ear. (Reproduced with permission of Professor A. Wright, University College London.)

pocket in the pars flaccida and is associated with destruction of the outer attic wall and at a later stage erosion of the ossicular chain with associated conductive deafness. Cholesteatoma can occur in the pars tensa but results from a marginal, or unsafe, perforation or retraction pocket in the posterosuperior quadrant of the pars tensa. The resultant conductive deafness is due to destruction of the incudostapedial joint. If left untreated cholesteatoma will expand beyond the confines of the middle ear and mastoid air cell system, damaging other structures in the temporal bone. Facial nerve paralysis may occur, usually associated with the presence of granulation tissue and erosion of the facial nerve canal in the wall of the middle ear. Erosion of the lateral semicircular canal occurs, resulting in episodic vertigo and an increased risk of suppurative labyrinthitis. Involvement of the cochlea will produce a sensorineural hearing loss. Intracranial complications can arise due to erosion through the skull base into the middle or posterior cranial fossa creating a pathological route for the spread of infection; extradural abscess, subdural abscess, brain abscess and meningitis can all occur.

Syndromes

The association of cleft palate and middle ear pathology results in a conductive hearing loss. However, patients whose clefts form part of a recognized syndrome may have other types of hearing loss as well. Congenital conductive hearing loss can occur associated with atresia of the external and middle ear and/or ossicular anomalies, e.g. oto-palato-digital syndrome. Syndromes such as that described by Stickler manifest both conductive and sensorineural hearing loss. Patients with Goldenhar syndrome or hemifacial microsomia may sometimes have sensorineural hearing loss (see Lees, Chapter 6).

Effect of palatal surgery

The trend towards early palate repair has increased interest in its effect on Eustachian tube function. If Eustachian tube function could be improved by early palate repair, then the need for active intervention in the middle ear would be less. Certainly, contrast studies of the Eustachian tube have suggested that there is less functional obstruction of the tube after cleft repair (Bluestone et al., 1972b). Doyle et al. (1986) studied a group of 24 children (37 ears) before and after palatal repair, recording active and passive Eustachian tube function. All the children underwent ventilation tube insertion between three and six months of age irrespective of middle ear status and subsequently underwent palate repair between 14 and 18 months of age. They found that passive tubal function improved after palatal repair, postulating that this is due to the realignment of the levator palati muscle. Results for active tubal function were less convincing. A longitudinal study of the effect of early (under three years of age) versus late repair in Sri Lanka has shown a small, but statistically significant, improvement in otitis media with effusion with early repair (Mr D.M. Albert, personal communication).

ENT management

It has been recommended that all cleft palate teams should include an ENT surgeon. Their role is to diagnose and treat otitis media with effusion as well as excluding other types of hearing loss and other ENT problems. The severity and nature of any hearing loss needs to be established; in particular, the presence of a fluctuating hearing loss must not be overlooked. It is important to be familiar with the developmental milestones associated with normal hearing:

- By four months of age an infant becomes still and smiles in response to a parent's voice, even if the source is outside the visual field.
- By six months of age the infant can localize sound and will turn his head to the source of the sound. This forms the basis of distraction testing (see below).
- By nine months the child should be babbling and beginning to copy sounds; understanding of single words such as 'no' develops, and situational understanding.
- By one year double syllable babble such as 'dada' should be recognizable and some children will be attempting to say a few words.

- By 18 months many children can identify parts of the body, and name common objects.
- By the age of two the child can produce two word sentences and has a steadily increasing vocabulary.

Hearing loss of any cause can lead to delay in these milestones and is likely to contribute to the articulatory problems/language delay associated with a cleft palate (see Russell and Harding, Chapter 14). The specialist speech and language therapist will also be routinely reviewing these children, and will refer the infant to the ENT surgeon if concerned about hearing (see Sell and Grunwell, Chapter 16).

At the first consultation it is necessary to establish whether there are any predisposing factors for congenital hearing loss such as complications during pregnancy, a family history of hearing loss, birth asphyxia or hyperbilirubinaemia. It is also important to establish if there is a history of recurrent acute otitis media. This can present as an unexplained temperature, earache or discharge from the ear and there may be a history of repeated courses of antibiotics. A history of persistent smelly discharge from the ear should raise the suspicion of the presence of a cholesteatoma.

The presence of nasal obstruction with rhinorrhoea, sneezing and a family history of allergy is highly suggestive of the presence of allergic rhinitis. This is important to treat as it can also result in Eustachian tube dysfunction and otitis media with effusion. A history of unilateral nasal obstruction is often associated with deviated nasal septum in the cleft condition. It may, however, indicate the presence of atresia of one of the posterior choanae where the nose opens into the nasopharynx; this can be corrected surgically. Treatment may also be required for snoring and obstructive sleep apnoea. This is usually due to adenotonsillar hypertrophy. In non-cleft children, this is normally treated by adenotonsillectomy, but removal of the adenoids from a child with a repaired cleft palate may precipitate velopharyngeal dysfunction (see Mercer and Pigott, Chapter 17). It is essential, therefore, that these children undergo sleep studies to determine the severity of the airway obstruction and a decision to proceed is made in collaboration with the specialist speech and language therapist. If necessary, a limited removal of adenoid tissue can correct symptoms without compromising speech, but this should only be done by a surgeon experienced in the care of clefts.

Examination

Ear

This should include examination of the external ear for abnormalities often associated with a congenital syndromic hearing loss. The appearance of the tympanic membrane in otitis media with effusion is usually dull with increased vascularity of the handle of malleus (Figure 15.5). If the middle ear fluid is serous then it appears a golden colour. The drum may bulge or be retracted, with apparent shortening of the handle of malleus as the tip is pulled medially. A bulging erythematous drum indicates acute otitis media. If the drum is severely retracted, the incudostapedial joint appears more prominent and in more severe cases the drum appears to be draped over it. Retraction pockets and perforations need to be identified and their size and location noted. Finally, it is always important not to miss a cholesteatoma. This may not be obvious, appearing as an insignificant trail of keratin emerging from a retraction pocket or hidden behind an apparently harmless crust. The use of the outpatient microscope can be invaluable in these situations, although in the younger child it may be necessary to perform an examination under anaesthetic if there is a high index of suspicion.

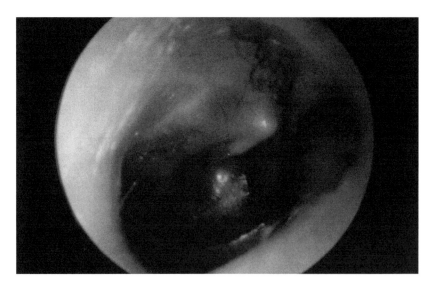

Figure 15.5. Otitis media with effusion in the right ear. The tympanic membrane appears dull due to the fluid behind it. (Reproduced with permission of Professor A. Wright, University College London.)

Nose

The palate forms the floor of the nose, which may therefore be involved in the cleft. Anterior rhinoscopy using a light, head-mirror and speculum to open the anterior nares allows visualization of the anterior nasal airway. Pale enlarged inferior turbinates indicate allergic rhinitis. Mucopus is present if the rhinitis is infective. The nasal airway can be roughly assessed by the size of the misting pattern on a mirror and in the older cooperative child it is possible to see enlarged adenoids with the head-mirror or flexible nasendoscope.

Investigations

Audiometry

Confirmation of the clinical diagnosis of glue ear can be made using tympanometry. This measures the compliance of the tympanic membrane as a function of mechanically varied air pressure in the external auditory canal. A graph of compliance versus air pressure is produced. Compliance of the tympanic membrane is maximal when the air pressure is equal on both sides of the tympanic membrane and appears as a peak on the graph. In normal ears this will be at atmospheric pressure. Negative middle ear pressure will shift the peak to the left. The presence of fluid in the middle ear produces a straight line.

The approach adopted to assess a child's hearing will depend on the developmental stage of that child. The involvement of an experienced paediatric audiologist is essential. Under the age of six months behavioural tests are not possible. A number of objective tests are available, although all have some limitations. Otoacoustic emissions (OAE) are useful to confirm the presence of normal cochlear (inner ear) function in the presence of normal middle ear function. Their absence does not indicate the type or severity of hearing loss, but is an indication for further testing and regular review. It is possible to obtain a hearing threshold with brainstem electrical tests carried out while a baby is asleep, but only in the higher (3–6 kHz) frequencies. The combination of absent OAE, normal middle ear function and a negative response with electrical tests suggests that the child may have a significant sensorineural hearing loss requiring some form of amplification and the involvement of the community services for hearing impaired children. By seven months head control is sufficient for distraction tests or visual reinforcement audiometry to be performed. Performance testing can be used by the developmental age of two and a half when the child is taught to perform a simple action such as dropping a brick into a box in response to a sound stimulus, either presented in the free field or through headphones. Standard pure tone audiometry using headphones is usually possible by the age of four.

Other investigations

These can include lateral X-rays of the nasopharynx to assess the size of the adenoids and degree of airway obstruction, as well as skin tests for perennial and seasonal allergy.

Management of OME

OME can be treated in both the cleft and non-cleft population by insertion of ventilation tubes. This requires a general anaesthetic, and, if the child is otherwise fit and well, is done as a day case procedure. A small hole or myringotomy is made in the anterior inferior quadrant of the tympanic membrane. Middle ear fluid may be cleared using suction and a ventilation tube is inserted into the tympanic membrane. This will ventilate the middle ear, preventing further effusion and giving time for the Eustachian tube function to recover. The commonest ventilation tubes are Shepherd or Shah grommets (Figure 15.6). These remain *in situ* for an average of nine months or one year respectively, and are then extruded by the tympanic membrane, which usually heals spontaneously. Infection, with discharge of pus through the grommet, may occur postoperatively. In the non-cleft population insertion of grommets has been shown to reduce the overall time that OME is present, although this is less marked in children under the age of two and a half (Maw and Bawden, 1993). There is a corresponding immediate improvement in the hearing. However, once the grommet extrudes this is not maintained fully and long-term hearing results are less satisfactory. It is possible to insert a more permanent ventilation tube; Goode T tubes or Permavent tubes are examples. However, these carry an increased risk of a persistent perforation and are generally reserved for the child who has required at least three grommet insertions. The alternative to surgical intervention is amplification using hearing aids, but this needs to be undertaken by an experienced paediatric audiologist with close liaison with the community services for hearing impaired children.

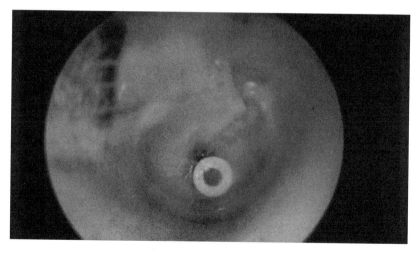

Figure 15.6. A Shah grommet inserted into the right tympanic membrane. (Reproduced with permission of Professor A. Wright, University College London.)

There are two approaches to the insertion of ventilation tubes in the cleft palate population. In many centres all children undergoing palate repair undergo myringotomy at the same time. As OME is almost universally present in these children insertion of grommets is advocated (Dhillon, 1988). As palate repair is usually carried out at around the age of six months this provides optimal hearing at a time when speech patterns are being recognized and imitated. A study of 24 matched pairs of children with repaired palates, in which one group underwent insertion of ventilation tubes at an average age of three months and the other at 30.8 months or not at all, suggests that early insertion of ventilation tubes results in marginally better hearing (Hubbard et al., 1985). However, the correlation was not statistically significant. Consonant articulation was better in this group, but comprehension, language and psychosocial development were not affected. In this study both groups had evidence of damage to the tympanic membrane, namely sclerosis or atrophy of the drum. Overall, children who have grommets inserted at an early stage often undergo more procedures than those who have grommets inserted at a later stage.

Despite the presence of OME, early grommet insertion may not be necessary. The degree of hearing loss is variable and may not justify insertion of grommets, particularly as spontaneous resolution with improvement in hearing is likely to occur from the age of six years (Moller, 1981). Some surgeons therefore prefer to 'watch and wait'. Insertion of grommets is indicated if there is a persistent conductive hearing loss of greater than 45 dB on distraction testing or greater than 35 dB on pure tone audiometry. In addition, surgeons will intervene if there is concern about the child's speech and language development, if the child is experiencing recurrent episodes of acute otitis media or there are concerns about irreversible damage to the tympanic membrane. Proponents of this approach argue that there is evidence that repeated insertion of ventilation tubes causes more otological damage than the middle ear effusion itself (Robson et al., 1992). Moreover these researchers were unable to demonstrate any improvement in speech development, and auditory thresholds were worse, in those children who underwent ventilation tube insertion.

Studies used to support either approach are now flawed in that the techniques of palatal repair are constantly evolving and it is now common to repair the palate at a much earlier age. Whichever approach is taken, it is important that every child with a cleft palate undergoes regular ENT review. Ideally this should be as part of a multidisciplinary cleft palate team. However, the frequency of ENT review, often six-monthly or even three-monthly, may be more than is required by the rest of the team and the child will therefore need to attend the ENT outpatients and paediatric audiology clinics as well.

Management of late sequelae

One of the indications for grommet insertion is to try to prevent the development of the late complications of chronic Eustachian tube dysfunction and otitis media with effusion. There are little recent data available on the true incidence of these complications in the cleft palate population, as most children will have had grommets inserted at some stage. In a study of 113 patients in Norway only 3% of ears were found to have persistent perforations and cholesteatoma was found in only 1% (Moller, 1975).

Repair of a safe (central) perforation can prevent recurrent discharge and may improve a conductive hearing loss. It is important to be sure that the Eustachian tube function of the ear is optimal before proceeding and even in the non-cleft population most surgeons will delay closure until the child is at least ten. A graft, taken from the patient through the same incision (temporalis fascia), is used to 'close' the hole allowing the tympanic membrane to heal across, repairing the defect. Cholesteatoma requires surgical exploration of the middle ear and the mastoid air cell system. This is termed a mastoidectomy and the surgery itself is associated with a small risk of sensorineural hearing loss, vertigo and facial nerve weakness.

Conclusion

The presence of a cleft palate results in a high incidence of OME in young children. This can cause a significant hearing loss, compromising speech and language development, and there is also a risk of irreversible damage to the middle ear. The management of these children therefore requires a multidisciplinary approach with the involvement of an ENT surgeon, paediatric audiologist, specialist speech and language therapist and close liaison with the community health services. OME in any child can be treated by grommet insertion. There remains some debate, however, about the indication and timing of grommet insertion in children with cleft palate. Further research is needed to establish whether earlier palate repair will improve Eustachian tube function sufficiently to reduce the need for grommet insertion in these children.

References

Alt A (1878) Ein Fall von gespattenem Gaumen mit acquirinter Taubstummheit Sta phyloraphie. Heilung. Archiv für Angenheilkunde 7: 211–215.

Bluestone CD, Wittel RA, Paradise JL (1972a) Roentgenographic evaluation of Eustachian tube function in infants with cleft and normal palates. Cleft Palate Journal 9: 93–100.

Bluestone CD, Paradise JL, Beery QC (1972b) Certain effects of cleft palate repair on Eustachian tube function. Cleft Palate Journal 9: 183–193.

Dhillon RS (1988) The middle ear in cleft palate children pre and post closure. Journal of the Royal Society of Medicine 81: 710–730.

Doyle WJ, Cantekin EI, Bluestone CD (1980) Eustachian tube function in cleft palate children. Annals of Otology, Rhinology and Laryngology 89: 34–39.

Doyle WJ, Reilly JS, Jardini L, Rovnak S (1986) Effect of palatoplasty on the function of the Eustachian tube in children with cleft palate. Cleft Palate Journal 23: 63–68.

Grant HR, Quiney RE, Mercer DM, Lodge S (1988) Cleft palate and glue ear. Archives of Disease in Childhood 63: 176–179.

Hubbard TW, Paradise JL, McWilliams BJ, Elster BA, Taylor FH (1985) Consequences of unremitting middle ear disease in early life. Otologic, audiologic and developmental findings in children with cleft palate. New England Journal of Medicine 312: 1529–1534.

Matsune S, Sando I, Takahashi H (1991a) Insertion of the tensor veli palatini muscle into the Eustachian tube cartilage in cleft palate cases. Annals of Otology, Rhinology and Laryngology 100: 439–446.

Matsune S, Sando I, Takahashi H (1991b) Abnormalities of lateral cartilaginous lamina and lumen of the Eustachian tube in cases of cleft palate. Annals of Otology, Rhinology and Laryngology 100: 909–913.

Maw R, Bawden R (1993) Spontaneous resolution of severe chronic glue ear in children and the effect of adenoidectomy, tonsillectomy, and insertion of ventilation tubes (grommets). British Medical Journal 306: 756–760.

Moller P (1975) Long term otologic features of cleft palate patients. Archives of Otolaryngology 101: 605–607.

Moller P (1981) Hearing, middle ear pressure and otopathology in a cleft palate population. Acta Otolaryngologica 92: 521–528.

Paradise JL, Bluestone CD, Felder H (1969) The universality of otitis media in 50 infants with cleft palate. Paediatrics 44: 35–42.

Robinson PJ, Lodge S, Jones BM, Walker CC, Grant HR (1992) The effect of palate repair on otitis media with effusion. Plastic and Reconstructive Surgery 89: 640–645.

Robson AK, Blanchard JD, Jones K, Albery EH, Smith IM, Maw AR (1992) A conservative approach to the management of otitis media with effusion in cleft palate children. Journal of Laryngology and Otology 106: 788–792.

Siegel MI, Sadler Kimes D, Todhunter SS (1988) Eustachian tube cartilage shape as a factor in epidemiology of otitis media. Proceedings of the 4th International Symposium. In: Lim DJ, Bluestone CD, Klein JO, Nelson JD (eds) Recent Advances in Otitis Media. Burlington, Ontario: BC Decker, pp. 114–117.

Van Cauwenberge PB, De Moor SEG, Dhooge I (1998) Acute suppurative otitis media. In: Ludman H, Wright T (eds) Diseases of the Ear, 6th edn. London: Arnold.

Zielhuis GH, Rach GH, Van Den Bosch AV, Van Den Broek P (1990) The prevalence of otitis media with effusion: a critical review of the literature. Clinical Otolaryngology 15: 283–288.

PART III
MANAGEMENT OF THE OLDER
CHILD, ADOLESCENT AND ADULT

CHAPTER 16

Speech Assessment and Therapy

D.A. SELL AND P. GRUNWELL

Introduction

The speech and language therapist is responsible for the screening, identification, assessment, interpretation, differential diagnosis leading to differential management, rehabilitation and prevention of communication problems associated with cleft lip and/or palate or other craniofacial problems as well as teaching and clinical research (Witzel, 1993). In particular, the therapist helps determine the relationship of structure to speech, whether the structure needs to be modified (usually through surgery but sometimes with prosthetics), the need for and timing of speech and/or language intervention, and the planning and undertaking of therapy.

This chapter focuses on the perceptual speech assessment in the older child, a brief consideration of some instrumental approaches to the measurement of speech, and a discussion regarding therapeutic management. This will be followed by a discussion of selected issues including the use of prosthetics in the management of velopharyngeal dysfunction, the timing of surgery/therapy/orthodontics and the older patient.

Perceptual speech assessment

Perceptual speech evaluation is at the centre of assessment. Although perceptual assessment has its limitations, Folkins and Moon (1991) stress that neither nasalance nor airflow measures in speech provide a good substitute for perceptual measures. The final decision as to whether an individual has nasality problems or not is still based on the listener's subjective judgement (Morley, 1970; McWilliams et al., 1990; Sweeney et al., 1996).

A fundamental problem for speech and language therapy has been the lack of an acceptable framework for measuring speech. Scheuerle (1993) argues how methods by which speech was judged were neither uniform nor comparable due to the variability of components evaluated and procedures applied to the evaluation process. Furthermore, there have been different emphases to different approaches to assessment. For example, the McWilliams and Phillips (1979) scale was designed to make an inference about velopharyngeal function. In contrast the Eurocleft Speech Group (1991, 1993, 2000) developed an assessment procedure that provided a detailed analysis of the phonetic and phonological characteristics of speech.

The potential speech problems consequent on the cleft palate condition can be predicted, and therefore routine speech assessment procedures should be adopted (Grunwell et al., 1993, and see Russell and Harding, Chapter 14). Dalston et al. (1988) proposed that as a minimum the following parameters of speech should always be reported: nasality (hypernasality and hyponasality), nasal air escape/emission, intelligibility and articulation. The assessment framework must also include nasal turbulence, nasal grimace, phonation (McWilliams et al., 1990; Sell et al., 1994, 1999) and the visual appearance of speech (Witzel, 1991). Grunwell et al. (1993) emphasize that the framework should be able to analyse all the parameters independently and yet acknowledge their interaction. McComb (1989) recommended that a standardized speech assessment should be developed at least on a national, and preferably, international basis, in order that inter-centre comparisons can be made. The Eurocleft Speech Group (1991, 1993) developed a framework that has potential as a cross-linguistic method of assessment of cleft palate speakers when used by trained listeners. Others have proposed frameworks for use internationally but to date there remains a lack of consensus (Henningsson and Hutters, 1997; Hirschberg and Van Demark, 1997).

Historical perspectives on perceptual speech assessment

The main procedures that speech and language therapists have used to measure speech are judgements of the overall rating of articulatory ability, a quantitative approach detailing the correct number of responses, the articulation test and intelligibility ratings (McWilliams et al., 1990).

Ratings of articulatory ability

There is some evidence (Moll, 1968; Van Demark, 1974) to support the validity of ratings of articulation, such as the global rating scale with weighted values for speech symptoms developed by McWilliams and Phillips in 1979. The different speech parameters of nasal emission, facial grimace, nasal resonance, phonation and articulation performance are assessed and scored using weighted scores. A weighted score in excess of seven is interpreted as indicative of velopharyngeal dysfunction. It could be argued, however, that some of the characteristics may occur in the absence of velopharyngeal dysfunction, which casts some doubt on its overall validity. Furthermore, a rating scale does not provide information on patterns of misarticulation, and does not show how improvement occurs or its detail.

Correct number of responses

Another approach to analysis has been to compare the number of correct responses with normative data or the performance of a control group on the same test. This method provides information about the severity of the speech problem, but again gives no indication about the nature or pattern of errors, or the nature of the speech disorder. This type of assessment does not help to make decisions regarding speech therapy or surgery. In addition, averaged group results may be skewed by extreme individual results.

Articulation test

In an attempt to describe the pattern of sounds, and regularities in types of errors, articulation tests were designed to assess the speech of children with cleft palate, such as the Iowa Pressure Articulation Test (Morris et al., 1961) and the Bzoch Error Pattern Diagnostic Articulation Test (Bzoch, 1979). Each requires single word elicitation and a traditional type of error analysis based on the categories of distortion, substitution and omission. The Bzoch Error Pattern Test describes five categories of articulation error types on a continuum, from least severe to most severe: nasal emission, distortion, substitution, and gross substitution to omission. This approach does not require the examiner to transcribe responses phonetically. Such procedures examine single naming responses, in which the listener is usually interested in the consonant targets only.

This traditional framework of analysis has serious disadvantages. Grunwell (1987) pointed out the lack of information regarding the nature of a misarticulation using this approach. The types of articulation errors are ill-defined and potentially overlapping. A higher level of phonetic detail is required than the classification of an error simply as an oral or nasal distortion. To facilitate the understanding and interpretation of the nature of cleft palate speech, the types of oral and nasal distortions need to be identified.

A major difficulty of the traditional framework has been the inter-assessor reliability of examiners deciding the exact nature of an error. The same standards have not always been used for making articulatory judgements (Morris, 1979). McWilliams (1958) commented on how difficult it was to measure the degree of distortion. In contrast, Van Demark (1971) maintained that a distortion could be graded on a continuum of mild to severe, but this framework was not taken up by other researchers. Philips and Bzoch (1969) demonstrated insufficient inter-judge reliability of ten experienced speech pathologists when identifying type of error. They concluded that a satisfactory level of reliability was only achieved in calculations of the mean or averaged articulation scores. The Eurocleft study (1993) also reported similar difficulties of inter-judge reliability in the identification of error type, and in this research study a consensus approach to listening was adopted.

When the speech data for assessment are single word picture naming responses, the data obtained may not be typical of an individual's speech patterns. The degree to which such a sample is representative of conversational speech has been questioned (Shriberg and Kwiatkowski, 1982; Grunwell, 1985, 1987; Grunwell et al., 1993). There are additionally other problems with such an assessment technique. The target sounds (usually consonants) are only elicited once. The possibility that the same target may be produced differently in different contexts or that there may be developmental variability cannot be detected. This was recognized by McWilliams (1958), who urged that a sound be sampled more than once in a test. Furthermore, by recording errors on individual targets the presence of phonetic or phonological patterns cannot be appreciated, with the result that there is a dearth of information on the extent and nature of deviance and delay in the sound system.

Intelligibility ratings

It is well recognized that intelligibility is influenced by many variables other than the speech characteristics being assessed. For example, phoneme content, stress, accent, intonation and rate are all speaker variables influencing intelligibility. Listeners vary in their ability to resolve the ambiguities heard: this depends, for example, on how well the listener knows the speaker as well as his/her experience of speech disorders. External factors such as context, the message content, and background noise may also play a part. The difficulties of rater reliability and validity in this area are so great that Witzel (1991) stated that intelligibility alone should not be used to report speech results. However, when used by speech and language therapists who have undergone training and are aware of local accent and dialectal confounders and who are judging a controlled speech sample under controlled conditions, intelligibility ratings were found to correlate well with number of consonant errors (Sell et al., 2000).

Current perspectives on perceptual speech assessment

The nature of the speech assessment is determined by the age of the child, its purpose, and practical factors. For example, it is often appropriate to undertake a comprehensive detailed phonetic and phonological approach when planning therapy (Grunwell and Dive, 1988; Albery and Russell, 1994; Russell and Sell, 1998). However, in the interdisciplinary clinic a screening protocol is all that is possible (Sell et al., 1994, 1999). Assessment for audit purposes may also require a particular approach (Harding et al., 1997).

The Great Ormond Street SPeech ASSessment GOS.SP.ASS. (Sell et al., 1994, 1999) (Table 16.1) was developed as a comprehensive and standardized screening procedure for describing the speech characteristics commonly associated with cleft palate and/or velopharyngeal dysfunction, and which also facilitates the process of diagnosis and treatment planning. It evolved by drawing upon previous profiles (McWilliams and Philips, 1979; Bzoch, 1979). GOS.SP.ASS. was selected in a UK survey (Razzell and Harding, 1995) as the preferred clinical and research tool, but was considered too detailed to be recommended as a national audit protocol. A protocol was developed specifically for clinical audit purposes, known as the Cleft Audit Protocol for Speech CAPS (Harding et al., 1997). Since this used GOS.SP.ASS. as its foundation with a common set of sentence elicitation material, these protocols can be used independently with results that are comparable. The GOS.SP.ASS. protocol has subsequently been revised (Sell et al., 1999) based on the findings of the Razzell and Harding survey.

The major differences between GOS.SP.ASS. and CAPS occur in the use of intelligibility, the targets assessed, and the rating scales used for evaluating hypernasality, hyponasality, nasal air emission and nasal turbulence. Intelligibility is omitted in the GOS.SP.ASS. protocol. The CAPS protocol does not evaluate the /m, v, l, z, ng, h, th/ targets. The detail of the resonance and airflow description is condensed in the CAPS protocol; for example, consistency and severity ratings are described separately in GOS.SP.ASS. Grimace is described on a four-point scale in GOS.SP.ASS. but on a five-point scale in CAPS.

Both GOS.SP.ASS. and CAPS use a common set of sentences for speech sample elicitation (Table 16.2). Sentence repetition is a popular method of obtaining a speech sample in order to establish whether specific targets can be achieved, and thereby provide information on a child's phonetic repertoire. Van Demark (1964) found a high correlation between a task of sentence repetition and spontaneous speech. Sentence repetition is therefore a useful and economic, but controlled method of collecting a data

Table 16.1. GOS.SP.ASS.98

GOS.SP.ASS '98: SPEECH PROFILE FOR CHILDREN WITH CLEFT PALATE AND/OR
VELOPHARYNGEAL DYSFUNCTION (revised)

Name_____ Age _____ Hosp. No. _____ Date_____

Type of cleft _____ Tape Number _____

RESONANCE	Hypernasal	0 --- 1 --- 2 --- 3	a. inconsistent	b. consistent
	Hyponasal	0 --- 1 --- 2	a. inconsistent	b. consistent
	Mixed resonance	Cul de sac		

Mirror Test

	R	L
pa pa		
pi pi		
ka ka		
ki ki		
ssss		

NASAL EMISSION   0 --- 1 --- 2   a. inaudible   *and/or*   b. audible
                                              c. accompanying   *and/or*   d. replacing consonants
                                              e. inconsistent   f. consistent

NASAL TURBULENCE   0 --- 1 --- 2   a. accompanying   *and/or*   b. replacing consonants
                                              c. inconsistent   d. consistent

GRIMACE   0 --- 1 --- 2 --- 3   a. inconsistent   b. consistent

CONSONANT PRODUCTION

	Labial					Alveolar						Post-alveolar			Velar			Glottal	
	m	p	b	f	v	n	l	t	d	s	z	ʃ	tʃ	dʒ	ŋ	k	g	h	eʔ
SIWI															▨				
SFWF																			

Transcription of speech:

CLEFT TYPE CHARACTERISTICS (CTCS)

0	Dentalization..........................		5	Pharyngeal articulation ....
1	Lateralization/Lateral articulation .... *Anterior*		6	Glottal articulation ....
2	Palatalization/Palatal .... *Oral CTCs*		7	Active nasal fricatives ....
2/3	Double articulation		8	Weak/nasalized consonants ....
3	Backing to velar........................... *Posterior*		9a	Nasal realizations of fricatives ....
4	Backing to uvular......................... *Oral CTCs*		9b	Nasal realizations of plosives ....
			10	Absent pressure consonants.................................
			11	Gliding of fricatives/affricates ....

5 Pharyngeal articulation — 6 Glottal articulation — 7 Active nasal fricatives → *Non-Oral CTCs*

8 Weak/nasalized consonants, 9a Nasal realizations of fricatives, 9b Nasal realizations of plosives, 10 Absent pressure consonants, 11 Gliding of fricatives/affricates → *Passive CTCs*

DEVELOPMENTAL ERRORS e.g. ....

SUMMARY OF SPEECH PATTERN	0 Normal consonants	0-1 No CTCs	1 Anterior oral CTCs	2 Posterior oral CTCs
	3 Non-oral CTCs	4 Passive CTCs	5 Developmental errors	6 Other

SPEECH AND LANGUAGE THERAPY	0 Unnecessary	1 Waiting List	2 Therapy Ongoing	3 Regular Review
	4 Unavailable	5 No uptake		
Location	0 Specialist	1 Community		

RELEVANT INFORMATION FROM PARENTS

(contd)

Table 16.1. (contd)

VOICE	0 Normal	1 Dysphonic	2 Reduced volume

VISUAL APPEARANCE OF SPEECH

0 Unremarkable	2 Tongue tip appearing
1 Tight upper lip	3 Asymmetry of facial movement

ORAL EXAMINATION

1 Nose	0 Unremarkable	1 Deviated septum	2 Obstructed	
2 Lips	0 Unremarkable	1 Restricted movement	2 Open mouth posture	
3 Occlusion	0 Class I	1 Class II	2 Class III	3 Anterior open bite
4 Dentition	0 Unremarkable	1 Supernumerary	2 Missing teeth	3 Malaligned
5 Tongue	0 Unremarkable	1 Poor mobility	2 Abnormal posture	3 Tongue tie
6 Palatal Fistula	0 Absent	1 Present		
7 Fistula Size	1 Minute < than 2mm	2 Small between 2–5 mm	3 Medium between 5–8 mm	
	4 Large > 8 mm	5 Complete breakdown		
8 Fistula Location	1 Uvula	2 Soft palate	3 Junction soft/hard palate	
	4 Hard palate – post alveolus	5 Buccal sulcus	6 Other (describe)	
	7 Hard palate and buccal sulcus			
9 Palate Mobility	0 Marked	1 Moderate	2 Slight	3 None
10 Soft Palate	1 Bifid uvula	2 Notch	3 Blue/thin looking	
	4 Suspected incorrect muscle alignment		5 Apparently short	
11 Nasopharynx	1 Tonsils	....		
	2 Apparently deep pharynx	....		
	3 Pharyngeal wall movement	....		
	4 Pharyngeal flap	....		

LANGUAGE	0 Apparently normal	1 Delayed	2 Disordered

IDENTIFIABLE AETIOLOGY

1 Suspected VPI	7 Oral fistula	13 Other
2 Confirmed VPI	8 Cleft palate history	
3 Abnormal dentition	9 Intellectual deficit	
4 Malocclusion	10 Developmental	
5 Diagnosed hearing loss	11 Environmental	
6 Suspected hearing loss	12 Syndrome	

AREAS REQUIRING FURTHER ASSESSMENT ....

....

MANAGEMENT PLAN ....

....

Speech and Language Therapist ....

ADDITIONAL NOTES

Table 16.2. Sentences for use with GOS.SP.ASS.98

Sentences are presented verbally for imitation; pictures can be used to facilitate sentence imitation. A full set of colour pictures is now available (Harding et al., 1997; Sell et al., 1997).

Mum came home
The puppy is playing with a rope
Bob is a baby boy
The phone fell off the shelf
Dave is driving a van
Neil saw a robin in a nest
A ball is like a balloon
Tim is putting a hat on
Daddy mended a door
I saw Sam sitting on a bus
The zebra was at the zoo
Sean is washing a dirty dish
Charlie's watching a football match
John's got a magic badge
The bell's ringing
Karen is making a cake
Gary's got a bag of Lego
Hannah hurt her hand
This hand is cleaner than the other
The hamster scrambled up Stuart's sleeve

sample. Sentences have been chosen to be 'imageable', meaningful, and relevant whilst containing maximal numbers of each target consonant. Each sentence samples a target sound known to be particularly vulnerable to the effects of cleft palate, i.e. plosives, fricatives and affricates (see Grunwell and Sell, Chapter 5). The nasal consonants /m n/ are also included since errors of place can occur on this group of consonants (Philips and Harrison, 1969). These sentences have been designed not to include other vulnerable consonants, which might disturb production or perception of target consonants. Wherever possible, consonants other than the target consonant in each sentence were approximants. Final targets were followed by a vowel at every opportunity so that the final consonant was neither assimilated to the first consonant in the following word, or left unreleased being the last consonant in the sentence.

For a practical discussion of the general principles of speech assessment the reader is referred to Grunwell et al. (1993) and Trost-Cardamone and Bernthal (1993).

Great Ormond Street Speech Assessment GOS.SP.ASS.98

The Great Ormond Street SPeech ASSessment GOS.SP.ASS. (Sell et al., 1994, 1998, 1999) provides an evaluation of resonance, nasal emission, nasal turbulence, grimace, articulation characteristics and phonation together with a systematic approach to an oral examination, the mirror test and a description of the visual appearance of speech (Witzel, 1991). The rater is encouraged to identify aetiological factors and detail the management plan (Table 16.1).

Resonance and nasal airflow characteristics of nasal emission and nasal turbulence are assessed perceptually using scalar evaluations of presence of a characteristic, its consistency and degree of severity. Nasal emission and nasal turbulence may accompany and/or replace consonants. Nasal emission is classified as audible or inaudible.

Some comment is warranted about the speech cleft type characteristics adopted in this approach. Following phonetic transcription of the target consonants, the realizations are categorized according to the nature of the error into a speech cleft type characteristic category. Dentalization as a speech cleft type characteristic is a new concept probably reflecting the more recent trend to evaluate the visual appearance of speech using video speech recordings. Distinction should be made between fronting that occurs as a normal immaturity, and fronting that is a structurally related 'cleft type' characteristic (Eurocleft Speech Group, 1993). The presence of double articulation and backing has been confirmed by findings from electropalatography (Dent et al., 1992). A distinction is made between backing to velar and uvular place of articulation. It is possible that, when alveolar plosives are realized as velar plosives, this may precipitate further backing of targets /k g/ to uvular/pharyngeal place of articulation. This indicates that there is an appreciation of the need to signal a phonological contrast. It should be noted that the speech cleft type characteristic of weak/nasalized consonants is associated with reduced intraoral air pressure so that oral consonants are nasalized, and as a consequence there is weak oral air pressure. It is not necessarily the case that the articulatory stricture is weak.

Active nasal fricative is a category which identifies fricative targets realized by voiceless nasals with additional audible nasal emission. Articulation of active nasal fricatives [m̥ n̥] for targets /f s/ involves complete oral closure at the place of articulation, with the airstream directed exclusively nasally (Figure 16.1a). Where a backing pattern is present, [ɲ̃] is frequently a realization for targets /s ʃ/. It is important to identify realizations that are the result of an active compensatory strategy because these active nasal fricatives usually require speech therapy intervention and not surgery (see Grunwell and Sell, Chapter 5). The nasal fricative is usually specific to one or two phonemes. Where active nasal fricatives exist, there may be no additional nasal emission or hypernasality. Indeed these realizations are frequently produced by children who have no identifiable velopharyngeal insufficiency (VPI) or oral structural defect, and have been referred to, somewhat erroneously in the literature, as phoneme specific hypernasality when a more accurate description describes abnormal nasal airflow.

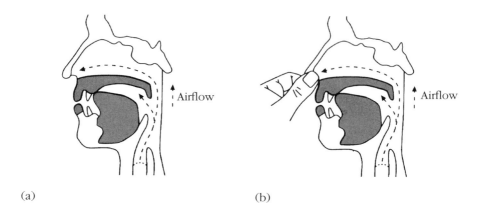

(a)   (b)

Figure 16.1. (a) Active nasal fricative: complete oral closure at the place of articulation with the airstream directed exclusively nasally: target /s/ is realized as [ñ̥]. (b) Noseholding does not facilitate target production, in contrast to passive nasal fricatives. No oral or nasal airflow occurs.

In contrast, nasal realization of fricatives involves a passive escape of air nasally. This distinction from active nasal fricatives involves establishing whether production of the target consonant, for example /s/, can be made normally when oral air pressure is facilitated by inhibition of nasal airflow through nose holding (Harding and Grunwell, 1998) (Figure 16.2a and b). If, for example, [s] can be produced with nose holding but is realized as a voiceless nasal without nose holding, then it is concluded that the nasal airflow is a passive loss of oral air during normal articulation of target /s/. In contrast, noseholding in the case of active nasal fricatives (Figure 16.1b) does not help the production of the target sounds

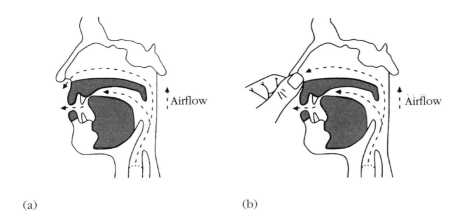

(a)   (b)

Figure 16.2. (a) Passive nasal fricative. (b) Oral air pressure is facilitated by inhibition of nasal airflow through nose holding.

Passive errors may co-occur with an absence of pressure consonants. This lack of pressure consonants is a strong indicator of velopharyngeal dysfunction (VPD), requiring investigations of the sphincter mechanism (Sell and Ma, 1996). Finally, gliding of fricatives/affricates, e.g. /ʃ/ or /tʃ/ realized as [j] or [w], is a relatively common characteristic but no research to date associates gliding of fricatives with either active compensatory characteristics or with passive VPD-related characteristics. It is possible that this characteristic may be a persisting developmental process which is perpetuated because of the cleft palate.

The importance of identifying developmental errors has already been alluded to (see Grunwell and Sell, Chapter 5) and, although not the focus of this chapter, a history of, or a current language problem should be recorded in order to alert the therapist to the possibility of a developmental phonological problem. It may also influence a child's ability to compensate for a structural defect. Furthermore, priorities for therapy may be different in the presence of an additional language problem. Children with cleft lip and/or palate are known to be at risk for language problems (Scherer and D'Antonio, 1995).

Aerodynamic and acoustic objective measures

In addition to perceptual assessment, instrumentation has been developed to provide aerodynamic and acoustic objective measures of the perceptual consequences of velopharyngeal dysfunction (Warren, 1975, 1979; Fletcher,

1970; Lubker and Moll, 1965; Moon, 1993). The reader is referred to Moon's chapter (1993) for a brief yet comprehensive overview of all the techniques.

Acoustic measures involve the movement of vibrational energy through the vocal tract, and include techniques such as spectrography, accelerometry and nasometry (Moon, 1993). Nasometry developed out of the premise that changes in the relative magnitudes of oral and nasal sound pressures reflect the degree to which the oral and nasal tracts are coupled during speech production (Moon, 1993). The Nasometer is a micro-computer based instrument and software-driven. It employs microphones on either side of a sound separator plate positioned on the upper lip. It detects sound from the nose and the mouth, and the resultant acoustic signal from each microphone is processed. A numeric ratio of nasal to nasal-plus-oral acoustic energy is calculated, and is expressed as a nasalance score (Dalston and Seaver, 1992). Studies have shown that there is a high degree of relationship between perceptual judgements of nasality and nasalance scores (Sweeney et al., 1999a), and therefore this makes nasometry an appealing method for the instrumental quantification of nasality. Furthermore, it is easy to use, providing graphical and numerical values. It has been reported that there are regional variations in normal scores ranging from 25 to 32% (Fletcher et al., 1989; Sweeney, personal communication). Unfortunately, to date there is limited normative data for most regions within the UK, a requirement for reliable and valid use of the nasometer on clinical populations.

Aerodynamics refers to the movement of a pressurized air stream. Aerodynamic methods include the measurement of airflows and air pressures. Techniques have ranged from simple sensing devices such as manometers and the mirror test, to combinations of pressure transducers and airflow meters. One of the most highly developed systems is that of PERCI: Palatal Efficiency Rating Computed Instantaneously (developed by Warren, 1979), which more recently has been refined further as the PERCI-SARS system. It makes use of pressure transducers for recording airway pressures within the vocal tract, and flowmeters for recording volume rates of airflow. Pressure difference on either side of the velopharyngeal port is measured during the production of /p/ using nasal and oral pressure transducers. An estimate of velopharyngeal port area is then calculated using the differential pressure and nasal airflow. Sweeney et al. (1999b) have shown a moderate to good relationship between the perceptual judgement of nasal emission and pressure flow measurements during the production of 'p' in hamper. This is additional evidence that the PERCI-SARS system is a potentially powerful tool (Moon, 1993).

Therapy

Changing philosophy in the healthcare system requires that clinical practice has its foundations in research evidence (Haines and Jones, 1994). In common with many areas of cleft palate, the literature relating to the efficacy of speech and language therapy in the treatment of cleft palate and velopharyngeal dysfunction is sparse in quantity and quality, and is mostly anecdotal and descriptive, with few randomized controlled trials (Enderby and Emerson, 1995). Howell and McCartney (1990) describe how 'speech and language therapists are remarkably successful in changing child speech patterns which deviate from the norm. Therapy evidence is based on clinical and anecdotal accounts rather than controlled experimental studies'. Enderby and Emerson (1995) caution that the randomized controlled trial may not always be appropriate because of the variations in the relationship between the therapist and patient, and the variation in the way in which therapists apply treatment, both of which may complicate treatment outcome. Furthermore, there are many variables in addition to the intervention which may influence results. For example, patients with different characteristics respond differently to a given treatment. Enderby and Emerson (1995) argue that a successful outcome of therapy should be seen in terms of the impact on communication in everyday life and its overall impact on the client.

Speech therapy for consonant production

Many of the therapy techniques advocated are based on the pioneering work of Morley (1970) and on principles of behaviour modification. Based on a comprehensive assessment the clinician needs to be prepared to adopt both a phonetic and phonological approach in therapy. It is important to look for patterns in which different speech sounds are influenced in a similar way. Therapy may be effective in favourably influencing a group of sounds simultaneously, rather than one target sound only (Trost-Cardamone and Bernthal, 1993; Harding and Grunwell, 1998; see Russell and Harding, Chapter 14). For example, within the GOS.SP.ASS. framework the lateral approximant [l] has been included as a consonant to assess. It is anticipated that where backing of alveolar plosive and/or nasal targets exists, target [l] may also be backed to [j] or [ŋ]. This is particularly important since identification and targeting all errors affected by a process is important in therapy. Determining the therapy programme depends on a comprehensive assessment (Golding-Kushner, 1995; Russell and Sell, 1998), stimulability testing, consistency of errors and a developmental evaluation of consonant production. Hoch et al. (1986) advocate that therapy begins with targets that are stimulable. Trost-Cardamone and Bernthal (1993) state that the clinician should select targets or several targets that focus on patterns which might contribute most to reduced intelligibility.

Estrem and Broen (1989) suggested that some speakers with cleft palate prefer to articulate at the peripheral ends of the vocal tract with little activity in the middle or posterior palate. Trost-Cardamone and Bernthal (1993) advocate the need for children to be taught directly the target sound. Trost (1981) suggests using techniques of mirror work, tactile cues, and the use of diagrams to teach simple phonetics. A general principle is working directly on place of articulation and the need to bring articulation more anterior (Trost, 1981). Often the focus should be on labial and tongue tip sounds. It is also important to work in parallel on auditory discrimination and self-monitoring skills in order to establish internal mechanisms for correct target selection (Morley, 1970; Russell and Sell, 1998) and perceptual-motor self-monitoring. Generalization and carryover are crucial aspects of the therapy programme.

Hoch et al. (1986) and Golding-Kushner (1995) describe the principles of treating glottal stops, based on whispering and sighing. Golding-Kushner (1995) stresses the importance of identifying glottal co-articulations. She has found that these occur in the speech of patients who have received therapy and have been instructed in correct lip/tongue placement, but not in airstream management. It is crucial that carers are trained to recognize the differences between the speech errors and correct targets. The reader is referred to Golding-Kushner (1995) for a detailed description of therapy techniques for eliminating glottal stops. Techniques are described such as gentle whispering to keep the vocal folds apart, over-aspiration, use of sustained /h/, multiple use of auditory, visual, phonetic, verbal, manual or tactile cues, use of nasal occlusion and release, and the use of correctly produced sounds as facilitators for error sounds.

Some authorities describe the need to increase the strength of articulatory contacts, to be direct and specific in instructing the child in how to place and move their articulators, to practise drilled multiple repetitions of the consonant–vowel syllable, and to build up a repertoire of correctly produced words by using only target words in which all sounds are produced correctly (Trost, 1981; Golding-Kushner, 1995). This is in contrast to Harding and Grunwell (1998), who advocate minimal articulatory effort and use of soft attack, and a more indirect approach described as 'deferred responsibility'. They advocate use of auditory training and caution against confronting the child with errors or risking his/her failure. The apparent differences in approach in part may relate more to the 'art' of therapy and to some extent depend on individual therapist style rather than scientific evidence. The approach adopted will also depend on patient characteristics.

Harding and Grunwell (1998) conclude that a combination of metaphono-logical (Grundy, 1989), phonological and articulatory approaches should be used, and provide useful examples of therapy principles. Russell and Sell (1998) emphasize the need for the therapy programme to have clear aims and specific goals and to be structured and focused. Parent/carer commit-ment is integral to the success of therapy, with homework, the use of 'benign misunderstanding' by the parents, and carryover, as important parts of the programme.

Importantly, it should be noted that improved articulation placement and airflow direction orally can reduce or even eliminate hypernasality and nasal emission.

Visual biofeedback for consonant production

A sophisticated and promising approach to assessment and treatment is electropalatography (EPG). This is a technique designed to record details of the timing and location of tongue contacts with the hard palate during continuous speech (Hardcastle and Gibbon, 1997). It is a powerful proce-dure in the clinical setting both for assessment and therapy purposes (Gibbon and Hardcastle, 1989). Hardcastle and Gibbon (1997) suggest that EPG is an additional strategy to therapy to be used in conjunction with other traditional approaches to improve speech intelligibility.

EPG has been found to be particularly effective in the treatment of children with cleft palate. McWilliams et al. (1990) described the resistance to conventional therapy for children who present with a posterior articula-tion pattern, and this was further substantiated by the findings of the UK national study of children with unilateral cleft lip and palate (CSAG Report, 1998; Sell et al., 2000). EPG is an appropriate technique for clients who have abnormally broad or increased posterior tongue placement often identified as palatal articulation, lateral/lateralized articulation and abnormal double articulations (Hardcastle et al., 1989a, 1989b; Michi et al., 1986; Gibbon and Hardcastle, 1987, 1989; Dent et al., 1992). Whitehill et al. (1996) attributed the use of an alveolar contact during velars to the tongue tip/blade being raised in an attempt to block the alveolar cleft. They found that establishing the anterior articulatory placement for /s/ and /t/ was associated with an improvement in nasal plosion and nasal emission, although neither were targeted in speech therapy. Further evidence of the effectiveness of EPG with patients with cleft palate is emerging (Gibbon et al., 1998).

Visual feedback for lingual–palatal contact may be more effective than for velopharyngeal contact due to the greater number of tactile and kinaes-thetic receptors in the tongue/hard palate region compared with the velopharyngeal region. Whitehill et al. (1996) also hypothesize that EPG visual biofeedback may be very useful if there is reduced oral sensation in the alveolar region. It is thought that visual biofeedback is effective because it makes tongue position and movement explicit and enables the development of conscious control of such clues (Hardcastle and Gibbon, 1997). An advantage of a computer mediated treatment is that clients tend to be more objective about their own performance when measured by a machine, rather than when judged by a therapist (Volin, 1993). Visual biofeedback, objective feedback allowing documentation of small changes, self-monitoring, client working independently, increased metalinguistic awareness, increased motivation, enjoyment, and the appeal of computer based equipment for young children are all factors which can be attributed to its success (Hardcastle et al., 1989b; Morgan Barry, 1989; Michi et al., 1993).

Speech therapy for hypernasality

Therapy for hypernasality has been undertaken for many years. The results, however, are generally disappointing. It is based on the assumption that if hypernasality is modified, velopharyngeal closure is improved. Starr (1993) reviewed comprehensively the three different approaches to therapy; these aim to change muscle behaviour, muscle control or listener perception. Activities that have been advocated include increasing strength of articulatory contacts, increased mouth opening, reduction of volume, palatal exercises, palatal massage, blowing, icing, sucking, interrupted swallowing, cheek puffing, gagging, palate strengthening, and stroking. He concludes, however, that the behavioural management of hypernasality and velopharyngeal problems is inappropriate for most patients with velopharyngeal problems, and this is a recurring theme through the literature (Ruscello, 1982; Shprintzen et al., 1974; Wolfaardt et al., 1993; McWilliams et al., 1990; Golding-Kushner, 1995). Many of these studies of therapy techniques have not been replicated and have not included direct visualization of the sphincter, which would be a method of documenting change. McWilliams et al. (1990) also caution that some of the techniques may result in the elevation of the larynx and in vocal hyperfunction leading to phonation disorders. Therapy for hypernasality per se should only be undertaken if the patient is capable of achieving velopharyngeal closure (McWilliams et al., 1990).

Speech therapy for persistent hypernasality following secondary management of the velopharyngeal sphincter is common practice (Pannbacker et al., 1984; CSAG Report, 1998). Sell and Ma (1996) examined the role of routine postoperative speech therapy based on the speech and postoperative nasopharyngoscopy of 68 patients who had had pharyngoplasty. Of those who had persistent symptoms of velopharyngeal dysfunction, endoscopy showed that 60% had structural problems, 20% had functional problems, and 20% had both structural and functional problems. Therefore the majority of persistent speech problems related to nasality and nasal airflow were a result of a persistent structural problem. In such cases, it is inappropriate for patients to *routinely* have speech therapy. For many of these patients the only option for removing the speech symptoms of velopharyngeal dysfunction are probably further surgery or prosthetics management. In contrast, in functional problems speech therapy may be appropriate. In combined problems it is unlikely that speech therapy alone will solve the problem of excessive hypernasality and/or nasal air emission.

Speech therapy aimed at eliminating hypernasality, nasal emission, nasal turbulence and nasal grimace per se should only be undertaken when there is clear evidence that the patient is able to achieve velopharyngeal closure during a speech task, usually from nasopharyngoscopy or multiview video-fluoroscopy. It is usually possible for therapy for articulation problems to be reinstigated three to four weeks after secondary surgery.

Visual biofeedback

There are several simple devices available which provide visual feedback regarding abnormal nasal airflow including the mirror test, the stethoscope, See-Scape, micronose, Exeter anemometry. Such devices are often easily available, of low cost and non-invasive. However, they do not provide quantitative information, and have questionable validity. For example, they also reflect nasal patency/resistance, nasal congestion and respiratory effort and depend on accurate placement of the device. There have been no efficacy studies. There have been some reports on the use of nasometry (Fletcher, 1972, 1978) to provide visual biofeedback which although promising must still be considered experimental (Starr, 1993).

There are a growing number of reports describing the use of fibreoptic nasopharyngoscopy as a technique to learn to increase or change velopharyngeal closure (Siegel-Sadewitz and Shprintzen, 1982; Witzel et al., 1989; Golding-Kushner 1995; Ysunza Pamplona and Femat, 1997). Witzel et al. (1989) state that it 'provides valuable information for revising the learning process, giving essential visual cues, that are missing in traditional techniques ... these emphasize auditory feedback'. Witzel describes how visual biofeedback makes use of the images of velopharyngeal movements to guide attempts at closure and observe changes in movements when attempting different tongue positions for articulation. The combined use of nasopharyngoscopy and videofluoroscopy in the treatment of borderline VPD and compensatory articulation is advocated by Kawano et al. (1997).

Prosthetic management of hypernasality

For some patients with velopharyngeal dysfunction, prosthetic management may be indicated (McGrath and Anderson, 1991; Leeper et al., 1993). Indeed

McGrath and Anderson (1991) even recommend that this should be considered as the first management option before surgery. In contrast, Marsh and Wray (1980) reported that the use of prosthetics was associated with non-compliance and consequent failure rate, a persistent sense of deformity and the need for secondary surgical conversions. Delgado et al. (1992) showed that the preferred management option is nowadays surgery and yet prosthetics should be part of the overall treatment armamentarium of the team.

There are three types of prosthetic appliances: the palatal training appliance (Tudor and Selley, 1974), the palatal lift (Gibbons and Bloomer, 1958; Gonzalez and Aronson, 1970; Turner and Williams, 1991) and the speech bulb obturator (Golding-Kushner et al., 1995). They can be used diagnostically, for prognostic purposes or treatment, reportedly in collaboration with a weaning or reduction programme. They depend on effective teamwork between the prosthodontist, dental technician, speech and language therapist, family and patient.

Many factors need to be carefully thought about when a prosthetic approach is under consideration. These include oral and patient characteristics including dental status, existing dentition, occlusal relationships, periodontal condition, oral hygiene, and factors such as age and health (Leeper et al. 1993; McGrath and Anderson 1991). The anterior portion of all three appliances can also function to obturate an oral–nasal fistula.

The palatal training appliance (Figure 16.3) consists of a wire loop attached to the back of an existing custom-built plate attached to the teeth.

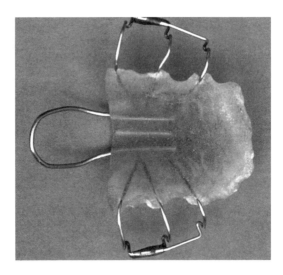

Figure 16.3. Palatal training appliance.

It has been suggested that this stimulates movement of the soft palate by sensory feedback, and assists in inhibiting the posterior bunching movement of the palatoglossus muscle. It has been advocated for use in patients with some existing movement and sensitivity of the palate. This was developed in the UK but is less used in recent times. Like many of the treatments used in this field there are considerable methodological flaws in the studies reporting effectiveness of this treatment. Studies were characterized by subjects with wide age ranges and mixed aetiologies, no separate reporting of speech parameters with no inter–intra rater reliability results reported, no standard times for evaluation, possible observer bias, and no visualization of the velopharyngeal sphincter before and after management.

The palatal lift aims to lift the soft palate in a posterior and superior direction by the use of an acrylic extension from the back of the plate. It has been advocated for use in patients with a long soft palate which is immobile on phonation, and particularly in neurological conditions. There is some evidence that this is an effective method of treatment (Gonzalez and Aronson, 1970; LaVelle and Hardy, 1979). Improved articulation is consistently reported with this treatment although Witt et al. (1995) found no evidence to support changes in neuromuscular function.

Speech bulbs (Figures 16.4, 16.5, 16.6, 16.7) were first introduced in the mid 1800s but have been re-popularized with the use of nasendoscopy and multiview videofluoroscopy permitting accurate fitting and evaluation (Karnell et al., 1987). The speech bulb consists of an oral plate with an extension which courses behind the palate and terminates in an acrylic ball or elliptical structure positioned in the velopharynx. They may be used as a permanent solution to velopharyngeal dysfunction, or on a trial basis to determine the benefits of possible surgery, or to improve lateral wall function usually prior to pharyngeal flap surgery. In the American literature, some clinicians have used the speech bulb obturator with severe problems of glottal and pharyngeal articulation to facilitate and expedite therapy, with reported improvement in lateral wall function, usually prior to velopharyngeal surgery. The therapeutic use of the speech bulb has encouraged the development of the speech bulb reduction programme (Israel et al., 1993; Golding-Kushner et al., 1995) but still such treatment should be regarded as experimental. Sell et al. (1997) found that speech bulb treatment can be an effective permanent solution for velopharyngeal dysfunction in patients with severe pathology for whom no other treatment option is available, such as occurs when there is a serious degree of tissue deficiency or complex medical condition, or anaesthetic contraindications to surgery exist.

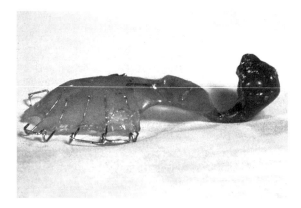

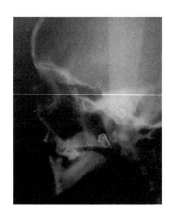

Figure 16.4. Speech bulb obturator.

Figure 16.5. Lateral X-ray of speech bulb obturator *in situ.*

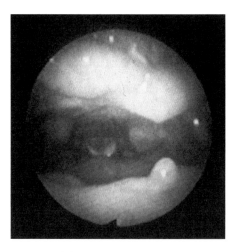

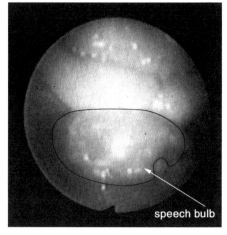

Figure 16.6. Nasendoscopic view during speech of the defect.

Figure 16.7. Nasendoscopic view during speech with the speech bulb obturator *in situ.*

Timing of speech interventions

Probably one of the most controversial and difficult decision-making areas with regard to management is the timing of an intervention, be it surgery, therapy or prosthetics. An example of this concerns the timing of velopharyngeal surgery versus therapy, when there are articulatory errors. This must be considered carefully and holistically in relation to a multitude of complex interacting factors. Traditionally it has been held that velopharyngeal dysfunction should be solved surgically or prosthetically before speech therapy for articulation errors is provided (McWilliams et al., 1990; Albery, 1986; Van Demark and Hardin, 1990). Recent reports have indicated that improvement of placement errors through speech therapy prior to surgery is not only possible but advisable in the case of speakers with VPD (Trost, 1981; Hoch et al., 1986; Hall et al., 1991; Henningsson and Isberg, 1991; Trost-Cardamone and Bernthal, 1993; Golding-Kushner, 1995; LeBlanc, 1996). This is particularly pertinent when the planned surgical management is velopharyngeal surgery such as a pharyngeal flap, on the basis that the extent of the pharyngeal flap may be reduced with improved articulation and, in some cases, the indication for this type of surgery even eliminated. On balance, a three to six month period of diagnostic articulation therapy is prudent, coupled with careful documentation of articulation change, until more is known about the effects of articulatory change on velopharyngeal closure (Albery, 1986; Bradley, 1979).

However, the issue of articulation errors and the timing of velopharyngeal surgery are less relevant if techniques such as palate re-repair or the Furlow technique are the first choice for managing velopharyngeal dysfunction (Sommerlad et al., 1994; Chen et al., 1994; D'Antonio, 1997) rather than pharyngoplasty. In this situation lateral videofluoroscopy and a perceptual speech assessment is the minimum standard of investigation required on which to base such surgery, and can be undertaken as young as three years. Even if this surgery does not result in complete elimination of hypernasality/nasal air emission/turbulence, it may increase the child's ability to achieve intraoral air pressure for consonant production, thereby facilitating articulation therapy. If need be a Hynes or sphincter-type pharyngoplasty can be undertaken at a later stage to eliminate the persistent abnormal resonance/airflow.

There may also be a conflict as to the timing of speech therapy intervention in relation to orthodontic treatment. If therapy is postponed until after the completion of orthodontics the patient will probably have entered puberty and may have passed through the critical period during which speech learning is easier. Furthermore, changing articulation in the presence of a structural deviation such as malocclusion, supernumerary or rotated teeth, protrusion of the premaxilla or maxillary collapse is often difficult or impossible and ill-advised (McWilliams et al., 1990). Articulation may also improve spontaneously following successful orthodontic correction or maxillary advancement. LeBlanc and Shprintzen (1994) advocate deferring speech therapy until after such treatment or surgery is completed. Each individual case depends on a clinical judgement as to the possibility of making changes in the context of the structural anomaly, the nature of the child's speech disorder, the child's stimulability, child and parental motivation, and possibly the availability of electropalatography.

Yet another issue is the timing of fistula repair. Usually it is preferable for a fistula to be repaired at the time of alveolar bone grafting, at 9–11 years of age (see Mars, Chapter 20). However, earlier repair may be necessary if speech is considered to be seriously affected by excessive hypernasality, weakness/nasalization/nasal air emission, and/or articulation disorders. The incorrect realization of alveolar consonants to a more posterior position may indicate that the speaker is trying to avoid contact with the fistula, thereby preventing loss of air pressure/abnormal nasal airflow. The presence of velopharyngeal dysfunction related to or in addition to the presence of a fistula may also be a complicating factor (Isberg and Henningsson, 1987; Henningsson and Isberg, 1990). The therapist must assess the effects of temporary obturation and make a differential diagnosis as to the source of hypernasality, weakness/nasalization/nasal air emission. This can be achieved by temporarily inserting gutta percha into the fistula and undertaking assessment under the two conditions of blocked and unblocked fistula. The assessment may involve perceptual assessment, nasopharyngoscopy, videofluoroscopy, and possibly nasometry and airflow studies. If fistula repair is indicated, with or without velopharyngeal surgical management, its timing needs to be considered in collaboration with the orthodontist. Temporary obturation with a small plate may be preferred until an alveolar bone graft can be undertaken as the appropriate long-term solution, or an 'early' bone graft may be advocated. Folk et al. (1997), in a review of the evaluation and management of fistulae, stress the need for a multidisciplinary approach.

It has also been stated that the outcome of velopharyngeal surgery is more disappointing in adults than in children. However, Hall et al. (1991) and Wu et al. (1997) stated that the success rate of removing VPI through surgery was not significantly different between children and adults. Successful outcome is more dependent on comprehensive assessment, the nature of the defect, surgical technique, experience and skill. Wu et al. (1997) studied 20 adult cleft palate patients with an average age of 28 years. They found that adults have the potential to acquire adequate articulation skills in controlled speech in the presence of a relatively competent velopharyngeal mechanism but they failed to maintain their newly learnt articulation pattern in spontaneous speech even when supported by group therapy. When palate repair is delayed into adulthood, Sell (1992) found that speech outcome and the incidence of velopharyngeal closure were extremely disappointing.

Even when surgery has been undertaken at conventional ages, there remains a small group of adolescents and adults who present with moderate to severe speech impairments that have been resistant to treatment, sometimes even with the provision of an adequate velopharyngeal mechanism (Noordhoff et al., 1987; Bzoch, 1989; McWilliams et al., 1990). Peterson-Falzone (1995) reported that 10.9% of 110 adolescents had severely deviant speech reflecting failed surgery and rehabilitation. The UK national study reported 15% of 12-year-olds with unilateral cleft lip and palate had serious errors of consonant production and appreciable hypernasality (CSAG Report, 1998). The adult with cleft lip and palate is often poorly-served by cleft palate teams, at least in part because of patterns of funding, service delivery and the perception that the rehabilitation process has been completed. However, adult clients may present with concerns that have not been addressed or are not resolved to their satisfaction. Furthermore, previous non-compliance as a result of burnout from repeated failed procedures, indifference to available treatments, peer pressure, or poor understanding of potential treatment (Riski, 1995; Witzel, 1991) may be replaced by renewed motivation in later years. New developments have recently become available which may be of assistance such as syndrome identification or electropalatography.

Speech and maxillary advancement

When patients are being considered for maxillary osteotomy, the speech/language pathologist must evaluate speech production, particularly velopharyngeal function, and counsel the patient and other team members regarding the possibility of a deterioration in resonance and speech quality following the procedure (see Lello, Chapter 21).

It is generally recognized that consonant articulation often spontaneously improves following maxillary advancement, particularly in the production of targets /sz, pb, fv, ∫, t∫, ʤ/ (Schwartz and Gruner, 1976; Witzel et al., 1980; Ruscello et al., 1985; Kummer et al., 1989).

Several studies have questioned the effect of advancing the maxilla on the velopharyngeal mechanism and speech (Schwarz and Gruner, 1976; Epker and Wolford, 1976). Whilst there is evidence that there are no adverse effects on speech and the velopharyngeal mechanism (Bralley and Schoeny, 1977; McCarthy et al., 1979; Schendel et al., 1979; Kummer et al., 1989) there are reports of speech deterioration following Le Fort I osteotomy (Witzel and Monro, 1977; Witzel et al., 1980; Shprintzen et al., 1979; Witzel, 1981; Watzke et al., 1990; Okazaki et al., 1993). There would appear therefore to be a growing body of more recent evidence to substantiate the adverse effects of standard osteotomy on speech production. Sell et al. (1993) reported that the transpalatal osteotomy does not adversely disturb speech or velopharyngeal function based on a consecutive series of 16 cleft palate patients, but this technique is considered difficult, often associated with large anterior fistulae.

Conclusion

This chapter begins with a critique of the traditional approach to speech assessment and presents an approach to perceptual speech assessment in keeping with increased understanding of speech production in children with cleft palate/velopharyngeal anomalies. It summarizes some of the well-established therapy techniques for treating errors of consonant production, and reviews the role of therapy and prosthetics in the treatment of nasality and nasal airflow. It reflects on some of the difficulties faced in the decisions regarding the timing of interventions, and in so doing demonstrates the key position of the speech and language therapist in the multidisciplinary team.

References

Albery E (1986) The management of cleft palate speech. In: Albery E, Hathorn I, Piggott RW (eds) Cleft Lip and Palate: A Team Approach. Bristol: Wright, pp. 58–62.

Albery E, Russell J (1994) Cleft Palate Sourcebook. Winslow: Winslow Press.

Bradley DP (1979) Congenital and acquired velopharyngeal inadequacy. In: Bzoch KR (ed.) Communicative Disorders Related to Cleft Lip and Palate: Boston: Little, Brown, pp. 106–122.

Bralley RC, Schoeny ZG (1977) Effects of maxillary advancement on the speech of a submucosal cleft palate patient. Cleft Palate Journal 14: 98–101.

Bzoch KR (1979) Measurement and assessment of categorical aspects of language, voice and speech disorders. In: Bzoch KR (ed.) Communicative Disorders Related to Cleft Lip and Palate. Boston: Little, Brown, pp. 161–191.

Bzoch KR (1989) Communicative Disorders Related to Cleft Lip and Palate, 3rd edn. Boston: Little, Brown (College-Hill publication).

Chen PK, Wu JT, Chen VR, Noordhoff MS (1994) Correction of secondary velopharyngeal insufficiency in cleft palate patients with the Furlow palatoplasty. Plastic and Reconstructive Surgery 7: 933–941.

CSAG Report - Clinical Standards Advisory Group (1998) Cleft Lip and Palate. London: HMSO.

Dalston RM, Seaver EJ (1992) Relative values of various standardised passages in the nasometric assessment of patients with velopharyngeal impairment. Cleft Palate–Craniofacial Journal 29: 17–21.

Dalston RG, Marsh JL, Vig KW, Witzel MA, Bumstead MA (1988) Minimal standards for reporting the results of surgery on patients with cleft lip, cleft palate or both: a proposal. Cleft Palate Journal 25: 3–7.

D'Antonio L (1997) Correction of velopharyngeal insufficiency using the Furlow Double-opposing Z-plasty. Western Journal of Medicine 167: 101–102.

Delgado AA, Schaff NG, Emrich L (1992) Trends in prosthodontic treatment of cleft palate patients at one institution: A twenty-one year review. Cleft Palate–Craniofacial Journal 29: 425–428.

Dent H, Gibbon F, Hardcastle W (1992) Inhibiting an abnormal lingual pattern in a cleft palate child using electropalatography (EPG). In: Lahey MM, Kallen JL (eds)

Interdisciplinary Perspectives in Speech and Language Pathology. Dublin: School of Speech and Language Studies, pp. 211–221.

Enderby P, Emerson J (1995) Does Speech and Language Therapy Work? A review of the literature. London: Whurr.

Epker BN, Wolford LM (1976) Middle-third facial osteotomies: their use in the correction of congenital dentofacial and craniofacial deformities. Journal of Oral Surgery 34: 325–343.

Estrem T, Broen PA (1989) Early speech production of children with cleft palate. Journal of Speech and Hearing Research 32: 12–23.

Eurocleft Speech Group: Grunwell P, Brondsted K, Henningsson G, Jansonius K, Karling J, Meijer M, Ording U, Sell D, Wyatt R, Vermeij-Zieverink E (1991) The Eurocleft Speech Group: a phonetic framework for the cross-linguistic analysis of cleft palate speech. Clinical Linguistics and Phonetics 8: 109–125.

Eurocleft Speech Group: Grunwell P, Brondsted K, Henningsson G, Jansonius K, Karling J, Meijer M, Ording U, Sell D, Wyatt R, Vermeij-Zieverink E (1993) Cleft palate speech in a European perspective: Eurocleft Speech Project. In: Grunwell P (ed.) Analysing Cleft Palate Speech. London: Whurr.

Eurocleft Speech Group: Grunwell P, Brondsted K, Henningsson G, Jansonius K, Karling J, Meijer M, Ording U, Wyatt R, Vermeij-Zieverink E, Sell D (2000) A six-centre international study of treatment outcome in patients with clefts of the lip and palate. Scandanavian J. of Plastic Reconstr Hand Surger 34(3): 1–11.

Fletcher SG (1970) Theory and instrumentation for quantitative measurement of nasality. Cleft Palate Journal 7: 601–609.

Fletcher SG (1972) Contingencies for bioelectric modification of nasality. Cleft Palate Journal 13: 31–44.

Fletcher SG (1978) Diagnosing Speech Disorders from Cleft Palate. New York: Grune and Stratton.

Fletcher SG, Adams LE, McCrutcheon MJ (1989) Cleft palate speech assessment through oral-nasal acoustic measures. In: Bzoch KR (ed.) Communication Disorders Related to Cleft Lip and Palate. Boston: Little, Brown.

Folk SN, D'Antonio LL, Hardesty RA (1997) Secondary cleft deformities. Clinics in Plastic Surgery 24: 599–610.

Folkins J, Moon J (1991) Approaches to the study of speech production. In: Bardach J, Morris HL (eds) Multidisciplinary Management of Cleft Lip and Palate. Philadelphia: Saunders.

Gibbon F, Hardcastle W (1987) Articulatory description and treatment of 'lateral s' using electropalatography: a case study. British Journal of Disorders of Communication 22: 203–217.

Gibbon F, Hardcastle W (1989) Deviant articulation in a cleft palate child following late repair of the hard palate: a description and remediation procedure using electropalatography (EPG). Clinical Linguistics and Phonetics 3: 93–110.

Gibbon F, Crampin L, Hardcastle, Nairn M, Razzell R, Harvey L, Reynolds B (1998) Cleft Net (Scotland): A network for the treatment of cleft palate speech using EPG. International Journal of Language and Communication 33 (Supplement: Proceedings of the conference of the Royal College of Speech and Language).

Gibbons P, Bloomer HH (1958) The palatal lift: a supportive-type speech aid. Journal of Prosthetic Dentistry 8: 362–369.

Golding-Kushner K (1995) Treatment of articulation and resonance disorders associated with cleft palate and VPI. In: Shprintzen RJ, Bardach J (eds) Cleft Palate Speech Management: A Multidisciplinary Approach. St Louis: Mosby, pp. 327–349.

Golding-Kushner KJ, Cisneros G, LeBlanc E (1995) Speech Bulbs. In: Shprintzen RJ, Bardach J (eds) Cleft Palate Speech Management: A Multidisciplinary Approach. St Louis: Mosby, pp. 352–363.

Gonzalez JB, Aronson AE (1970) Palatal lift prosthesis for treatment of anatomic and neurologic palatopharyngeal insufficiency. Cleft Palate Journal 7: 91–103.

Grundy K. (1989) Developmental Speech Disorders. In: Grundy K (ed.) Linguistics in Clinical Practice. London: Taylor & Francis.

Grunwell P (1985) Phonological assessment of child speech (PACS).Windsor: NFER.

Grunwell P (1987) Clinical Phonology, 2nd edn. London: Croom Helm.

Grunwell P, Dive D (1988) Treating 'cleft palate speech': combining phonological techniques with traditional articulation therapy. Child Language, Teaching and Therapy 4: 193–210.

Grunwell P, Sell D, Harding A (1993) Describing cleft palate speech. In: Grunwell P (ed.) Analysing Cleft Palate Speech. London: Whurr, pp. 6–15.

Haines A, Jones R (1994) Implementing findings of research. British Medical Journal 308: 1488–1492.

Hall CD, Golding-Kushner KJ, Argamaso RV, Strauch B (1991) Pharyngeal flap surgery in adults. Cleft Palate–Craniofacial Journal 28: 179–182.

Hardcastle WJ, Gibbon F (1997) Electropalatography and its clinical applications. In: Ball MJ and Code C (eds) Instrumental Clinical Phonetics. London: Whurr Publishers, pp. 149–193.

Hardcastle W, Jones W, Knight C, Trudgeon A, Calder G (1989a) New developments in electropalatography: a state-of-the-art report. Clinical Linguistics and Phonetics 3: 1–38.

Hardcastle WJ, Morgan Barry R, Nunn M (1989b) Instrumental articulatory phonetics in assessment and remediation: case studies with the electropalatograph. In: Stengelhofen J (ed.) Cleft Palate: The Nature and Remediation of Communication Problems. Edinburgh: Churchill Livingstone, pp. 136–164.

Harding A, Grunwell P (1998) Active versus passive cleft-type speech characteristics: implications for surgery and therapy. International Journal of Language and Communication Disorders 33: 329–352.

Harding A, Harland K, Razzell R (1997) Cleft Audit Protocol for Speech (CAPS). Available from Speech/Language Therapy Department, St Andrew's Plastic Surgery Centre, Broomfield, Chelmsford, Essex.

Henningsson G, Hutters B (1997) Perceptual assessment of cleft palate speech, with special reference to minimum standards for inter-centre comparisons of speech outcome. Paper presented at 8th International Congress on Cleft Palate and related Craniofacial Anomalies, Singapore.

Henningsson G, Isberg A (1990) Oronasal fistulas and speech production. In: Bardach J, Morris HL (eds) Multidisciplinary Management of Cleft Lip and Palate. Philadelphia: Saunders, pp. 787–791.

Henningsson G, Isberg AM (1991) A cineradiographic study of velopharyngeal movements for deviant versus nondeviant articulation. Cleft Palate–Craniofacial Journal 28: 115–118.

Hirschberg J, Van Denmark DR (1997) A proposal for standardisation of speech and hearing evaluations to assess velopharyngeal function. Folia Phoniatrica et Logopaedica 49: 158–167.

Hoch L, Golding-Kushner K, Sadewitz VL, Shprintzen RJ (1986) Speech Therapy. Seminars in Speech and Language 7: 311–323.

Howell J, McCartney E (1990) Approaches to remediation. In: Grunwell P (ed.) Developmental Speech Disorders. Edinburgh: Churchill Livingstone.

Isberg AM, Henningsson G (1987) Influence of palatal fistulas on speech and resonance. Folia Phoniatrica 39: 183–191.

Israel JM, Cook TA, Blakeley RW (1993) The use of a temporary oral prosthesis to treat speech in velopharyngeal incompetence. Facial Plastic Surgery 9: 206–212.

Karnell MP, Rosenstein H, Fine L (1987) Nasal videoendoscopy in prosthetic management of palatopharyngeal dysfunction. Journal of Prosthetic Dentistry 58: 479–484.

Kawano M, Isshiki N, Honjo I, Kojima H, Kurata K, Tanokuchi F, Kido N, Isobe M (1997) Recent progress in treating patients with cleft palate. Folia Phoniatrica Logopaedica 49: 117–138.

Kummer AW, Strife JL, Grau WH, Creaghead NA, Lee L (1989) The effects of Le Fort 1 Osteotomy with maxillary movement on articulation, resonance and velopharyngeal function. Cleft Palate Journal 26(3): 193–200.

LaVelle WE, Hardy JC (1979) Palatal lift prostheses for treatment of palatopharyngeal incompetence. Journal of Prosthetic Dentistry 42: 308–315.

LeBlanc EM (1996) Fundamental principles in the speech management of cleft lip and palate. In: Cleft Lip and Palate with an Introduction to other Craniofacial Anomalies. Perspectives in Management. San Diego: Singular, pp. 75–84.

LeBlanc EM, Shprintzen RJ (1994) Speech and the maxillofacial complex. A structural-functional perspective for diagnosis and management. Oral and Maxillofacial Surgery in Children and Adolescents 6: 113–120.

Leeper HA, Sills PS, Charles DH (1993) Prosthodontic management of maxillofacial and palatal defects. In: Moller KT, Starr CD (eds) Cleft Palate. Interdisciplinary Issues and Treatment. Austin, TX: Pro-ed, pp. 145–188.

Lubker J, Moll K (1965) Simultaneous oral-nasal air flow measurements and cinefluorographic observations during speech production. Cleft Palate Journal 2: 257–242.

Marsh JL, Wray RC (1980) Speech prosthesis versus pharyngeal flap: a randomized evaluation of the management of velopharyngeal incompetency. Plastic and Reconstructive Surgery 65: 592–594.

McCarthy JG, Coccaro PJ, Schwartz MD (1979) Velopharyngeal function following maxillary advancement. Plastic and Reconstructive Surgery 64: 180–189.

McComb H (1989) Cleft lip and palate: new directions for research. Cleft Palate Journal 26: 145–147.

McGrath CO, Anderson MW (1991) Prosthetic treatment of velopharyngeal incompetence. In: Bardach J, Morris HL (eds) Multidisciplinary Management of Cleft Lip and Palate. Philadelphia: Saunders, pp. 809–814.

McWilliams BJ (1958) Articulation problems of a group of cleft palate adults. Journal of Speech and Hearing Research 1: 68–74.

McWilliams BJ and Phillips BJ (1979) Velopharyngeal Incompetence: Audio Seminars in Speech Pathology. Philadelphia: Saunders.

McWilliams BJ, Morris HL, Shelton RL (1990) Cleft Palate Speech, 2nd edn. Philadelphia: BC Decker.

Michi K, Suzuki N, Yamashita Y, Imai S (1986) Visual training and correction of articulation disorders by use of dynamic palatography: serial observation in a case of cleft palate. Journal of Speech and Hearing Disorders 51: 226–238.

Michi K, Yamashita Y, Imai S, Suzuki N, Yoshida H (1993) Role of visual feedback in the treatment for defective /s/ sounds in patients with cleft palate. Journal of Speech and Hearing Research 36: 277–285.

Moll KL (1968) Speech characteristics of individuals with cleft lip and palate. In: Spreistersbach DC, Sherman D (eds) Cleft Palate and Communication. New York: Academic Press, pp. 61–118.

Moon JB (1993) Evaluation of velopharyngeal function. In: Cleft Palate. Interdisciplinary Issues and Treatment. Austin, TX: Pro-ed, pp. 251-306.

Morgan Barry RA (1989) EPG from square one: an overview of electropalatography as an aid to therapy. Clinical Linguistics and Phonetics 3: 81-91.

Morley ME (1970) Cleft Palate and Speech, 7th edn. Baltimore: Williams & Wilkins.

Morris HL (1979) Evaluation of abnormal articulation patterns. In: Bzoch KR (ed.) Communicative Disorders Related to Cleft Lip and Palate. Boston: Little, Brown, pp. 192–201.

Morris HL, Spreistersbach DC, Darley FL (1961) An articulation test for assessing competency of velopharyngeal closure. Journal of Speech and Hearing Research 4: 48–55.

Noordoff MS, Kuo J, Wang F, Huang H, Witzell MA (1987) Development of articulation before delayed hard-palate closure in children with cleft palate: a cross-sectional study. Plastic and Reconstructive Surgery 80: 518–524.

Okazaki K, Satoh K, Kato M, Iwanami M, Ohokubo F, Kobayashi K (1993) Speech and velopharyngeal function following maxillary advancement in patients with cleft lip and palate. Annals of Plastic Surgery 30(4): 304–311.

Pannbacker M, Lass NJ, Middleton GF, Crutchfield E, Trapp DS, Scherbick KA (1984) Current clinical practices in the assessment of velopharyngeal closure. Cleft Palate Journal 21: 33–37.

Peterson-Falzone SJ (1995) Speech outcomes in adolescents with cleft lip and palate. Cleft Palate–Craniofacial Journal 32(2): 125–128.

Philips BJ, Bzoch KR (1969) Reliability of judgements of articulation of cleft palate speakers. Cleft Palate Journal 6: 24–34.

Philips BJ, Harrison RJ (1969) Articulation patterns of preschool cleft palate children. Cleft Palate Journal 6: 245–253.

Razzell RE, Harding A (1995) A review of cleft palate speech assessment methods in the UK. Paper presented at International Association of Logopaedists and Phoniatrists, Cairo.

Riski JE (1995) Speech assessment of adolescents. Cleft Palate–Craniofacial Journal 32: 109–113.

Ruscello D (1982) A selected review of palatal training procedures. Cleft Palate Journal 22: 181–193.

Ruscello DM, Tekieli ME, Sickels JE (1985) Speech production before and after orthognathic surgery: a review. Oral Surgery, Oral Medicine, Oral Pathology 59: 10–14.

Russell VJR, Sell DA (1998) Training video of therapy techniques for children with cleft palate and/or velopharyngeal dysfunction. Available from the Department of Medical Illustration, Great Ormond Street Hospital.

Schendel SA, Oeschlaeger M, Wolford LM, Epker BN (1979) Velopharyngeal anatomy and maxillary advancement. Journal of Oral and Maxillofacial Surgery 7: 116–124.

Scherer NJ, D'Antonio LL (1995) Parent questionnaire for screening early language development in children with cleft palate. Cleft Palate–Craniofacial Journal 32: 7–13.

Scheuerle J (1993) Cleft palate speech – an opinion. Journal of Craniofacial Surgery 4: 122–123.

Schwarz C, Gruner E (1976) Logopaedic findings following advancement of the maxilla. Journal of Maxillofacial Surgery 4: 40–55.

Sell D (1992) Speech in Sri Lankan cleft palate subjects with delayed palatoplasty. Unpublished PhD, De Montfort University.

Sell D, Ma L (1996) A model for the management of velopharyngeal dysfunction. British Journal of Oral and Maxillofacial Surgery 34: 357–363.

Sell D, Ma L, James DR, Mars M, Sherif PD (1993) A pilot study to investigate the effects of transpalatal Le Fort 1 maxillary osteotomy on velopharyngeal function in cleft palate patients. Paper presented at Seventh International Congress on Cleft Palate and Related Craniofacial Anomalies, Broadbeach, Australia.

Sell D, Harding A, Grunwell P (1994) GOS.SP.ASS. A screening assessment of cleft palate speech. European Journal of Disorders of Communication 29: 1–15.

Sell D, Mars M, Worrell E (1997) Speech bulb treatment for velopharyngeal dysfunction. Paper presented at the annual meeting of the Craniofacial Society of Great Britain, Writtle, Essex.

Sell D, Harding A, Grunwell P (1998) Training Video GOS.SP.ASS (98): Speech assessment profile for children with cleft palate and/or velopharyngeal dysfunction. Available from the Department of Medical Illustration, Great Ormond Street NHS Trust, London.

Sell D, Harding A, Grunwell P (1999) Revised GOS.SP.ASS (98): Speech assessment for children with cleft palate and/or velopharyngeal dysfunction. International Journal of Disorders of Communication 34(1): 7–33.

Sell D, Grunwell P, Mildinhall S, Murphy T, Cornish TC, Bearn D, Shaw WC, Murray J, Williams A, Sandy J (2000) Cleft lip and palate care in the United Kingdom (UK) – The Clinical Standards Advisory Group (CSAG) Study. Part 3 - Speech outcomes. Cleft Palate-Craniofacial Journal (in press).

Shprintzen RJ, Lencione RM, McCall GN, Skolnick ML (1974) A three dimensional cinefluoroscopic analysis of velopharyngeal closure during speech and nonspeech activities in normals. Cleft Palate Journal 11: 412–428.

Shprintzen RJ, Lewin ML, Croft CB, Daniller AI, Argamaso RV, Ship AG, Strauch B (1979) A comprehensive study of pharyngeal flap surgery: tailor made flaps. Cleft Palate Journal 16: 46–55.

Shriberg LD, Kwiatkowski J (1982) Phonological disorders II: a conceptual framework for management. Journal of Speech and Hearing Disorders 47: 242–256.

Siegel-Sadewitz V, Shprintzen R (1982) Nasopharyngoscopy of the normal velopharyngeal sphincter: an experiment of biofeedback. Cleft Palate Journal 19: 194–200.

Sommerlad BC, Henley M, Birch M, Harland K, Moiemen N, Boorman JG (1994) Cleft palate re-repair –a clinical and radiographic study of 32 consecutive cases. British Journal of Plastic Surgery 47: 406–410.

Starr CD (1993) Behavioural approaches to treating velopharyngeal closure and nasality. In: Cleft Palate. Interdisciplinary Issues and Treatment. Austin, TX: Pro-ed, pp. 337–356.

Sweeney T, Grunwell P, Sell D (1996) Describing types of nasality. Paper presented at the annual meeting of the Craniofacial Society of Great Britain, Egham.

Sweeney T, Sell D, Grunwell P (1999a) The relationship between perceptual ratings of nasality, the nature of the speech sample and nasometry. Paper presented at the European Craniofacial Meeting, Manchester.

Sweeney T, Sell D, Grunwell P (1999b) The relationship between nasal airflow errors and pressure/flow measurements. Paper presented at the European Craniofacial Meeting, Manchester.

Trost JE (1981) Articulatory additions to the classical description of the speech of persons with cleft palate. Cleft Palate Journal 18: 193–203.

Trost-Cardamone JE, Bernthal JE (1993) Articulation assessment procedures and treatment decisions. In: Cleft Palate. Interdisciplinary Issues and Treatment. Austin, TX: Pro-ed, pp. 307–335.

Tudor C, Selley W (1974) A palatal training appliance and a visual aid for use in the treatment of hypernasal speech. British Journal of Disorders of Communication 9: 117–122.

Turner GE, Williams WN (1991) Fluoroscopy and nasoendoscopy in designing palatal lift prostheses. Journal of Prosthetic Dentistry 66: 63–71.

Van Denmark DR (1964) Misarticulations and listener judgements of the speech of individuals with cleft palates. Cleft Palate Journal 1: 232–245.

Van Demark DR (1971) Clinical research methodology in evaluating the therapeutic process. Cleft Palate Journal 8: 26–35.

Van Demark DR (1974) Assessment of articulation for children with cleft palate. Cleft Palate Journal 11: 200–208.

Van Demark DR, Hardin MA (1990) Speech therapy for the child with cleft lip and palate. In: Bardach J, Morris HL (eds) Multidisciplinary Management of Cleft Lip and Palate. Philadelphia: Saunders, pp. 799–805.

Volin RA (1993) Clinical applications of biofeedback. American Speech-Language-Hearing Association 35: 43–44.

Warren D (1975) The determination of velopharyngeal incompetence by aerodynamic and acoustical techniques. Clinics in Plastic Surgery 2: 299–304.

Warren D (1979) PERCI: A method for rating palatal efficiency. Cleft Palate Journal 16: 279–285.

Watzke I, Turvey TA, Warren DW, Dalston R (1990) Alterations in velopharyngeal function after maxillary advancement in cleft palate patients. American Association of Oral and Maxillofacial Surgeons 48: 685–689.

Whitehill TL, Stokes SF, Man YHY (1996) Electropalatography treatment with an adult with late repair of cleft palate. Cleft Palate–Craniofacial Journal 33: 160–165.

Witt PD, Rozelle AA, Marsh JL, Marty-Grames L, Muntz HR, Gay WD, Pilgram TK (1995) Do palatal lift prostheses stimulate velopharyngeal neuromuscular activity? Cleft Palate–Craniofacial Journal 32: 469–475.

Witzel MA (1981) Orthognathic defects and surgical correction: The effects on speech and velopharyngeal function. Doctoral dissertation. The University of Pittsburgh, PA.

Witzel MA (1991) Speech evaluation and treatment. Oral and Maxillofacial Surgery Clinics of North America 3: 501–516.

Witzel MA (1993) Cleft Lip and Palate and Craniofacial Treatment. American Speech-Language Hearing Association, pp. 42–43.

Witzel MA, Munro IR (1977) Velopharyngeal insufficiency after maxillary advancement. Cleft Palate Journal 14: 176–180.

Witzel MA, Wu J (1989) Compensatory articulation – techniques for assessment and treatment. Paper presented at the Sixth International Congress on Cleft Palate and Related Craniofacial Anomalies, Jerusalem, Israel.

Witzel MA, Ross, RB, Munro IR (1980) Articulation before and after facial osteotomy. Journal of Maxillofacial Surgery 8: 195–202.

Witzel M, Tobe J, Salyer K (1989) The use of videonasopharyngoscopy for biofeedback therapy in adults after pharyngeal flap surgery. Cleft Palate Journal 26: 29–34.

Wolfaardt JF, Wilson FB, Rochet A, McPhee L (1993) An appliance based approach to the management of palatopharyngeal incompetency: a clinical pilot project. Journal of Prosthetic Dentistry 69: 186–195.

Wu J, Chen YR, Noordhoff MS (1997) Total management of speech problems in adult cleft palate patients. In: Scientific Programme Summary and Book of Abstracts. Singapore. Eighth International Congress on Cleft Palate and Related Craniofacial Anomalies.

Ysunza A, Pamplona M, Femat T (1997) Videonasopharyngoscopy as an instrument for visual biofeedback during speech in cleft palate patients. Paper presented at the Eighth International Congress on Cleft Palate and Related Craniofacial Anomalies.

CHAPTER 17

Assessment and Surgical Management of Velopharyngeal Dysfunction

N.S.G. MERCER AND R.W. PIGOTT

Introduction

Easily intelligible speech requires that a stream of air is either forced past the tongue and palate, teeth and lips or allowed to pass through the nose, so that they may modulate it into the sounds we can recognize. To provide these alternative air streams, the velopharyngeal isthmus must be able to close firmly and open rapidly. Failure to produce adequate oral pressure can prevent the production of normal sounds, resulting in abnormal articulation. Intelligibility is impaired and patients can experience frustration, loss of confidence and reduced achievement. Even for those individuals who do not substitute inappropriate sounds, hypernasality, loss of volume and reduced continuity of speech can impair the quality of life. The change in a child who has been successfully treated can be dramatic. While the commonest cause of loss of oral air pressure is disordered function of the velopharyngeal isthmus, air can also be lost through oronasal fistulae.

The terminology of disorders of velopharyngeal function in speech (Pigott, 1994) remains unresolved and for simplicity will be referred to in this chapter under the commonly used acronym VPI (velopharyngeal insufficiency).

In velopharyngeal dysfunction from whatever cause, air resonates in the nose and nasopharynx when this should not normally occur. This is called hypernasal resonance (see Grunwell and Sell, Chapter 5), as opposed to reduced or hyponasal resonance which is heard in the common cold or where adenoidal hyperplasia reduces the nasopharyngeal space. Frequently air can be heard hissing, bubbling or snorting from the nose (nasal escape, turbulence or emission). Patients may also grimace by using their nasal or facial musculature in an attempt to prevent air escaping down the nose (see Sell and Grunwell, Chapter 16).

The act of closure between palate and pharynx normally takes place out of sight above the palate, so oral examination is of limited value in assessing the size, site or timing of a failure to close. The gap size can vary from a pinhole to a totally immobile velopharynx resulting in a large defect.

Correction of VPI is usually surgical. The aim of the operation is to correct the specific defect in the individual, obturating the defect which remains on attempted velopharyngeal closure but leaving a sufficient resting gap to permit nasal resonance to occur normally on the sounds 'm', 'n' and 'ng', to allow comfortable nasal breathing while eating and sleeping, and normal drainage of the nasal cavity. Excessively obstructive operations must be avoided. In addition, surgery will fail to produce a total correction if muscular activity of the palate or pharyngeal walls is absent or mistimed. Recognition of these groups of patients prior to offering surgery is important for, whilst reducing the resting velopharyngeal gap may be beneficial, a normal speech result is unlikely to be achieved (Davison et al., 1990).

Assessment of the patient for consideration of surgery is complex and must be carried out by a specialist speech and language therapist and surgeon together. Awareness of the specific characteristics of each patient and of the procedures available which have the potential to correct the disorder offers the best chance of success without over-treatment and allows the surgeon and speech and language therapist to provide the patient and family with a realistic prognosis. In some situations surgery will not be necessary. For example, when a patient has intermittent closure, speech therapy alone may be effective. In others, surgery will be contraindicated (e.g. in the presence of tonsillar hypertrophy and some cardiac and neurological conditions). A prosthesis can sometimes help in these cases (see Griffiths, Chapter 22, and Sell and Grunwell, Chapter 16). Speech therapy may be required before a valid assessment of velopharyngeal function can be made, for example when a patient only has consonants which do not require velopharyngeal closure during speech. This may occur when all sounds are articulated in the glottis and oropharynx (e.g. glottal stops and pharyngeal fricatives). However, therapy prior to surgery should not be continued if patients are unable to make progress, because they are likely to become discouraged and their cooperation will decline (see Sell and Grunwell, Chapter 16). It is sometimes necessary to operate and give additional speech therapy postoperatively to correct residual articulatory errors. If patients have normal intelligibility but have residual traces of nasal escape they may require no further treatment if the patient and family are not concerned. To report results of surgery simply in terms of 'speech improvement' is not now acceptable scientifically and ratings of nasal escape and nasal resonance should be cited together with articulation and intelligibility (Sell et al., 1994, 1999; Hirschberg and Van Demark, 1997; see Sell and Grunwell, Chapter 16).

Pharyngoplasty rates have often been reported as an assessment of outcome after primary palatal surgery, but they say as much about the levels of expectation of patient and family, surgeon and speech and language therapist as they do about surgical outcome.

Functional anatomy

There are many detailed descriptions of the anatomy of the velopharyngeal isthmus (see Sommerlad, Chapter 3). During closure of the isthmus the levator veli palatini muscles contract, lifting and lengthening the soft palate upwards and backwards. The palate may be further lengthened by the horizontal fibres of palatopharyngeus. Lateral and posterior pharyngeal wall movement contribute to closure to a variable extent (Figure 17.1). In addition, contraction of the musculus uvulae may assist closure (Pigott, 1987) by adding to the bulk of the midline dorsal ridge over the levator eminence and also probably by lifting the free border of the palate into deeper contact with the posterior wall (Kuehn et al., 1988).

The introduction of the complementary investigations of nasopharyngoscopy (Pigott 1969, Pigott et al., 1969) and multiview videofluoroscopy (Skolnick, 1970) allowed three-dimensional imaging of the isthmus to be obtained during connected speech. Croft et al. (1981) compared closure patterns between subjects with normal and cleft palates. They showed that in normal subjects 55% had a coronal closure pattern (palate to posterior pharyngeal wall across most or all of the isthmus) but that this was reduced to 45% in patients with a cleft palate and that there was a higher incidence of the next commonest, sphincteric, pattern of closure in subjects with cleft palate. Asymmetrical closure attempts and bilateral defects were also noted (Pigott et al., 1969, Witzel and Posnick, 1989). Different levels of complete or incomplete closure of the velopharyngeal isthmus were reported by Shprintzen et al. (1983; Shprintzen, 1986) with maximal lateral wall movement observed on frontal X-rays to occur at a variable level below the plane of the hard palate (Shprintzen et al., 1975). Passavant's ridge (Figure 17.2) is the visible posterior part of a sphincteric contraction of superior constrictor and is believed to be a compensatory movement (Calnan, 1954, 1957; Finkelstein et al., 1993b).

Aetiology of VPI

The aetiology of VPI has been extensively discussed by Trost-Cardamone (1989). She defined local structural, neurological and behavioural diagnoses. Overlapping categories occur such as hypoplasia of the soft palate in some neurological conditions and residual phoneme-specific errors of misarticulation after correction of VPI.

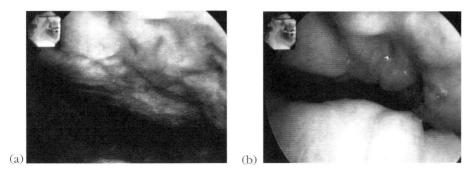

(i) Coronal closure. Maximal palatal excursion with minimal lateral wall adduction in attempted closure. (a) At rest. (b) On attempted closure.

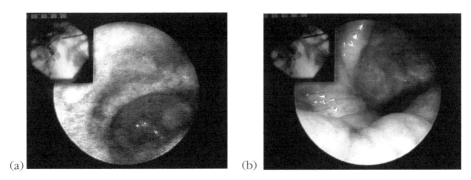

(ii) Sphincteric closure. Moderate movement of the palatal, lateral and posterior walls. (a) At rest. (b) On closure.

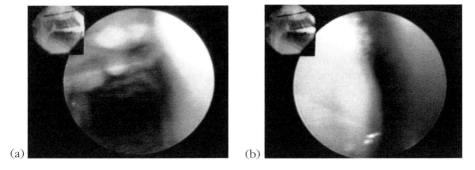

(iii) Sagittal closure. Maximal lateral wall adduction with minimal palatal excursion to achieve closure. (a) At rest. (b) On closure.

Figure 17.1. Endoscopic views with an inset simultaneous lateral videofluoroscopic view showing different types of closure of the velopharyngeal isthmus.

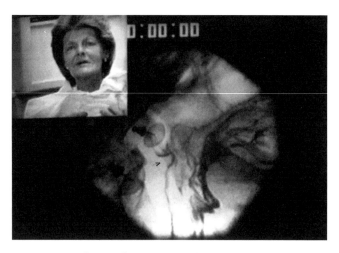

Figure 17.2. Passavant's ridge on the posterior pharyngeal wall shown on lateral coated X-ray.

The analysis of 100 cases of patients treated for VPI reported in 1982 (Albery et al., 1982) showed 28 had repaired complete clefts of the palate, 25 clefts of the secondary palate, 11 submucous clefts, 23 with pharyngeal disproportion and 13 were of neurological aetiology. By comparison, the diagnoses for 100 consecutive referrals in 1992–1993 (Pigott, 1994) were 24 overt cleft palates, 14 submucous clefts, 32 neurological, 8 post adenoidectomy, 4 hypoplasia of the adenoids, 3 tonsillar hypertrophy and the remainder included trauma, post tumour resection or radiotherapy, post infection, sarcoid, scleroderma and 4 cases only of pharyngeal disproportion. Six patients were inappropriate referrals and the velopharyngeal mechanism closed normally. The marked drop in the proportion of patients with cleft palate in the second series is only in part due to improvement in results from primary surgery, and mainly due to improved awareness of other diagnostic categories. A number of cases included under the portmanteau of pharyngeal disproportion in the first series would now be allocated to another category. Most of the repaired clefts showed a midline gutter on the dorsum of the palate on nasopharyngoscopy, as is seen in a submucous cleft of the palate. Various combinations of palate, lateral and posterior wall movement resulted in coronal, sphincteric or sagittal patterns of attempted closure, and asymmetrical movement was occasionally seen.

Almost half of the group of 32 'neurological' patients were misdiagnosed prior to investigation by nasopharyngoscopy and videofluoroscopy. These patients were shown to have a flat upper surface to their soft palate, a sign of an occult submucous palate. An important subgroup in this category were those with velocardiofacial syndrome (see below).

In the remainder of the 'neurological' group, the muscles often appeared hypoplastic, with a long thin palate, the movement of which was slow or of poor amplitude with a failure of the posterior and lateral walls to close on either side of a normal, midline dorsal eminence.

Velocardiofacial syndrome

Sedlackova described a group of patients with submucous cleft palate and an associated seventh cranial nerve involvement (Sedlackova, 1955, 1967, 1973). She suggested that there was dual innervation of levator veli palatini. Nishio et al. (1976) lent this support by sectioning the seventh nerve inter-cranially in rhesus monkeys which resulted in reduced lift of the soft palate. The nerve fibres responsible were traced to the greater superficial petrosal nerve. The patients are characterized by hypodynamic facies associated with a hypodynamic palate and pharynx. Others (Calnan, 1959; Shprintzen et al., 1978) have reported patients with these features of a syndrome which is now described as the velocardiofacial syndrome (see Lees, Chapter 6). Expression of the syndrome is variable and not all patients with a cardiac defect will have a submucous cleft nor will all those with a submucous cleft palate have a cardiac defect.

The syndrome is frequently associated with characteristic facies (a square looking lower nose, small nostrils, mouth and palpebral apertures) which makes a provisional 'spot' diagnosis possible, a submucous cleft palate and a hypodynamic pharynx, which in combination can result in a large velopharyngeal gap. Repair of the palate does not necessarily enable velopharyngeal closure to occur and a pharyngoplasty may be required. The surgeon must, however, remember that these patients may have medially displaced internal carotid arteries which can be seen pulsating under the posterior pharyngeal wall. Ross et al. (1996) confirm that the pulsations can be seen on nasopharyngoscopy and conclude that a superi-orly based pharyngoplasty would be safe in 52% of cases, 28% would require a 'customized' flap and in 20% there would be a severe risk of damage to the vessels. Mitnick et al. (1996) have shown that in a series of 20 patients all had anomalies of the carotid arteries, but it must be borne in mind that 10% of the normal population may have medially displaced or 'C' shaped carotid arteries (Mercer and MacCarthy, 1995a). There have been no reports of damage to the vessels during surgery, presumably because they are covered by the carotid sheath, but care must be taken in the planning of these patients' surgical treatment. Apart from concerns about the carotid arteries, the presence of a hypodynamic pharynx and a large velopharyn-geal gap makes a successful outcome difficult to achieve. Complete closure would require a wide pharyngeal flap which would almost obstruct the nasopharynx, increasing the risk of postoperative obstructive symptoms, including sleep apnoea. If there is a coexisting cardiac problem such symptoms are dangerous and must be avoided. Witt et al. (1999) report a series of nineteen cases of VCF syndrome in which eighteen were managed successfully by a sphincter pharyngoplasty.

Post-adenoidectomy VPI

VPI occurs in 1 out of 1500 patients who undergo adenoidectomy, of whom 50% will require further surgery (Donnelly, 1994). The VPI occurs by the unmasking of an underlying velopharyngeal problem such as a 'box' like pharynx in which the palate is unable to reach the posterior wall, or a submucous cleft palate, or by leaving behind an irregular adenoid remnant or by large tonsils physically obturating the velopharyngeal isthmus (Ren et al., 1995). Half of the children who develop VPI will require surgical intervention but conservative treatment should be continued for a year to allow the possibility of spontaneous resolution (Fernandes et al., 1996). Children should always be examined for the stigmata of submucous cleft palate before adenoidectomy. Surgery for patients who have large velopharyngeal gaps or who fail to respond to speech therapy following adenoidectomy should be planned as for cleft related VPI. It is imperative that the patient and family are carefully counselled if a posterior pharyngeal flap is required because of the potential for complications such as snoring, mouth breathing, catarrh and difficulty in blowing the nose, the same symptoms for which the adenoidectomy was undertaken (Lesavoy et al., 1996). Occasionally, the adenoids can be congenitally absent and very large tonsils can physically obstruct the palate because they prolapse through the isthmus resulting in a characteristic 'hot potato' voice (Finkelstein et al., 1993a, Kummer et al., 1993).

Investigation of VPI

There are several indirect methods of studying VPI. Analysis of pressure and airflow studies and acoustic analysis give confirmation of speech assessments performed by a specialist speech and language therapist and can give objective information about the results of treatment. However, they do not provide information that is valuable to the surgeon when planning which operation to choose for a patient (Hutters and Brondsted, 1992; Warren et al., 1993, 1994; Hinton and Warren, 1995; Tassone et al., 1995; Vallino-Napoli and Montgomery, 1997; Fischer and Swank, 1997). MRI scanning may prove valuable in the future but still remains too slow for real time VPI studies, and the patient must lie down rather than sit (McGowan et al., 1992, Yamawaki et al., 1993.). The development of non-invasive techniques is the way forward in the investigation of VPI, particularly of the very young child. However, at the present time only nasopharyngoscopy and multiview videofluoroscopy provide direct evidence of the shape, size and range of movement of each of the walls of the isthmus. The two investigations are complementary, endoscopy showing what structures are involved and radiology showing how much movement takes place. The former is largely qualitative, provided that the correct viewing point and angle of view are achieved. Videofluoroscopy can be quantitative provided that some form of scale of magnification is included and the interpretation of the image is correct.

Nasopharyngoscopy

Pigott et al. first described the use of nasopharyngoscopy for the investigation of VPI in 1969. Details of techniques, instrumentation, problems and pitfalls of endoscopy have been published by a number of authors, including Pigott and Makepeace (1982) and Shprintzen and Golding-Kushner (1989). Instrument quality continues to improve. The 3.5 mm diameter 70 degree oblique Storz-Hopkins rigid endoscope gives the best view but can be difficult to pass in the presence of gross septal deviation. A 2.2 mm rigid nasendoscope is also available, but is fragile and gives a restricted view. Fibreoptic endoscopes (e.g. Olympus ENFP) are easier to pass. End viewing instruments are commercially available at the present time but it may sometimes be difficult to position these correctly to obtain a good view, particularly in the older patient with a horizontal closure plane. A 2 mm flexible scope (Wolff) is even easier to pass and is more reassuring to small children, but its relatively low light-carrying capacity makes it less valuable in a large nasopharynx. The endoscopes and recording equipment used in our clinic (the Bristol Cleft and Craniofacial Unit) are shown in Figure 17.3. The side-viewing Olympus flexible endoscope has been found useful by A.C.H. Watson (personal communication) for the older patient but it can be difficult to elevate the tip sufficiently to see the full circumference of the pharynx at the attempted plane of closure in the restricted space of the small child's nasopharynx.

The inability to judge size and movement, wide angle distortion and oblique view distortion are problems with all types of endoscopes. Although correction factors for these distortions have been worked out, they do not provide a ready basis for clinical practice (Kouwenhoven et al., 1993), and endoscopy cannot be safely considered a quantitative technique.

Multiview radiology

The technique described by Skolnick and co-workers (1970, 1973, 1975) has gained widespread acceptance. The videofluoroscopic views show movement; only limited information can be gained from still photographs

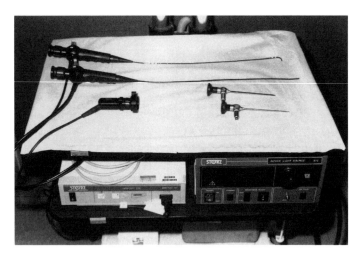

Figure 17.3. Storz camera, xenon light system and endoscopes. From top to bottom: Wolff 3 mm end-viewing flexible, Wolff 2 mm end-viewing flexible, Storz 3.6 mm rigid and Storz 2.2 mm rigid.

taken from the video monitor. The lateral view is most valuable for assessing the range of palate and posterior wall movement, including Passavant's ridge formation (Figures 17.2, 17.4). Frontal views demonstrate the extent of lateral wall motion at the level of the arch of the atlas, where most pharyngeal flaps will be sited. The submento-vertex (basal) view gives an equivalent image to the 70 degree endoscopic view in an adult but the fronto-occipital (Townes) view is used in children with a relatively horizontal isthmus (Figure 17.5). Oblique views have been said to be helpful, but we have found that they are not required when endoscopy is carried out at the same time. Very occasionally, lateral X-rays, taken first with the head neutral and then hyperextended, may reveal restricted palatal lift in a case where tightness of the posterior faucial pillars is suspected, such as after tonsillectomy.

The plain radiological view can be enhanced by the use of a contrast medium (Figure 17.6). Barium gives the best contrast but it can pool in crevices and cast confusing double shadows. Improved electronics now give better images, reducing the need for contrast and the radiation exposure to the patient. In our clinic barium is now used only when the plane of closure is obscure, for example when evaluating a patient who has persistent VPI after a pharyngoplasty. It can, however, prove impossible to align the ports to the X-ray beam after pharyngeal flap surgery and in this situation we find that endoscopy is more reliable (Sinclair et al., 1982). Training in the procedure and interpretation of the findings is required (D'Antonio et al., 1993).

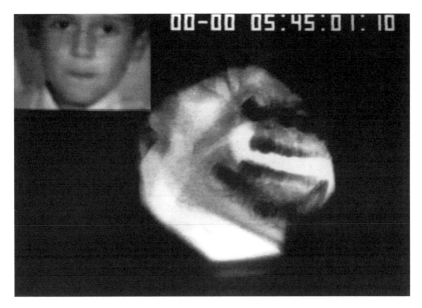

(a)

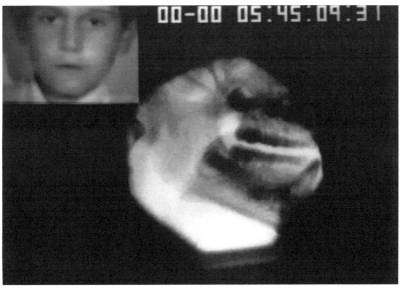

(b)

Figure 17.4. Stills from lateral videofluoroscopy, without barium. (a) At rest. (b) Maximum palatal elevation.

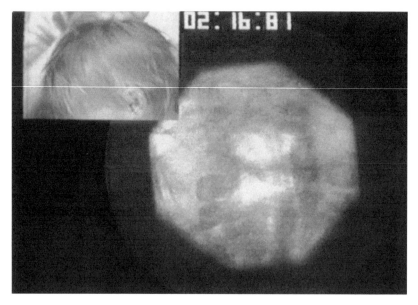

(a)

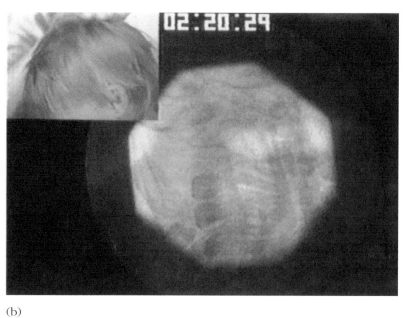

(b)

Figure 17.5. Fronto-occipital view in a child with a repaired cleft lip and palate. (a) At rest. (b) On closure.

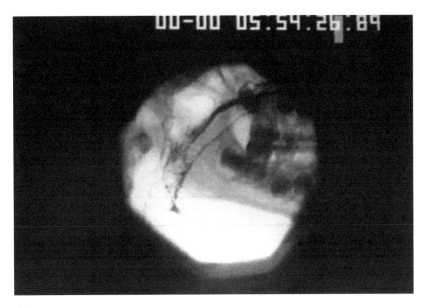

(a)

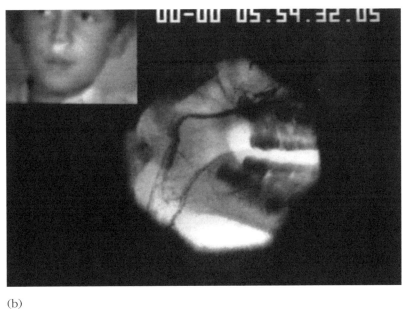

(b)

Figure 17.6. Stills from lateral videofluoroscopy, using barium. (a) At rest. (b) Maximum palatal elevation.

The magnification of the X-ray image can be established by placing an object of known size in the field. If synchronous nasopharyngoscopy is used the diameter of the nasopharyngoscope can be used, allowing direct measurements to be made from the videofluoroscopic image. Sommerlad et al. (1994a) have devised an ingenious piece of apparatus using a children's Viewmaster both to keep the child's attention and its head still at the same time. A wire ring of known circumference (2 cm) positioned on the midline of the apparatus enables absolute measurements to be made.

Either the screening facility of an X-ray department or an image intensifier can be used for the investigation. We advocate the use of simultaneous videofluoroscopy and nasopharyngoscopy and find the mobility provided by the C arm image intensifier useful in obtaining a correctly orientated view. A Philips BV25 machine is used in our clinic. A suitable chair and recording equipment are required (Figure 17.7).

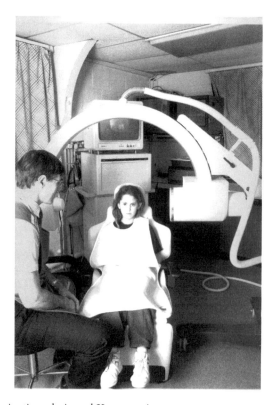

Figure 17.7. Examination chair and X-ray equipment.

The technique of recording investigations simultaneously

We perform simultaneous recording on videotape using a set sequence of speech sounds and views. Following speech assessment, the nasal cavity and nasopharynx are anaesthetized. Convenient methods are by a spray of 4% lignocaine and 0.5% phenylephrine or by direct application of the mixture using a modified suction catheter and cotton wool, depending on the patient's preference. It must be remembered that both endoscopy and radiology are invasive and the minimum time required to obtain adequate views for formulating a treatment plan must be used. The combined investigation gives a radiation dose equivalent to three skull films. A standardized speech sample must be obtained in all patients. Comparisons between pre- and postoperative status can then be made.

The images produced by endoscopy and videofluoroscopy should give detailed information on the movement of the velum and pharyngeal walls and of the site, size and shape of any gap.

Choice of operation

It is not uncommon to find that a surgeon was trained in and has undertaken one type of operation for virtually all patients, and other operations rarely if ever. The majority of defects will benefit from any of the popular operations performed competently but the same design of operation done by the same surgeon does not always produce the predicted result. One reason for this is the differing nature of the velopharyngeal gap from patient to patient.

Tailoring the operation to the patient

Since it is now reasonably simple to establish the size and shape of the defect and the range of movement of any component of the isthmus, it should be possible to choose an operation that has the best potential to correct the deficiency in any individual patient. Fitting the operation to the patient in this way seems logical and attractive in theory and ought to reduce the numbers of failures. However, more evidence is needed to establish whether this is indeed the case.

Palate re-repair

Undoubtedly, the most physiological operation is to improve palatal function without interfering with the lateral and posterior pharyngeal walls and avoiding constriction of the resting isthmus. This may be indicated if there is evidence of a poorly repaired levator veli palatini in a repaired cleft palate or an unrepaired submucous cleft palate, particularly if the velopharyngeal gap is small. Sommerlad's approach to re-repairing the palate (Sommerlad et al., 1994b, Sommerlad, 1995) is a logical and effective procedure. An alternative procedure in this situation is a Furlow palate repair, as recommended by Chen et al. (1994). Both procedures can be expected to correct a residual dorsal midline gutter on the nasal surface of the palate which can occur after cleft palate repair (Figure 17.8).

Pharyngoplasty

Unfortunately, there are some patients for whom palate re-repair is not appropriate, particularly those whose VPI is not due to a cleft and those with severe tissue deficiency. For these patients, whose palatal function cannot be adequately improved, a number of operations have been devised which alter the shape of the nasopharynx to reduce its size and make closure easier. These operations are called pharyngoplasties. They can be divided into two main types: midline pharyngeal flaps and sphincter pharyngoplasties.

Midline pharyngeal flaps

These involve the raising of a flap of muscle and mucosa from the posterior pharyngeal wall and attaching it to the soft palate to form a bridge

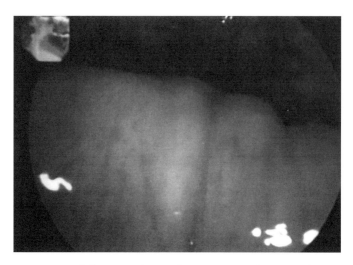

Figure 17.8. Diastasis of the musculus uvulae seen on endoscopy after a palate repair indicating conversion of an overt cleft palate into a submucous cleft.

separating the naso- from the oropharynx. The flap may be inferiorly or superiorly based (Schoenborn, 1876; Rosenthal, 1932; Sanvenero-Roselli, 1933) and may be set into the palate in a variety of ways. It may be lined with palatal flaps in an attempt to prevent tubing and shrinkage, or the procedure may be combined with palatal lengthening (Honig, 1967) (Figure 17.9).

In the presence of poor palatal movement, midline pharyngeal flaps may allow complete closure of the velopharyngeal isthmus if there is sufficient lateral wall movement (i.e. attempted sagittal or sphincteric closure) to close or approximate to the flap where it spans the velopharynx (Figure 17.10). If there is little or no lateral wall movement (i.e. attempted coronal closure), it is unlikely that a midline pharyngeal flap will achieve competence unless it is made so wide that it will cause obstruction of the airway.

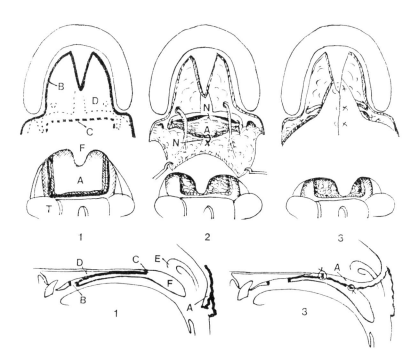

Figure 17.9. Modified Honig pharyngoplasty.
1. Superiorly-based posterior wall muco-muscular flap (A) incised. Hard palate incision marked in continuous line (B). Nasal layer incision (C) about 1 cm behind hard palate (D) marked in dotted line (T) tongue (F) Uvula (E) Eustachian cushion.
2. Mucoperiosteal flaps turned back. Nasal layer (N) divided. Tip of pharyngeal flap sutured to anterior cut edge of nasal layer. Palatal oral layer sutured to pharyngeal flap about 1.5–2.0 cm from tip.
3. Oral layer mucoperiosteal flaps sutured to central v about 1.5–2.0 cm back.

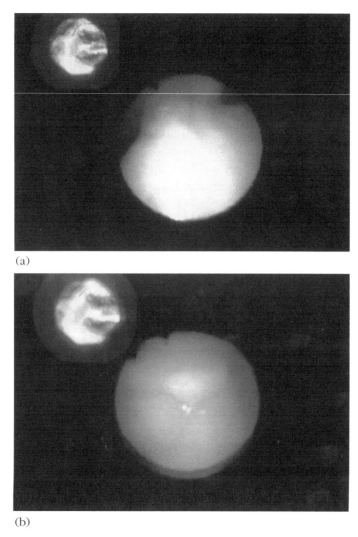

(a)

(b)

Figure 17.10. The appearance of a superiorly based pharyngeal flap on endoscopy. (a) Open. (b) Closed.

Sphincter pharyngoplasty

An alternative approach is to reduce the size of the nasopharynx by raising superiorly based flaps from the posterior pillars of the fauces and lateral pharyngeal walls and insetting them into the posterior pharyngeal wall (Hynes, 1953, 1967). Orticochea in 1968 emphasized the inclusion of the palatopharyngeus muscles and demonstrated that they could achieve complete sphincteric closure of the resulting aperture. Jackson and Silverton (1977) set the flaps into the posterior wall as high as possible, as described originally by Hynes (Figures 17.11, 17.12). Georgantopolou et al. (1996) have shown that part of the success of the sphincter pharyngoplasty can be due to an improvement in the range of palatal movement by altering the vector of the palatopharyngeus which normally acts as a depressor of the palate. Some surgeons use a sphincter pharyngoplasty for all patients with VPI but, in the context of selective surgery, it is more appropriate than a midline posterior pharyngeal flap for patients with a coronal pattern of attempted closure.

Patients with little or no movement of the palate or pharyngeal walls would require an operation that completely separates the nasopharynx from the oropharynx to eliminate the nasal emission of air; however, this would cause unacceptable obstruction (Davison et al., 1990). The aim must be a compromise, and these patients and their parents must be made aware that the prognosis for 'normal' velopharyngeal function is poor, though worthwhile improvement can be achieved. A speech bulb which can be removed at night may be the best option for many of these patients, particularly if they have a 'neurological' diagnosis (Shifman et al., 2000), if a cleft palate has been repaired as part of the Robin sequence where obstructive sleep apnoea is more likely (Abramson et al., 1997), or where there is a severe shortage of tissue as, for example, after cancer treatment (see Sell and Grunwell, Chapter 16).

Patients in whom midline contact of the palate leaves bilateral defects, or who have asymmetrical closure, may be successfully treated by a modified Hynes or Orticochea sphincter pharyngoplasty, or by an offset pharyngeal flap.

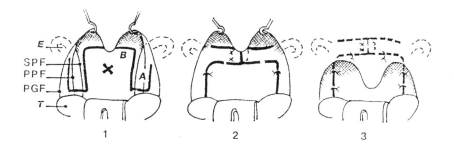

Figure 17.11. Modified Hynes pharyngoplasty.
1. Flaps outlined. X, Arch of atlas vertebra; E, Eustachian tube cartilage; A, superiorly based muco-muscular flap; B, Transverse mucosal incision; SPF, salpingopharyngeal fold; PPF, palatopharyngeal fold; PGF, palatoglossal fold. T, tongue.
2. Flaps transposed. Mucosa and muscle of tips of flaps sutured end to end.
3. Transverse ridge hidden behind soft palate.

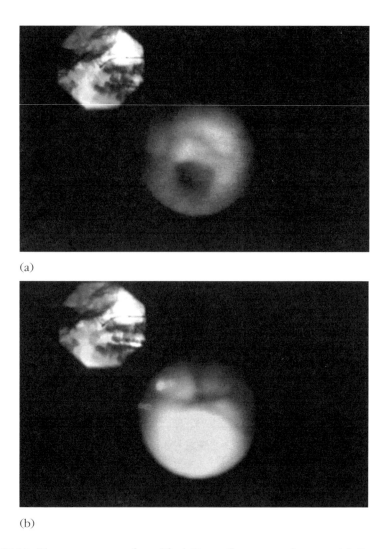

(a)

(b)

Figure 17.12. The appearance of modified Hynes flaps on endoscopy. (a) Open. (b) Closed.

Much has been made of the need to place a pharyngoplasty at a high level, at the plane of attempted closure. For this reason, superiorly based flaps have been favoured over inferiorly based flaps and the various modifications of the Hynes type of pharyngoplasty should also be placed as high as possible. However, most small children attempt closure against the adenoids, and unfortunately there is no pharyngoplasty that can be placed high enough to complete closure at this level where the defect is smallest. A pharyngeal flap is designed to allow the side walls to abut against it to gain closure but the site of maximum lateral wall movement is lower than the adenoids, lying at the level of the upper fibres of superior constrictor, which is 8 mm from the basisphenoid in an adult. Similarly, modified Hynes flaps are placed at the level of the inferior border of the adenoidal pad, which is also below the plane of closure in a child.

In cases where the adenoids are congenitally absent or where they have been removed surgically, the nasopharynx may have a vertical posterior wall described as a 'box pharynx' (Nieman et al., 1975). Some children compensate for this with marked velar stretch but others maintain a simple lift and develop VPI. For these children, a very substantial procedure may be needed, such as a V–Y pushback and wide pharyngeal flap (Honig, 1967), or a tight sphincter pharyngoplasty.

Posterior pharyngeal wall implants

An alternative to operations which cut through and realign parts of the pharyngeal wall is the insertion of an implant behind the posterior pharyngeal wall to bring it forward. The positioning and size of the implant can be determined by nasopharyngoscopy and videofluoroscopy if this method of treatment is chosen. In the past foreign materials such as silicone, Teflon, Proplast and collagen have been used but they have proved unreliable because they are frequently extruded (Blocksma, 1963; Lewy et al., 1965; Ward et al., 1966; Bluestone et al., 1968; Blocksma and Braley, 1969; Sturim and Jacob, 1972; Brauer, 1973; Evans and Ardran, 1977; Smith and McCabe, 1977; Kuehn and van Demark, 1978; Furlow et al., 1982; Wolford et al., 1989; Remacle et al., 1990). Autogenous materials such as costal cartilage have also been used. However, Witt et al. (1997) have concluded that they confer little advantage.

The uppermost fibres of superior constrictor show a dehiscence in the midline extending 0.8 cm from the skull base. This point corresponds to the level of the arch of the atlas (Mercer and MacCarthy, 1995a) and implants placed high enough to allow closure against the raised soft palate would therefore be covered only by mucosa, explaining the likelihood of extrusion.

Reliability of procedures

The discussion of pharyngoplasties and how they can be tailored to the needs of the individual patient has perhaps implied that these surgical procedures can be made more precise than is really the case. Unfortunately, due to scar contraction and variations in wound healing, predictions of the exact size and position of flaps cannot be certain. At postoperative follow-up, stringy low-based pharyngeal flaps and even total loss of the flap have been reported. A recent unpublished study has shown that shrinkage of posterior pharyngeal flaps varies from 45 to 80% (Vandervort and Mercer, 1998). Considerable variation in projection of Hynes flaps used to augment the posterior wall has also been documented (as has their sphincteric activity) (Moss et al., 1987; Pigott, 1993). One reason for this is probably the random blood supply of posterior pharyngeal flaps and, whilst modified Hynes flaps have a better axial supply, if they are raised above the superior pole of the tonsil they too will become 'random' (Mercer and MacCarthy, 1995a). There is a minimum length-to-breadth ratio of the flap to ensure its complete survival and if this is exceeded, the flap will atrophy due to its inadequate vascular supply. Variations in the sphincter activity of the so-called sphincter pharyngoplasties occur (Witt et al., 1998a and b); this may be related to the original activity of the palatopharyngeus during speech or damage to its nerve or blood supply.

Any type of pharyngoplasty may cause obstructive symptoms; for example, the Iowa group have reported an 89.2% risk of snoring after pharyngeal flap (Morris et al., 1995). At worst, obstruction may give rise to obstructive sleep apnoea, which can be severely disabling and potentially fatal (Wells et al., 1999). It is for these reasons that wide posterior flaps, which were effective in correcting hypernasality, have fallen out of favour and attempts are now made to use a less obstructive and more appropriate operation for the individual patient. However, because of the variation in results which occur for the reasons described above, this can mean a lower success rate in terms of complete correction of hypernasality. The need for such compromises clearly gives rise to controversies and it means that any future reports on the success of procedures to correct VPI must include information on obstructive symptoms as well as speech results.

If there were no articulatory faults preoperatively, surgery may result in normal speech. Even if there is a small residual gap after surgery, good progress towards normal articulation can often be made with speech therapy. If in the opinion of the patient, family and speech and language therapist, the level of residual VPI is unacceptable, further surgery can only be reliably planned using videofluoroscopy and nasopharyngoscopy.

Assessment of results

Speech assessment

Assessment of speech results should be carried out by independent specialist speech and language therapists. In the United Kingdom there are now agreed criteria and inter-centre comparisons are the norm (Sell et al., 1994, 1999; Harding et al., 1996 see Sell and Grunwell, Chapter 16).

Standardization of measurements from investigations

In an analysis of the difficulties of recording the findings of endoscopic and radiological investigation, Sinclair et al. (1982) and Golding-Kushner et al. (1990) proposed that movement should be recorded as a ratio of the resting position, but this gives no indication of true size; it is not 'quantitative'. Making measurements from X-rays is difficult but it is possible to calculate gap size with a degree of accuracy that is sufficient for the surgeon (Birch et al., 1994). There is a significant difference between the procedure required to correct a defect of 5 and one of 50 square millimetres, but in view of the relative unpredictability of the operations at present available (Vandervort and Mercer, 1998), any errors in measurement due to magnification and optical distortion are insignificant.

Does matching the operation to the defect improve results?

Boorman and Ray (1994) have reported a review of 298 consecutive operations undertaken by various surgeons, in which nasopharyngoscopy was performed prior to surgery. The surgeons did not vary their technique dependent on the results of these investigations. Regardless of technique or experience, about 70% of patients were considered to have been successfully treated on the basis that no further surgery was undertaken.

Other studies, however, support the use of preoperative planning. It has been postulated that knowledge of the extent of lateral pharyngeal wall movement before surgery should aid treatment planning (Shprintzen et al., 1977). Others have corroborated this hypothesis (Kelsey et al., 1972; Argamaso et al., 1980), concluding that preoperative assessment of the lateral pharyngeal wall motion was the prime determinant of success after pharyngeal flap surgery. A study by Albery et al. (1982) of 100 patients selected for surgery on the basis of combined nasopharyngoscopy and videofluoroscopy showed that 97% were cured of 'unacceptable' nasal escape (63% normal, 19% slight/occasional and 15% slight) and 93% of 'unacceptable' nasal resonance. Witt et al. (1994) studied a group of patients after sphincter pharyngoplasty and found that only 18% had their hypernasality and nasal escape corrected and 30% were rendered hyponasal after surgery. Riski et al. (1992) analysed 30 cases in whom a sphincter pharyngoplasty had failed and concluded that improved preoperative planning would have improved the outcome of surgery. In another study (Peat et al., 1994) patients were allocated to one of the following: a posterior wall augmentation/sphincter operation (Hynes), a V–Y pushback/superiorly base flap (Honig), a superiorly based flap alone (Roselli) or a dorsal surface reconfiguration (Fish flap) depending on the findings on endoscopy and X-ray. It was found, in a consecutive series of 132 pharyngoplasties, that hypernasal resonance was corrected in 85%, although 6.8% (9/132) required some degree of reversal for obstructive symptoms. These studies suggest that a lack of planning does adversely affect the outcome of surgery and suggest that tailoring operations to preoperative findings can be beneficial, but further research is needed to establish whether this is indeed so and a multicentre randomized trial is now in progress.

Key points for clinical practice

1. There is considerable variation in the range of movement of the velum and pharyngeal walls and of the size and shape of an incompetent velopharyngeal gap when it occurs.
2. Not every patient referred with presumed VPI requires surgery.
3. Examination of attempted closure patterns suggests that about two-thirds to three-quarters of patients could be successfully treated by any pharyngoplasty performed well.
4. Preoperative investigation by endoscopy and multiview radiology should reduce the risk that treatment will be unsuccessful.
5. The surgeon should choose the least obstructive operation with the highest probability of cure for each patient.
6. Recording on video tape or computer the fluoroscopic, nasendoscopic, speech and facial movements of the patient before and after operation is mandatory and allows audit of results and research to be conducted.

References

Abramson DL, Marrinan EM, Mulliken JB (1997) Robin sequence: obstructive sleep apnea following pharyngeal flap. Cleft Palate–Craniofacial Journal 34(3): 256–260.

Albery EH, Bennett JA, Pigott RW, Simmons RM (1982) The results of 100 operations for velopharyngeal incompetence selected on the findings of endoscopic and radiological examination. British Journal of Plastic Surgery 35: 118–126.

Argamaso RV, Shprintzen RJ, Strauch B, Lewin ML, Ship AG, Croft CB (1980) The role of lateral pharyngeal movement in pharyngeal flap surgery. Plastic and Reconstructive Surgery 66: 214–219.

Birch M, Sommerlad BC, Bhatt A (1994) Image analysis of lateral velopharyngeal closure in repaired cleft palates and normal palates. British Journal of Plastic Surgery 47(6): 400–405.

Blocksma R (1963) Correction of velopharyngeal insufficiency by silastic pharyngeal implant. Plastic and Reconstructive Surgery 31: 268–274.

Blocksma R, Braley S (1969) Present status of retropharyngeal implantation for velopharyngeal insufficiency. Plastic and Reconstructive Surgery 44: 242–247.

Bluestone CD, Musgrave RH, McWilliams BJ, Crozier PA (1968) Teflon injection pharyngoplasty. Cleft Palate Journal 5: 19–22.

Boorman J, Ray A (1994) Presented at the Annual Meeting of the Craniofacial Society of Great Britain.

Brauer RO (1973) Retropharyngeal implantation of gel pillows for velopharyngeal incompetence. Plastic and Reconstructive Surgery 51(3): 254–262.

Calnan JS (1954) The error of Gustav Passavant. Plastic and Reconstructive Surgery 13: 275–289.

Calnan JS (1957) Modern views on Passavant's Ridge. British Journal of Plastic Surgery 10: 89–113.

Calnan JS (1959) The surgical treatment of nasal speech disorders. Annals of the Royal College of Surgeons of England 25: 119–141.

Chen PK, Wu JT, Chen YR, Noordhoff MS (1994) Correction of secondary velopharyngeal insufficiency in cleft palate patients with the Furlow palatoplasty. Plastic and Reconstructive Surgery 94(7): 933–941.

Croft CB, Shprintzen RJ, Rakoff SJ (1981) Patterns of velopharyngeal valving in normal and cleft palate subjects: a multiview videofluoroscopic and nasendoscopic study. Laryngoscope 91: 265–271.

D'Antonio LL, Achauer BM, Vander Kam VM (1993) Results of a survey of cleft palate teams concerning the use of nasendoscopy. Cleft Palate–Craniofacial Journal 30(1): 35–39.

Davison PM, Razzell RE, Watson ACH (1990) The role of pharyngoplasty in congenital neurogenic speech disorders. British Journal of Plastic Surgery 43: 187–196.

Donnelly MJ (1994) Hypernasality following adenoidectomy. Irish Journal of Medical Science 163(5): 225–227.

Evans DM, Ardran GM (1977) Silastic implant pharyngoplasty: Radiographic planning and evaluation. British Journal of Plastic Surgery 30: 206–211.

Fernandes DB, Grobbelaar AO, Hudson DA, Lentin R (1996) Velopharyngeal incompetence after adentonsillectomy in non-cleft patients. British Journal of Oral and Maxillofacial Surgery 34(5): 364–367.

Finkelstein Y, Bar-Ziv J, Nachmani A, Berger G, Ophir D (1993a) Peritonsillar abscess as a cause of transient velopharyngeal insufficiency. Cleft Palate–Craniofacial Journal 30(4): 421–428.

Finkelstein Y, Lerner MA, Ophir D, Nachmani A, Hauben DJ, Zohar Y (1993b) Nasopharyngeal profile and velopharyngeal valve mechanism. Plastic and Reconstructive Surgery 92(4): 603–614.

Fischer KV, Swank PR (1997) Estimating phonation threshold pressure. Journal of Speech, Language and Hearing Research 40(5): 1122–1129.

Furlow LT, Williams WN, Eisenbach CR, Bzoch KR (1982) A long term study on treating velopharyngeal insufficiency by Teflon injection. Cleft Palate Journal 19: 47-56.

Georgantopoulou AA, Thatte MR, Razzell RE, Watson ACH (1996) The effect of sphincter pharyngoplasty on the range of velar movement. British Journal of Plastic Surgery 49: 358–362.

Golding-Kushner KJ, Argamaso RV, Cotton RT, et al. (1990) Standardisation for the reporting of nasopharyngoscopy and multi view videofluoroscopy. A report from an international working group. Cleft Palate Journal 27: 337–347.

Harding A, Harland K, Razzell RE (1996) Cleft Audit Protocol for Speech (CAPS). Available from Speech/Language Therapy Department, St Andrew's Plastic Surgery Centre, Broomfield, Chelmsford, Essex.

Hinton VA, Warren DW (1995) Relationships between integrated oral-nasal differentiated pressure and velopharyngeal closure. Cleft Palate–Craniofacial Journal 32(4): 306–310.

Hirschberg J, Van Demark DR (1997) A proposal for standardization of speech and hearing evaluations to assess velopharyngeal function. Folia Phoniatrica et Logopedica 49(3-4): 158–167.

Honig CA (1967) The treatment of velopharyngeal insufficiency after palate repair. Archivum Chirurgium Nederlandicum 19: 71–81.

Hutters B, Brondsted K (1992) A simple nasal anemometer for clinical purposes. European Journal of Disorders of Communication 27(2): 101–109.

Hynes W (1953) The results of pharyngoplasty by muscle transplantation in failed cleft palate cases. Annals of the Royal College of Surgeons 13: 17–35.

Hynes W (1967) Observations on pharyngoplasty. British Journal of Plastic Surgery. 20: 244–256.

Jackson IT, Silverton JS (1977) The sphincter pharyngoplasty as a secondary procedure in cleft palates. Plastic and Reconstructive Surgery 59: 518–524.

Kelsey CA, Ewanowski SJ, Crummy AB, Bless DM (1972) Lateral pharyngeal wall motion as a predictor of surgical success in velopharyngeal insufficiency. New England Journal of Medicine 287(2): 64–68.

Kouwenhoven E, Mast F, van Rijk-Zwikker GI (1993) Geometrical reconstruction of images obtained with electronic endoscopy. Physics in Medicine and Biology 38: 13–24.

Kuehn DP, Van Demark DR (1978) Assessment of velopharyngeal competency following Teflon pharyngoplasty. Cleft Palate Journal 15: 145–149.

Kuehn DP, Folkins JW, Linville RN (1988) An electromyographic study of the musculus uvulae. Cleft Palate Journal 25: 348–355.

Kummer AW, Billmire DA, Meyer CM 3d (1993) Hypertrophic tonsils: the effect on resonance and velopharyngeal closure. Plastic and Reconstructive Surgery 91(4): 608–611.

Lesavoy MA, Borud LJ, Thorson T, Riegelhuth ME, Berkowitz CD (1996) Upper airway obstruction after pharyngeal flap surgery. Annals of Plastic Surgery 36(1): 26–30.

Lewy R, Cole R, Wepman J (1965) Teflon injection in the correction of velopharyngeal insufficiency. Annals of Otology, Rhinology and Laryngology 74: 874–879.

McGowan JC, Hatabu H, Yousems DM, et al. (1992) Evaluation of soft palate function with MRI: Application to the cleft palate patient. Journal of Computer Assisted Tomography 16: 877–883.

Mercer NSG, MacCarthy P (1995a) The arterial basis of pharyngeal flaps. Plastic and Reconstructive Surgery 96: 1026–1037.

Mercer NSG, MacCarthy P (1995b) The arterial supply of the palate: Implications for closure of cleft palates. Plastic and Reconstructive Surgery 96: 1038–1044.

Mitnick RJ, Bello JA, Golding-Kushner KJ, Argamaso RV, Shprintzen RJ (1996) The use of magnetic resonanace angiography prior to pharyngeal flap surgery in patients with velocardiofacial syndrome. Plastic and Reconstructive Surgery 97(5): 908–919.

Morris HL, Bardach J, Jones D, Christianssen JL, Gray SD (1995) Clinical results of pharyngeal flap surgery: The Iowa experience. Plastic and Reconstructive Surgery 95(4): 652–662.

Moss AL, Pigott RW, Albery EH (1987) Hynes pharyngoplasty revisited. Plastic and Reconstructive Surgery 79: 346–355.

Nieman GS, Peterson SJ, Prusansky S (1975) Delayed pharyngeal flap success: report of a case. Cleft Palate Journal 12: 244–246.

Nishio J, Matsuya T, Machida J, Miyazaki T (1976) The motor nerve supply of the velopharyngeal muscles. Cleft Palate Journal 13: 20–30.

Orticochea M (1968) Construction of a dynamic muscle sphincter in cleft palates. Plastic and Reconstructive Surgery 41: 323–327.

Peat B, Albery EH, Jones K, Pigott RW (1994) Tailoring velopharyngeal surgery: The influence of aetiology and type of operation. Plastic and Reconstructive Surgery 93: 948–953.

Pigott RW (1969) The nasendoscopic appearance of the normal palato-pharyngeal valve. Plastic and Reconstructive Surgery 43(1): 19–24.

Pigott RW (1987) Objectives for cleft palate repair. Annals of Plastic Surgery 19: 247–259.

Pigott RW (1993) The results of pharyngoplasty by muscle transplantation. British Journal of Plastic Surgery 46: 440–442.

Pigott RW (1994) Velopharyngeal (speech) disorder (VP(S)D) without overt cleft palate. British Journal of Plastic Surgery. 47: 223-229.

Pigott RW, Makepeace APW (1982) Some characteristics of endoscopic and radiological systems used in elaboration of the diagnosis of velopharyngeal incompetence. British Journal of Plastic Surgery 35: 19–32.

Pigott RW, Bensen JF, White FD (1969) Nasendoscopy in the diagnosis of velopharyngeal incompetence. Plastic and Reconstructive Surgery 43(2): 141–147.

Remacle M, Bertrand B, Eloy P, Marrbaix E (1990) The use of injectable collagen to correct velopharyngeal insufficiency. Laryngoscope 100: 269–274.

Ren YF, Isberg A, Henningsson G (1995) Velopharyngeal incompetence and persistent hypernasality after adenoidectomy in children without palatal defect. Cleft Palate–Craniofacial Journal 32(6): 476–482.

Riski JE, Ruff GL, Georgiade GS, Barwick WJ (1992) Evaluation of failed sphincter pharyngoplasties. Annals of Plastic Surgery 28(6): 545–553.

Rosenthal W (1932) Pathologie und therapie der gaumendefecte. Fortschritte Zahnheilkunde 8: 890.

Ross DA, Witzel MA, Armstrong DC, Thompson HG (1996) Is pharyngoplasty a risk in velocardiofacial syndrome? An assessment of medially displaced carotid arteries. Plastic and Reconstructive Surgery 98(7): 1182–1190.

Sanvenero-Roselli G (1933) Restaurazioni plastiche del viso e del palato. Atti e memorie della societ‡ lombarda di chirurgia 1: 1–26.

Schoenborn K (1876) Ueber eine neue methode der staphylorrapie. Archiv f¸r Klinische Chirugie 19: 527–531. [Trans. Stellmach RK (1972) Plastic and Reconstructive Surgery 49: 558–562.]

Sedlackova E (1955) Insuicience patrohltanoveho zaveru jako vyvojova porucha. Casopis Lekaru Ceskych 94: 1304–1307.

Sedlackova E (1967) The syndrome of the congenitally shortened velum. The dual innervation of the soft palate. Folia Phoniatrica 19: 441–450.

Sedlackova E (1973) Contribution to knowledge of soft palate innervation. Folia Phoniatrica 25: 434–441.

Sell D, Harding A, Grunwell P (1994) A screening assessment of cleft palate speech (GOSSPAS). European Journal of Disorders of Communication 29: 1–15.

Sell D, Harding A, Grunwell P(1999) Revised GOS.SP.ASS (98): Speech assessment for children with cleft palate and/or velopharyngeal dysfunction. International Journal of Disorders of Communication 34: 17–33.

Shifman A, Finkelstein Y, Nachmani A and Ophir D (2000) Speech aid prostheses for neurogenic velopharyngeal incompetence. Journal of Prosthetic Dentistry 83(1): 99.

Shprintzen RJ (1986) Evaluating velopharyngeal incompetence. Journal of Children's Communication Disorders 10: 51–66.

Shprintzen RJ, Golding-Kushner KJ (1989) Evaluation of velopharyngeal insufficiency. Otolaryngological Clinics of North America 22: 519-536.

Shprintzen RJ, McCall G, Skolnick ML, Lencione RM (1975) Selective movements of the lateral aspects of the pharyngeal walls during velopharyngeal closure for speech, blowing and whistling in normals. Cleft Palate Journal 12: 51–58.

Shprintzen RJ, Rakoff SJ, Skolnick ML, Lavorato AS (1977) Incongruous movements of the velum and lateral pharyngeal walls. Cleft Palate Journal 14: 148–157.

Shprintzen R J, Goldberg R, Lewis M, Sidell E, Berkmann M, Argamaso R et al. (1978) A new syndrome involving cleft palate, cardiac anomalies, typical facies and learning disabilities: velo cardio facial syndrome. Cleft Palate Journal 15: 56–62.

Shprintzen RJ, Ibuki K, Karrell MP, Morris HL (1983) Commentary on reliability of the nasopharyngeal fibrescope (NPF) for assessing velopharyngeal incompetence. Cleft Palate Journal 20: 105–107.

Sinclair SW, Davies DM, Bracka A (1982) Comparative reliability of nasal pharyngoscopy and videofluorography in the assessment of velopharyngeal incompetence. British Journal of Plastic Surgery 35: 113–117.

Skolnick ML (1970) Videofluoroscopic examination of the velopharyngeal portal during phonation in lateral and base projections. A new technique for studying the mechanisms of closure. Cleft Palate Journal 7: 803–816.

Skolnick ML, McCall GN, Barnes M (1973) The sphincteric mechanism of velopharyngeal closure. Cleft Palate Journal 10: 286–305.

Skolnick ML, Shprintzen RJ, McCall GN, Rakoff S (1975) Patterns of velopharyngeal closure in subjects with repaired cleft palate and normal speech: a multi-view videofluoroscopic analysis. Cleft Palate Journal 12: 369–376.

Smith JK, McCabe BF (1977) Teflon injection in the nasopharynx to improve velopharyngeal closure. Annals of Otology, Rhinology and Laryngology 86: 559–563.

Sommerlad BC (1995) Towards a more functional palate repair. In: Jackson IT, Sommerlad BC (eds) Recent Advances in Plastic Surgery 5. Edinburgh: Churchill Livingstone.

Sommerlad BC, Rowland N, Harland K (1994a) Lateral videofluoroscopy: a modification to aid in velopharyngeal assessment and measurement. Cleft Plalate–Craniofacial Journal 31(2): 134–135.

Sommerlad BC, Henley M, Birch M, Harland K, Moieman N, Boorman (1994b) Cleft palate re-repair – a clinical and radiographic study of 32 consecutive cases. British Journal of Plastic Surgery 47(6): 406–410.

Sturim HS, Jacob CT (1972) Teflon pharyngoplasty. Plastic and Reconstructive Surgery 49(2): 180–185.

Tassone G, Massari MG, Ottaviani F (1995) Phonorhinorheometric study and laryngeal sonography in subjects affected by velopharyngeal insufficiency. Acta Otorhinolaryngologia Italica 15(3): 205–213.

Trost-Cardamone JE (1989) Coming to terms with VPI. Cleft Palate Journal 26(1): 68–70.

Vallino-Napoli LD, Montgomery AA (1997) Examination of standard deviation of mean nasalance scores in subjects with cleft palate. Cleft Palate–Craniofacial Journal 34(6): 512–519.

Vandervort M, Mercer N (1998) Shrinkage in pharyngeal flaps. Paper presented at the Annual Meeting of the Craniofacial Society of Great Britain.

Ward PH, Goldman R, Stoudt RJ (1966) Teflon injection to improve velopharyngeal insufficiency. Journal of Speech and Hearing Disorders 31: 267–273.

Warren DW, Dalston RM, Mayo R (1993) Hypernasality in the presence of 'adequate' velopharyngeal closure. Cleft Palate–Craniofacial Journal 30(2): 150–154.

Warren DW, Dalston RM, Mayo R (1994) Hypernasality and velopharyngeal impairment. Cleft Palate–Craniofacial Journal 31(4): 257–262.

Wells MD, Vuta EA, Luce EA (1999) Incidence and sequelae of nocturnal respiratory obstruction following posterior pharyngeal flap operation. Annals of Plastic Surgery 43(2): 252–257.

Witt PD, D'Antonio LL, Zimmerman GJ and Marsh JL (1994) Sphincter pharyngoplasty: a preoperative and postoperative analysis of perceptual speech characteristics and endoscopic studies of velopharyngeal function. Plastic and Reconstructive Surgery 93(6): 1154–1168.

Witt PD, O'Daniel TG, Marsh JL, Grames LM, Muntz HR, Pilgram TK (1997) Surgical management of velopharyngeal dysfunction: outcome analysis of autogenous posterior pharyngeal wall augmentation. Plastic and Reconstructive Surgery 99(5): 1287–1296.

Witt PD, Marsh JL, Arlis H, Grames LM, Ellis RA, Pilgram TK (1998a) Quantification of dynamic velopharyngeal port excursion following sphincter pharyngoplasty. Plastic and Reconstructive Surgery 101(6): 1457–62.

Witt PD, Myckatyn T, Marsh JL, Grames LM, Pilgram TK (1998b) Does pre-existing posterior pharyngeal wall motion drive the dynamism of sphincter pharyngoplasty? Plastic and Reconstructive Surgery 101(6): 1457–62.

Witt PD, Cohen D, Grames LM, Mark J (1999) Sphincter pharyngoplasty for the surgical management of speech dysfunction associated with velocardiofacial syndrome. British Journal of Plastic Surgery 52(8): 613–618.

Witzel MA, Posnick JC (1989) Patterns and location of velopharyngeal valving problems: Atypical findings on video nasopharyngoscopy. Cleft Palate Journal 26: 63–70.

Wolford LM, Oelschlaeger M, Deal R (1989) Proplast as a pharyngeal wall implant to correct velopharyngeal insufficiency. Cleft Palate Journal 26: 119–126.

Yamawaki Y, Sawada M, Isshiki N, et al. (1993) Diagnostic value of dynamic MRI for velopharyngeal function. Presented at 7th International Congress on Cleft Palate. Broadbeach Australia. Abstract 134.S.

CHAPTER 18

Secondary Surgery of Lip and Nose Deformities and Palatal Fistulae

A.C.H. WATSON

Ideally, the primary operations to close clefts of the lip and palate should be all that are needed, although in complete alveolar clefts bone grafting is usually planned for when the child is nine or ten years old (see Mars, Chapter 20). Primary nasal tip surgery may be deliberately delayed, particularly with a bilateral cleft lip, until just before the child goes to school. Unfortunately, primary surgery is not always entirely successful and secondary operations are often required (CSAG, 1998). These may be to the lip or nose, to improve appearance, lip function or nasal airways, or because of palatal fistula or velopharyngeal insufficiency (see Mercer and Pigott, Chapter 17). As the child grows, new deformities may become apparent, particularly due to restriction of maxillary growth, which may need to be corrected by orthognathic surgery once growth is complete (see Lello, Chapter 21). Deviation of the nasal bridge may only become obvious during adolescence, requiring rhinoplasty. In early childhood middle ear effusions (glue ear) often need intervention by the otolaryngologist (see Lennox, Chapter 15). This chapter deals with those secondary operations to the lip and nose and closure of palatal fistulae.

If there are significant residual deformities of lip or nose, it is desirable that they be corrected as far as possible before the child goes to school. Sometimes, however, minor deformities may be left and dealt with only if they attract teasing. Each child must always be considered as an individual, keeping in mind social and other factors which may influence decisions regarding treatment, and it must be remembered that hospital admissions and surgical operations are traumatic experiences (see Bradbury, Chapter 23).

Secondary deformities vary widely and, if surgery is indicated, the operation must be tailored to the particular problem. There is space here to consider only a selection of procedures which this author has found valuable in dealing with the commoner deformities.

Lip revision

After a competent cleft lip repair, abnormalities are usually minor, but several may coexist and their correction can challenge the artistic eye and technical ingenuity of the plastic surgeon.

Unilateral clefts

The most frequent residual deformities are an asymmetry of the cupid's bow or of the free margin of the upper lip. The Millard rotation-advancement repair may result in a lip that is too short on the cleft side, with drawing up of the peak of the cupid's bow; it is rarely too long. There may be a malalignment of the mucocutaneous junction, or of the white roll. Minor irregularities of this type can be corrected by small Z-plasties (Figures 18.1 and 18.2) but if there is a serious discrepancy it may be necessary to take down the whole lip repair and refashion it. Unfortunately the scar, which is usually pale and inconspicuous after a primary repair in infancy, is more likely to be red and noticeable after a secondary repair in later childhood.

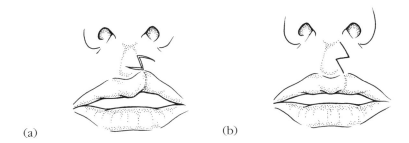

(a)   (b)

Figure 18.1. Z-plasty to correct raised peak of cupid's bow. (a) Flaps incised; (b) flaps transposed.

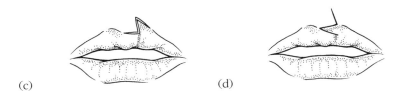

(c)   (d)

Figure 18.2. Technique for correcting misaligned mucocutaneous junction. (a) Flaps incised; (b) flaps transposed.

A notch at the free margin of the lip can often be corrected by an elliptical excision of vermilion and mucosa and freeing and suturing of the underlying muscle (Figure 18.3). Accurate approximation of the junction of vermilion and wet mucosa is as important as that of the mucocutaneous junction, and for this reason Z-plasties at the free margin must be viewed with caution. If the mucosa needs to be adjusted it should usually be done out of sight, inside the free margin, where fusiform incisions can be carried out for mucosal excess and transposition or V–Y advancement flaps to build up deficiencies (Figures 18.4 and 18.5). It is important when planning such surgery to the lip to examine it not only from directly in front, but also from above, below and from the side. Muscle deficiencies particularly, may be apparent only on one of these views. Movement of the lip should be assessed, particularly smiling and pursing. A lip may look symmetrical at rest but, if the muscle has not been properly mobilized and rotated downwards, asymmetry will become obvious on movement. If it has not been freed from the alar base, an ugly bulge will become apparent on the cleft side as it contracts. To correct these functional deformities the muscles need to be widely freed and repositioned. This can often be done from the mucosal aspect of the lip to avoid interfering with an inconspicuous cutaneous scar.

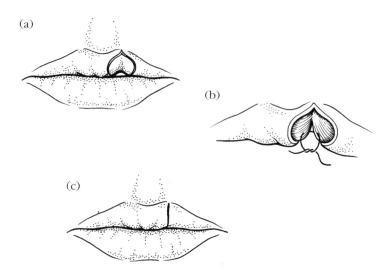

Figure 18.3. Correction of notch at free margin. (a) Elliptical excision of vermilion around notch; (b) suturing of the mobilized muscle; (c) closure.

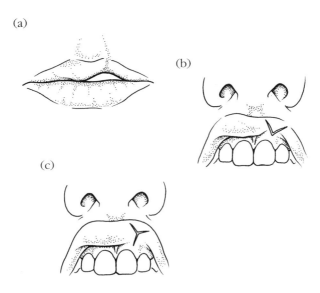

Figure 18.4. Correction of mild whistle deformity by V–Y advancement of mucosa. (a) Deformity; (b) V-shaped flap on buccal aspect of lip; (c) flap advanced after undermining to be closed as a Y.

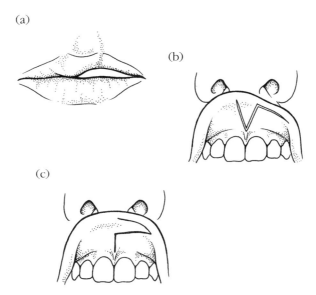

Figure 18.5. Correction of more severe vermilion deficiency by transposition flap of mucosa inside lip. (a) Deformity; (b) flap raised in continuity with incision along buccal aspect of defect; (c) flap transposed after undermining.

Bilateral clefts

Because the bilateral cleft lip deformity is more difficult to correct, secondary deformities are more common. A deficiency of vermilion in the midline – the so-called 'whistle deformity' – is frequently found; the lip can be tethered to the underlying premaxilla and there may be no muscle union across the midline. Muscle bulges may be very prominent on each side, and the lip may be immobile. These deformities can often be corrected at the same time and, if the original cutaneous scars are good, they can be left undisturbed. Enough mucosa can usually be found in or adjacent to the midline to line the premaxilla, and more can be advanced from laterally to deepen the sulcus and cover the muscle. This muscle can be mobilized and sutured to that from the opposite side behind the prolabium. It may sometimes be difficult to get enough muscle bulk and vermilion to correct the whistle deformity fully. Advancement of wet mucosa to replace midline vermilion is unsatisfactory, and Kapetansky (1971) has described 'pendulum flaps' from the lateral elements in this situation (Figure 18.6).

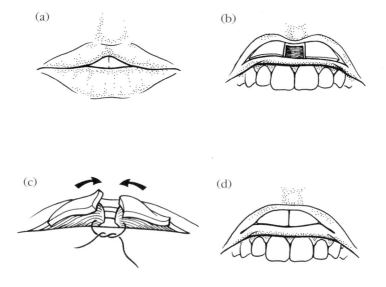

Figure 18.6. Kapetansky pendulum flaps for midline whistle deformity. (a) Deformity; (b) Island mucosal flaps marked, based on underlying muscle; (c) Mucosa and muscle mobilised, advanced medially and sutured; (d) V–Y closure.

Abbe flap

Abbe of New York in 1898 described a flap transferred from the midline of the lower lip on a narrow pedicle to fill a defect in the upper lip. This flap has proved invaluable to augment a tight, deficient lip, particularly following repair of a bilateral cleft. It is not often required nowadays, due to improved primary surgery, but can still on occasion be useful, either in its original form or modified so that it may only include vermilion, muscle or mucosa as required (Figure 18.7).

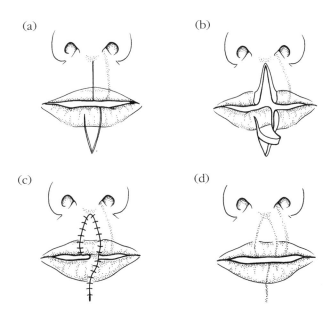

Figure 18.7. Abbe flap. (a) Tight upper lip with midline incision marked; flap marked on lower lip with narrow pedicle containing coronal vessels; (b) upper lip incised and flap raised; (c) flap sutured; (d) flap divided and inset after 10 days.

Nasal deformities

Most surgeons now carry out some degree of nasal correction at the time of primary lip surgery (see Watson, Chapter 12) and many children may not require any secondary nasal surgery, at least until adolescence. However, the cleft nasal deformity is difficult to correct, as it is based on underlying bony deformities which may remain after primary surgery, and it is the feature that most commonly gives rise to teasing. The bilateral cleft lip nose will almost always need tip advancement – indeed, this is usually part of the original plan, but the unilateral may also sometimes need to be revised during early childhood if bullying at school is to be avoided.

The secondary unilateral cleft lip nasal deformity is a very complex one which has many facets, but bony displacement underlies them all. First, the deviation of the anterior nasal spine towards the non-cleft side takes with it the septum and columella, which contains the medial crura of the alar cartilages. At the same time, the lateral element of the maxilla and the attached alar base tends to be displaced posteriorly and laterally. The alar cartilage is put on the stretch and rotates downwards, becoming flattened and sometimes kinked, and the nose on the cleft side is lengthened (Figure 18.8). These deformities are present before primary repair, and are often not fully corrected at that time. Among other abnormalities, the nostril margin may be slumped, the nostril oriented more transversely than the other side, and the nostril floor may be too wide (or occasionally too narrow) or it may be deficient.

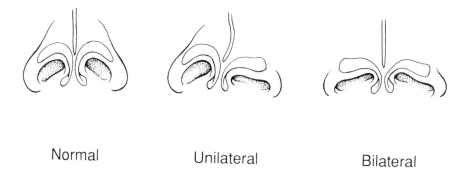

Normal   Unilateral   Bilateral

Figure 18.8. Cleft lip nasal deformity.

Many methods have been described to correct the nasal deformity – suggesting that none are completely effective. Unfortunately the underlying bony defect cannot be corrected without risk to growth until the time of alveolar bone grafting, usually at about nine or ten years (see Mars, Chapter 20) and if nasal surgery is thought advisable at a younger age for social reasons, its success must therefore be limited. The main aims of any secondary surgery in childhood are to raise the slumped nostril, correct any nasal floor discrepancy, lengthen the columella on the cleft side and perhaps to straighten the distal septum. This last can be done by dividing its attachment to the anterior nasal spine and scoring it on the concave side. Of the many methods of correcting the alar deformity, the author has had greatest success with a modification of the Tajima 'reverse U' operation (Tajima and Maruyama, 1977) (Figure 18.9). In this procedure, both the

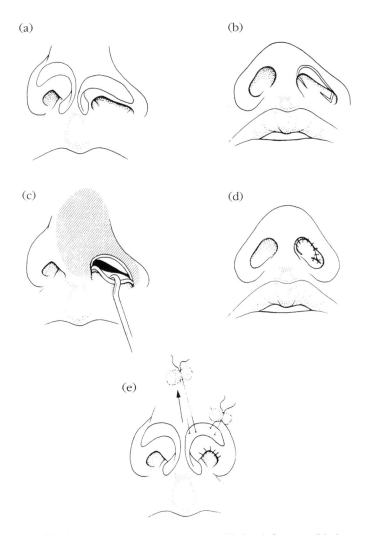

Figure 18.9. Modified Tajima 'reverse U' operation. (a) the deformity; (b) the 'reverse U' incision with back-cut; (c) incision and undermining; alar cartilage freed from skin and other cartilages; (d) the incision sutured with V–Y advancement of lateral crus; (e) mattress sutures tied over boluses to elevate alar cartilage as in McComb's primary correction.

medial and lateral crura of the alar cartilage are separated from the overlying skin and the other cartilages, and are elevated with mattress sutures through the dome. The most important point seems to be the release of the lateral end of the lateral crus, which is advanced forwards and medially. This technique has resulted in significantly less relapse than a series in which the lateral release was not done (Coghlan and Boorman, 1996, Rider and

Watson, 1997). A nasal floor that is too wide or deficient can be corrected by raising a de-epithelialized flap from the nostril floor, attached to the alar base, and advancing it medially under the skin (Figure 18.10).

The nasal deformity associated with the bilateral cleft lip is shown in Figure 18.8. The columella is short or absent and the alar cartilages are splayed with wide separation of the medial crura. The nostril floors are wide. There are many ways of lengthening the columella, but none will produce a good result unless the medial crura are sutured together, the alar domes elevated and the lateral crura released laterally (Figure 18.11).

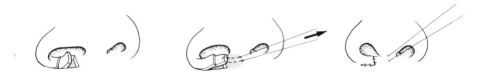

Figure 18.10. Correction of wide nostril floor.

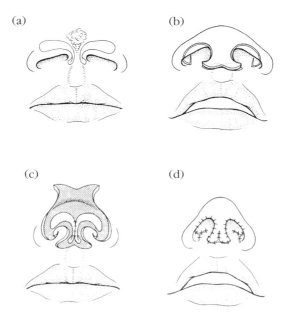

Figure 18.11. Open tip rhinoplasty for bilateral cleft lip nose. (a) Bilateral cleft lip nasal deformity. (b) Incisions similar to the modified Tajima procedure, joined across the columellar base with two nostril floor flaps. (c) Columellar flaps raised; fat pad excised and medial crura sutured together with fine non-absorbable sutures. (d) Incisions sutured; V–Y advancement of lateral crura; nostril floor flaps sutured together to lengthen columella. Mattress sutures are also inserted to elevate the alar domes.

Surgery to the nose in early childhood is usually limited to the nasal tip. Alveolar bone grafting at the age of nine or ten will give support to the nostril floor and to the alar base on the cleft side, which may itself improve the symmetry. However, as the nose grows during adolescence, deviation of the bony bridge towards the non-cleft side may become more apparent. Obstruction of one or both nasal airways may be due to the anterior septum obstructing the nostril on the non-cleft side while, further posteriorly, it can bulge into the airway and obstruct the cleft side. Spurs of bone along the nasal floor, probably the result of raising vomer flaps in the primary operation, may often contribute to nasal airway obstruction. It is usually felt unwise to interfere with the septum other than at its very anterior end until facial growth is complete but, at the age of about 16, it is common for septorhinoplasty to be required. If the septal deviation is not marked, it may be possible to straighten it adequately simply by scoring the cartilage on the concave side but, if it is more severe, a submucous resection of the septum may be needed (Figure 18.12). At the same operation the nasal bones may be fractured and the nasal bridge brought to the midline. If a hump is present, as is frequently the case in bilateral clefts, this can be reduced and any final work done on the nasal tip to improve its symmetry.

Figure 18.12. Septoplasty and limited submucous resection of septal cartilage.

Palatal fistulae

Sometimes the hard palate or alveolus is deliberately left open at the first operation (see Watson, Chapter 12) and its repair at a second stage is usually straightforward. However, if an attempted repair breaks down, this is usually due to necrosis of tissue, and closure of the resulting fistula is made difficult by the scarring and tissue loss. Often such a fistula is small and, if the edges are apposed, it may not cause any significant symptoms and may not warrant operation. If closure is necessary, it is better delayed for as long as possible, as further palatal surgery will cause more scarring which will result in even more interference with maxillary growth. Fistulae occur most commonly in or just behind the alveolar cleft or at the junction of the hard and soft palate. The former can often be left until the time of alveolar bone grafting (see Mars, Chapter 20).

Sometimes fistulae cause troublesome symptoms which call for early closure. Food and drink may leak into the nose and out of the nostril, which is embarrassing. If air leaks into the nose during speech, it may interfere with articulation and/or cause audible nasal emission. This can be confused with velopharyngeal insufficiency (which may coexist) and careful assessment will be required (see Sell and Grunwell, Chapter 16 and Mercer and Pigott, Chapter 17).

Surgical closure of fistulae should, if possible, be in two layers with the suture lines not superimposed. This means that flaps have to be raised and raw areas left behind (Figure 18.13). Very large fistulae may require tissue to be brought in from elsewhere, e.g. a tongue flap (Figure 18.14) (Guerrero-Santos and Altamirano, 1966).

Occasionally the best efforts of the surgeon to close a fistula fail, and the patient will require an obturator (see Griffiths, Chapter 22).

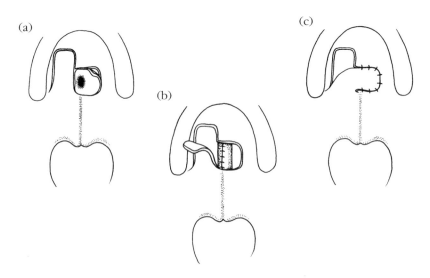

Figure 18.13. Closure of palatal fistula. (a) Hinged flap marked, based on fistula margin, for nasal lining. Veau type flap for oral closure; (b) flap raised; nasal closure; (c) Veau flap transposed to complete oral closure. Residual raw area.

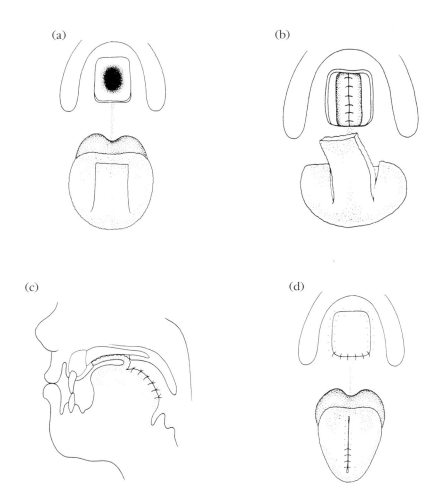

Figure 18.14. Tongue flap to close large palatal fistula. (a) Hinge flap raised around the fistula to close nasal layer. Tongue flap outlined; (b) nasal layer closed; tongue flap raised; (c) lateral view of tongue flap inset into palatal defect; (d) after division of tongue flap at two to three weeks.

References

Abbe R (1898) A new plastic operation for relief of deformity due to double hare lip. Medical Record 53: 477.

Clinical Standards Advisory Group (CSAG) (1998) Report. Cleft Lip and/or Palate. London: HMSO.

Coghlan B, Boorman JG (1996) Objective evaluation of the Tajima secondary cleft lip nose correction. British Journal of Plastic Surgery 49: 457–461.

Guerrero-Santos J, Altamirano JT (1966) The use of lingual flaps in repair of fistulas of the hard palate. Plastic and Reconstructive Surgery 38: 123–128.

Kapetansky KI (1971) Double pendulum flaps for whistling deformities in bilateral cleft lips. Plastic and Reconstructive Surgery 47: 321.

Rider M, Watson ACH (1997) Outcome analysis of a modified Tajima procedure. British Journal of Plastic Surgery 50: 590–594.

Tajima S, Maruyama M (1977) Reverse U incision for secondary repair of cleft lip nose. Plastic and Reconstructive Surgery 60: 256.

CHAPTER 19

Orthodontics

G. SEMB AND W.C. SHAW

Introduction and treatment goals

The orthodontic specialist responsible for the care of children with cleft lip and palate must have an appreciation of the overall burden of care that children with clefts endure. The nature of dental development in repaired clefts is such that there may be temptations to intervene at almost any point between birth and end of the teens. Consequently clear choices must be made and orthodontic treatment that does not significantly contribute to the end result should be eliminated from the programme of care.

The orthodontist will aim to provide a dentition that functions well and is capable of lifetime maintenance by routine oral hygiene and dental care. The anterior maxillary dentition should align symmetrically around the facial midline. However, without osteotomy, it must be appreciated that the underlying skeletal morphology (Figure 19.1) that reflects intrinsic variation and the consequences of surgery severely restricts occlusal change (Semb and Shaw, 1996).

Thus orthodontic treatment for children with clefts should:

- achieve an optimal occlusion and dentofacial aesthetics within the constraints imposed by the underlying skeletal pattern;
- keep the duration of treatment to a minimum;
- accomplish as much as possible during periods of active treatment;
- be sympathetic to individual needs and circumstances.

In many countries children from underprivileged backgrounds would not commonly receive orthodontics. When affected by clefts, however, such children may become orthodontic patients. Their need for special assistance in maintaining good oral hygiene and additional support for completing lengthy complex treatment must be recognized. It must also be remembered

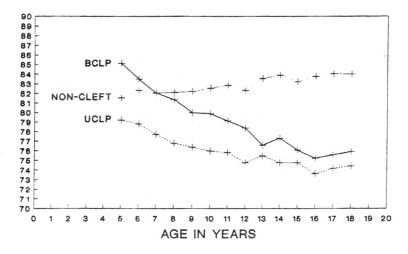

Figure 19.1. Changes in maxillary prominence (S/N/SS; degrees) for a sample of 257 patients with UCLP (Semb, 1991a) and 90 patients with BCLP (Semb, 1991b) followed longitudinally. The non-cleft sample is derived from the Bolton Standards (Broadbent BH, Broadbent BH Jr, Golden WH. Bolton Standards of Dentofacial Developmental Growth. St Louis: CV Mosby, 1975).

that the prevalence of dental cavities in children with clefts is higher than in non-cleft children (Bokhout et al., 1996) and so regular dental check-ups and use of flouride supplements must be available.

The orthodontists will with other members of the multidisciplinary team monitor the patient's general well-being, particularly during the years of greater involvement, e.g. 7-16 years.

Dental development

Failure of union of the embryonic facial processes leads to discontinuity and disorientation of the cells of the primordial dental lamina. These distur-bances produce variations in number, morphology, enamel formation and eruption of teeth in the cleft area, with the lateral incisor being most affected (Bøhn, 1963; Ranta, 1972, 1986, 1990).

Lateral incisor

In the primary dentition the lateral incisor is congenitally missing in 12–14% of cases (Bøhn, 1963; Ranta, 1972), while in the permanent dentition the lateral incisor is missing in about 50% of cases (Bøhn, 1963; Ranta, 1986, Suzuki et al., 1992). When present, the lateral incisors may be found on either side of the alveolar cleft or, in case of supernumerary incisors, on both sides. Supernumerary lateral incisors are more common in the primary dentition (Bøhn, 1963). In a sample of 360 clefts involving the alveolus the lateral incisor was found to be impacted in 1% (Semb and Schwartz, 1997).

Central incisor

The permanent central incisor on the cleft side is on average 10% narrower than the other central incisor, and its shape is often abnormal. In a sample of 360 clefts involving the alveolus the central incisor was found to be so malformed in 1% of patients that it had to be removed (Semb and Schwartz, 1997).

The central incisors of patients with bilateral cleft lip and palate (BCLP) (and in some instances the cleft side central incisor in unilateral cleft lip and palate (UCLP)) often have an unusual crown–root angulation and are retroclined. In BCLP they are frequently malformed and have a short root length.

Canine

The morphology of the canine does not appear to be affected by the occurrence of a cleft, but this tooth is commonly impacted. In at least one report canine impaction is reported to occur 10 times more often in patients with complete CLP than in non-clefts, especially in UCLP (Semb and Schwartz, 1997).

Other variations

Alterations of tooth development in areas distant from the cleft also occur more frequently in patients with CLP than in the non-cleft population. In the deciduous dentition, the frequency of congenitally missing, fused and peg-shaped posterior teeth has been reported to be four times more common; a slight tendency to delayed eruption has been also been demonstrated (Pöyry, 1987; Kramer, 1994). In the mixed dentition stage there is a general delay in tooth formation and eruption of approximately 6 months, especially on the cleft side (Fishman, 1970; Ranta, 1986).

The prevalence of congenital absence of permanent teeth (excluding the cleft side maxillary lateral incisor and third molars) in a population of children with complete CLP has been reported to be as high as 50% (Ranta, 1990). The permanent teeth most affected outside the cleft region are the non-cleft lateral incisor and the second premolars, especially in the maxilla (Ranta, 1972, 1986). The development of the second premolars may be delayed for many years, and their presence cannot be ruled out on X-rays before the age of nine years (Ranta, 1990). When they are present, they are frequently small and deformed (Bøhn, 1963; Ranta, 1983, 1986). A higher frequency of first molar impaction has been reported, (Bjerklin et al., 1993). Finally the teeth in patients with CLP are generally smaller than those in the non-cleft population (Foster and Lavelle, 1971; Ranta, 1986; McCance et al., 1990).

Occlusal development

Before surgery the maxillary segments may assume a variety of positions, related perhaps, to tongue posture and function, and fetal moulding. After lip and palate closure medial movement of the maxillary lateral segment(s) is often found and segments that have been apart usually contact each other by four years of age (Harvold, 1947; Pruzansky and Aduss, 1967; Vargervik, 1990). The form of the alveolar process is determined to a large extent by the number, position, size and shape of the teeth in the area. Early removal of teeth is therefore contraindicated (Vargervik, 1990).

In the primary dentition in UCLP, crossbite of one or more teeth on the cleft side is the commonest deviation from normal dental arch form. In some instances anterior crossbite may also be found. A mandibular displacement may be associated with crossbites (though this can often be corrected by reduction of the cusps of the primary teeth that interfere with each other). An open bite in the cleft region may be apparent.

In BCLP the premaxilla is usually quite prominent during the primary dentition stage, but recedes over time (Figure 19.1). Since mandibular growth will later catch up with the premaxilla, it is important to resist the temptation to set back the premaxilla surgically. Bilateral crossbites are quite common.

The transition from deciduous to the mixed dentition is characterized by a worsening of the anterior occlusion due to the palatal path of eruption and the rotation of the central incisor(s) adjacent to the cleft (Ross, 1970; Bergland and Sidhu, 1974).

As further development of the permanent dentition takes place, scar tissue in the palate may cause the permanent canines and premolars to erupt in a palatal direction (Ross and Johnston, 1972). Even where an expanded maxillary arch is retained with a palatal archwire, premolars and canines may occasionally erupt palatal to the archwire. As a consequence of the shorter dental arches, especially in UCLP, crowding commonly develops in the posterior dentition when all teeth are present. Lack of space may also be a factor in tooth impaction. In UCLP the maxillary dental midline tends to be displaced to the cleft side, exaggerating the asymmetry of the face. In patients with BCLP the midline tends to be more centrally placed.

With unfavourable skeletal development, the possibility of anterior crossbite over time becomes more likely, and given the tendency to posterior rotation of the mandible, reduced overbite is common except in a few patients with BCLP. In some patients open bite in the cleft region may be evident from an early age. The incisors in both jaws are usually retroclined.

Complete cleft lip and palate – treatment

Principles

Formerly, the aims of the orthodontic treatment for children with complete clefts were limited to tooth alignment and arch expansion, followed by permanent artificial retention in the form of fixed bridgework or other prostheses. This was often linked with artificial restoration of the lateral incisor space as the alveolar bony defect made orthodontic space closure impossible. This approach, however, had several disadvantages, for in addition to the general undesirability of artificial teeth for long-term aesthetics and dental health (Nordquist and McNeill, 1975), lack of investing bone often precluded the correction of the anterior tooth irregularities. Lack of supporting bone could also lead to so much loss of attachment of teeth adjacent to the cleft that they were lost after some years, and in patients with bilateral clefts, the mobility of the premaxilla made the retention of bridge-work difficult.

With the advent of a successful alveolar bone grafting technique in the early 1970s (Boyne and Sands, 1972, 1976), the aims of treatment have been revised so that the alveolar bony defect is restored before the time of canine eruption. Subsequent orthodontic treatment can then achieve alignment and space closure in the majority of cases. The following simplified approach to treatment has provided satisfactory results in a large series of consecutive cases (Åbyholm et al., 1981; Bergland et al., 1986; Enemark et al., 1987, 1990; Paulin et al., 1988). Because of the doubtful benefits of presurgical orthopaedics (see Hathorn, Chapter 11), deciduous dentition treatment and attempted skeletal protraction, and the unnecessary burden of care they impose, these interventions will not be recommended. We do not recommend the use of removable appliances.

Orthodontics prior to bone grafting

Incisor alignment

By age seven to eight years an increased awareness of dental appearance and motivation for orthodontic treatment often becomes evident (see Bradbury, Chapter 23). Incisor alignment can be provided at this stage if requested for aesthetic reasons. It is also possible that a correction of anterior crossbite at this stage will maximize the forward development of the maxillary dentoalveolar process (Ross and Johnston, 1972; Vargervik, 1990). Orthodontic movement of maxillary anterior teeth at this time must, however, be done with great caution because of the closeness of the roots to the bony defect (Figure 19.2) and in a few patients treatment is better postponed until after the alveolar process has been completely restored by bone.

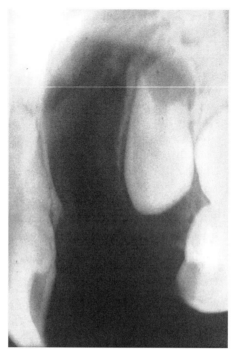

Figure 19.2. Radiograph of an alveolar cleft defect. Note the very thin bone lamellae distal to the central incisor that limits orthodontic tooth movement.

If treatment is to be undertaken, and anterior crossbite and maxillary incisor rotation coexist, treatment should be directed to the simultaneous correction of both. The appliance shown in Figure 19.3 incorporates the upper second deciduous molars (or first permanent molars) and the incisors that are present. A push-coil is used on the cleft side(s) for incisor advancement and elastic chains for derotation. The arch wire should be adjusted to lie below the incisal edge so that, when engaged in the brackets, it tends to increase overbite and sets up anchorage in the molars to resist posterior displacement forces. It is important that the archwire is adapted closely to the alveolar process since the repaired lip and a low buccal sulcus are more easily irritated. Looped archwires are generally inappropriate for this reason. It is often advantageous to open the bite while correcting a negative overjet and, for this purpose, a composite build-up on the lower deciduous molars is used (Figure 19.3a). As soon as the anterior crossbite is corrected the composite is removed. Correction of inverted and rotated incisors will take between three and six months. Detailed alignment of teeth is not attempted, if this would prolong treatment. A small bonded retainer is placed on the palatal aspects of the corrected incisors and is kept in place until the start of permanent dentition treatment.

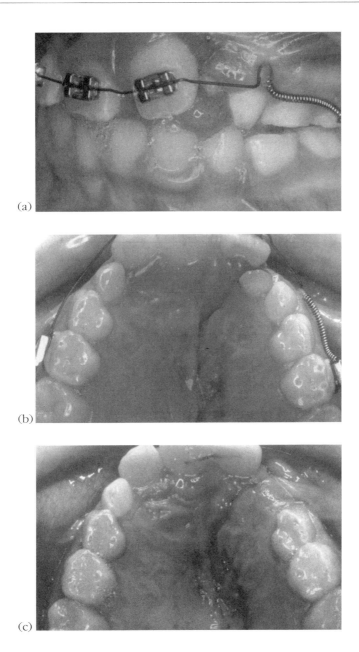

Figure 19.3. (a) Orthodontic appliance for proclination of incisors. Three incisors and the second deciduous upper molars are bonded. A passive archwire with a push-coil is fitted. Composite build-up of the buccal cusps of the lower second deciduous molars makes proclination of the inverted incisor easier. (b) Occlusal view. It is important that the archwire is adapted closely to the alveolar process to reduce the risk of trauma. (c) A small twistflex retainer is bonded on the central incisors.

The same design of archwire in BCLP can achieve substantial anterior rotation of the premaxilla and an improved interincisal angle. Most movement takes place around the premaxillary–vomerine suture so that considerable improvement in the inter-incisal relationship is achieved without applying heavy torquing forces to the retroclined incisors. As noted above, incisor root development is often impaired in BCLP and excessive and lengthy application of force should be avoided.

Transverse expansion

If possible, transverse expansion can be combined with the correction of incisor irregularities but expansion prior to bone grafting should not be regarded as essential for all crossbites. Only cases with significant segmental displacement require pre-bone graft expansion to rotate the lateral segment(s) outward and facilitate placement of the graft. Segmental rotation cannot be obtained after grafting (Vargervik, 1978).

Expansion may produce a slight widening of the nasal cavity in the antero-inferior region, but there is no evidence that this is permanently maintained. It is therefore likely that a significant improvement in nasal airflow occurs in only a small number of patients (Ross and Johnston, 1972). However, expansion of a severely constricted maxilla in the mixed dentition period may provide greater space for the tongue and improve speech artic-ulation and masticatory function.

Most often a removable quad-helix or palatal arch with lateral expansion spring is used for segment repositioning as selective expansion anteriorly is required (Figure 19.4). Segment repositioning will take approximately six to eight months. Rapid maxillary expansion screws are unnecessary.

In patients with complete BCLP, the premaxilla may be mobile and stabi-lization of the premaxilla immediately before grafting has been found to improve the success of bone grafting (Bergland et al., 1986). A heavy rectan-gular archwire is used for this and kept in place for three months after surgery.

Timing of bone grafting

The optimum time of bone grafting will be decided individually (see also Mars, Chapter 20). In patients with a well-formed lateral incisor that is not too displaced from the arch, bone grafting is usually done quite early, around seven to eight years. Since the majority of patients have a missing ectopic or deformed lateral incisor, bone grafting may be postponed until 10 to 11 years. This allows the canine's root-development to progress more and may reduce canine impaction (Sindet-Pedersen and Enemark, 1993). However, grafting should still be performed prior to canine eruption.

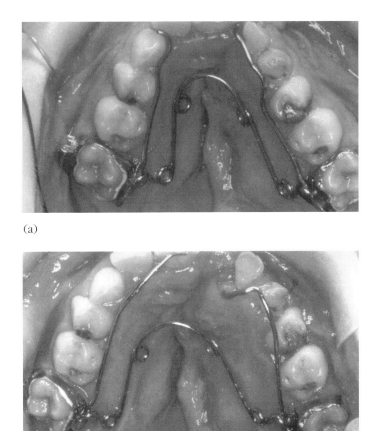

(a)

(b)

Figure 19.4. A removable quad-helix used for segment repositioning. The expansion took six months; (a) before, and (b) after expansion.

Postsurgical stabilization

The quad-helix and/or stabilizing archwire used in BCLP may be removed during the bone grafting procedure for improved surgical access, but these appliances should be replaced before the patient leaves the operating theatre, and left in place for three months. When a substantial outward movement of the lateral segment(s) has been necessary, clinical experience suggests that bone grafting alone cannot be relied upon to maintain the expansion. In these circumstances stabilization in the form of a simple palatal arch would be advisable until the permanent dentition has erupted (Figure 19.5).

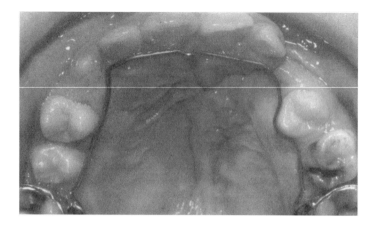

Figure 19.5. Removable palatal archwire for the retention of segment repositioning.

Post-bone graft observation

Resting the patient from appliance therapy is highly desirable at this stage. Occasional observation is generally all that is necessary in the years between bone grafting and eventual eruption of the permanent dentition. The status of unerupted teeth, especially the cleft side canine, does, however, need careful monitoring.

Permanent dentition orthodontics

A number of special considerations make orthodontic treatment of children with complete clefts distinctive from general orthodontics.

Deteriorating class III skeletal pattern

Early determination of the eventual need for maxillary osteotomy is the most difficult and important decision for the orthodontist (See also Lello, Chapter 21). Where the likelihood of osteotomy is high, simple alignment of the upper arch may be all that is required until the end of the teens, when presurgical orthodontics is performed. Extracting teeth to permit the retroclination of lower incisors that will later be proclined during 'decompensation' is clearly unwise.

Since deterioration of the skeletal pattern, especially in males, is the rule, borderline cases in the early teens should be assessed most carefully. Plotting jaw growth on longitudinal cephalometric radiographs against norms for cleft patients is advisable. Non-cleft norms are not appropriate for patients with clefts (Enemark, 1993).

Where extractions are necessary to relieve lower incisor crowding, the greater likelihood of absence of the second premolars should be borne in mind. Loss of a lower incisor may also be considered where local relief of crowding is required or where a modest amount of lower incisor retroclination is desirable to secure a better overjet and overbite in non-osteotomy cases.

Ectopic lateral incisors

When present, maxillary lateral incisors on the distal side of the cleft are often palatally displaced with the root in an extreme palatal position (Figure 19.6). Firm attachment of the supragingival fibres of the periodontal ligament may only become obvious when alignment is attempted and tooth movement may be resisted until the tissues actually rupture. Lateral incisors on the distal side of the cleft are especially difficult to align and more than two-thirds of lateral incisors are ultimately extracted (Bergland et al., 1986).

Absent lateral incisors

When maxillary lateral incisors are absent, two options present – space closure, or space preservation for a replacement of various kinds.

In the authors' opinion space closure so that the canine occupies the lateral incisor's position is generally the first choice since the natural dentition has the best prognosis for long-term health of the dentition. Composite build-up of the canine may be necessary to modify its shape (Figure 19.7). Successful space closure relieves the patient of the burden of prosthodontics and the associated lifetime maintenance (Figure 19.8).

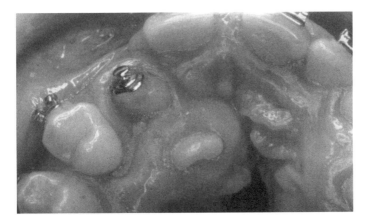

Figure 19.6. A palatally displaced lateral incisor.

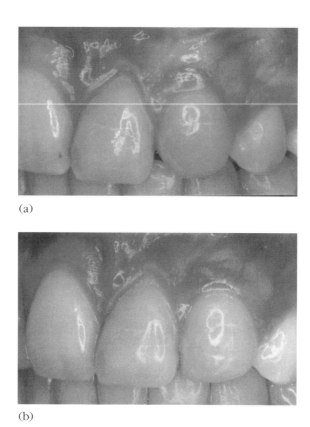

(a)

(b)

Figure 19.7. (a) Before, (b) after composite build-up of canine in the lateral incisor position.

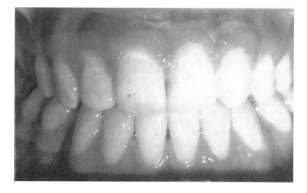

Figure 19.8. A patient where the space related to a congenitally missing upper left lateral incisor was closed by moving the canine medially into contact with the central incisor. No prosthodontic replacement was therefore necessary.

However, in patients with severely impaired maxillary growth and multiple missing teeth, orthodontic space closure may not be feasible. Despite the advent of bone grafting, 10% of patients with UCLP still require some form of prosthesis (Ramstad and Semb, 1997).

When full coverage abutment crowns are anticipated, the orthodontist should finish treatment with the abutment teeth in a slightly intruded and palatal position so that excessive grinding can be avoided (Ramstad, 1998). Even with adhesive bridges the prosthodontist should be consulted about the positioning of abutments beforehand (see Griffiths, Chapter 22).

Surgical transplantation of teeth can now be regarded as a treatment with high reliability in suitable cases (Andreasen, 1992). Premolars in a crowded lower jaw are suitable candidates for transplantation to the upper arch (Figure 19.9). Periodontal and pulp healing is best achieved if transplantation is carried out when root development is half to three-quarters complete. Experimental research suggests that simultaneous bone grafting and tooth

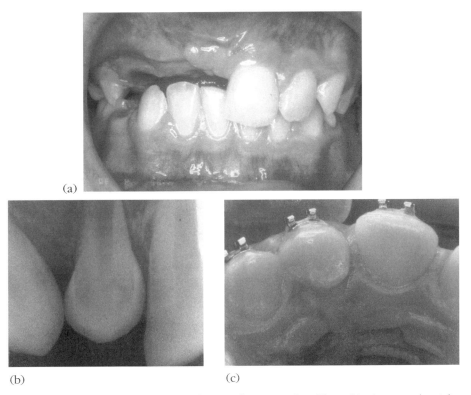

(a)

(b)   (c)

Figure 19.9. (a) Patient where both the maxillary central and lateral incisors on the right side were missing. The alveolar cleft had been bone grafted six months before. (b) A lower second premolar was transplanted to the right central incisor region. (c) The teeth were bonded and aligned.

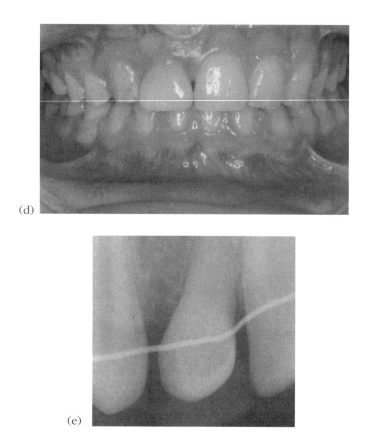

(d)

(e)

Figure 19.9. (d) The transplanted premolar had a composite build-up to obtain the shape of an incisor. The upper canine has been orthodontically moved to the lateral incisor position. (e) Eight years after tooth transplantation. The pulp seems obliterated, but the tooth is still vital.

transplantation should not be performed (Stenvik et al., 1989). Instead a six-month period should be allowed for graft consolidation. Cryopreservation may be considered when a useful tooth is removed during bone grafting (Schwartz, 1992). Transplantation of ectopic teeth is also possible.

Unfortunately, the maxillary lateral incisor region may be an unsuitable site for single tooth implant (J. O. Andreasen, personal communication, 1996). Even in non-cleft patients one study found that only 31.8% of implants in the maxillary incisal, canine and premolar region survived more than eight years (Haas et al., 1996). Continued growth precludes the placement of an implant until the end of growth, during which time the alveolar process reduces in height and volume, often requiring a further bone graft. For these reasons implants are especially unsuited to the lateral incisor region and their use in this setting should await further long-term follow-up studies.

Maxillary extraction choice

The maxillary arch is difficult to assess accurately when there is a superimposed contraction and anteroposterior discrepancy, so that it is often preferable to begin alignment, expansion and incisor correction before deciding on maxillary extractions. Frequently a great deal of space becomes available.

Extraction of teeth may be required in UCLP in the non-cleft quadrant, either because of crowding, or to allow correction of the dental midline. The tooth most commonly removed is the non-cleft second premolar, as this tooth is frequently malformed. Removal of the first premolar before the eruption of the second premolar is contraindicated. In some patients removal of the non-cleft lateral incisor allows the rapid restoration of symmetry (Figure 19.10). However, it should only be considered when compliance with space closure is assured.

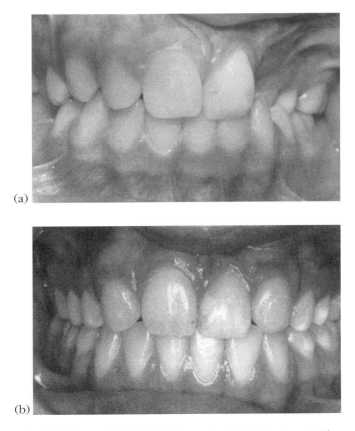

(a)

(b)

Figure 19.10. (a) Patient with UCLP before orthodontic treatment. The upper dental midline is displaced to the cleft side. The cleft side lateral incisor is congenitally missing. (b) The non-cleft lateral incisor was removed so that the midline deviation could be corrected. Reasonable symmetry in the upper dental arch was obtained.

Since the maxillary lateral incisor is often missing and the central incisor on the cleft side is often smaller than the other one, composite build-up of maxillary incisors may be necessary to achieve harmonization of the upper and lower arches.

Anchorage

Facial aesthetics takes precedence over 'normal' tooth positioning and it may be desirable to place the incisors in a slightly anterior position to improve lip relations. The upper incisors are often better carefully extruded since patients with a repaired upper lip often show little of their upper incisors, and a deep overbite is some compensation against the vertical growth pattern. Constant monitoring of the anterior position of the maxillary incisors is necessary, since they can very readily slip back into an anterior crossbite. Generally speaking, a stopped maxillary archwire will be used to maintain arch length, and elastic chain should be used only with caution. Bilateral class II elastics or headgear are clearly inappropriate. However, in patients where arch symmetry is being restored a combination of class II elastics on the non-cleft side and class III on the cleft side may be used with caution.

Protraction headgear (facemask) can be a valuable source of anchorage for retaining the incisor position while advancing posterior teeth during space closure (Figure 19.11a). The attachment hooks should be placed in the lateral incisor region to avoid molar extrusion (Figure 19.11b), and the mask used at night for 8–12 months. The side effects of protraction must be recognized, however. Retrusion of the lower incisors and occasional damage to the lower incisor gingiva may occur, while bite opening and increase in the lower facial height is unavoidable. These changes often create the false impression that anteroposterior skeletal change has been achieved. However, the normal facial skeleton is barely amenable to maxillary advancement without surgery (Profitt, 1993), and the maxilla with a repaired cleft is not amenable at all. Protraction of the cleft maxilla, even at an early stage, has nowhere been shown to provide lasting skeletal benefit or to reduce the frequency of maxillary osteotomy.

Canine impaction

In a series of 56 impacted canines in patients with alveolar clefts about two-thirds of impacted canines were found to lie on the palatal aspect of the arch and one-third high up in the alveolus (Semb and Schwartz, 1997). As their alignment may take a considerable length of time after exposure, this should be commenced first if possible. A palatal arch can often serve as anchorage for traction of the canine, allowing the placement of brackets on the other teeth to be delayed.

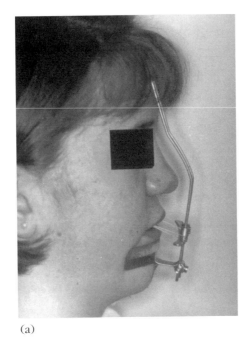

(a)

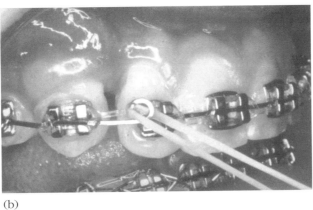

(b)

Figure 19.11. (a) Face mask, Delaire type. (b) The attachment hooks for the elastics are paced distal to the lateral incisors.

Extreme premaxillary prominence or displacement

Though the premaxilla in BCLP is often prominent in the early years of life, successful lip repair usually allows gradual moulding into a proper relationship. Integration of the premaxilla is completed by bone grafting and thereafter even marked vertical discrepancies may level out spontaneously (Figure 19.12).

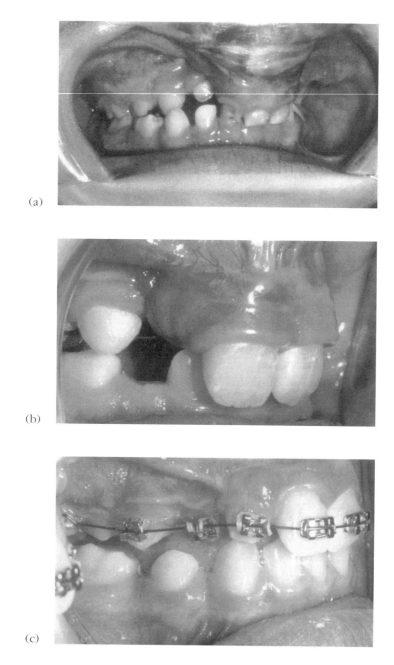

(a)

(b)

(c)

Figure 19.12. Patient with a vertically displaced premaxilla. (a) At age five years. (b) At age 10 years just prior to alveolar bone grafting. No intrusion of the incisors is attempted. (c) At 13 years of age. The upper teeth have just been bonded. The deep overbite has spontaneously improved. No special effort was made to intrude the incisors.

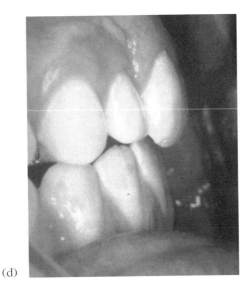

(d)

Figure 19.12 (contd) (d) At 18 years of age, three years after finishing orthodontic treatment. The overbite is 2 mm.

Persisting prominence of the premaxilla is usually the consequence of an unsuccessful primary lip repair and tethering of the lip above the premaxilla. In these circumstances the temptation to undertake surgical setback or orthodontic retraction should be resisted. Instead, successful sulcus deepening will allow the upper lip to start functioning in a more helpful way and bring about spontaneous alignment (Figure 19.13).

Retention

The relapse tendency in patients with clefts is great compared to non-clefts and is directly related to scar tissue from surgery. Thus a tight upper lip will prejudice the stability of proclined upper incisors and scars in the palate may encourage the migration of teeth into crossbite. However, apart from the use of a bonded retainer extending to at least two teeth either side of the cleft (Figure 19.14), we consider lifetime use of retainers undesirable. Where there has been an open bite in the cleft area, vertical relapse should also be anticipated.

The growth pattern and the above relapse tendencies will often combine to worsen the class III tendency, and it must be realized that perfect interdigitation of the teeth will not prevent this from happening. If at all possible it is therefore preferable, in cases with even a mild maxillary retrusion at age 10–12 years, to overcorrect the occlusion toward class II, especially in males, since they have a more adverse growth pattern than females (Ross, 1987; Paulin and Thilander, 1991; Semb, 1991a). In males a worsening of anteroposterior relations is almost certain and may be severe.

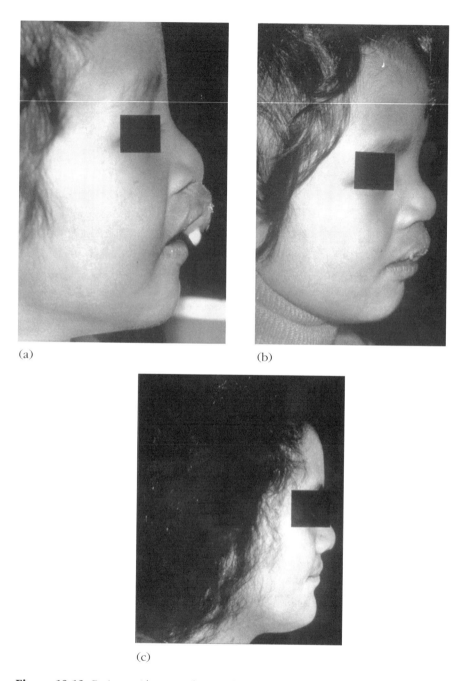

(a)

(b)

(c)

Figure 19.13. Patient with protruding and vertically displaced premaxilla after suboptimal lip closure. (a) At five years of age. (b) Four months after sulcusplasty, the profile is greatly improved as the lip covers the premaxilla. (c) Profile at 18 years of age.

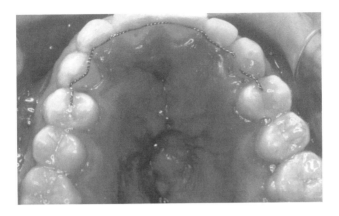

Figure 19.14. Bonded retainer including two teeth on either side of the cleft.

Unfavourable conditions for maxillary osteotomy

Orthognathic surgery in patients with repaired clefts requires especially careful planning between orthodontist, surgeon and speech therapist (see Lello, Chapter 21). Maxillary osteotomy is technically more challenging because of the underlying maxillary deformity, the presence of scarring, and the high relapse tendency – regardless of the means of fixation; the velopharyngeal mechanism may be adversely affected by maxillary advancement (Turvey et al., 1996).

It is important that the orthodontist is closely involved in the postoperative period. Elastics or even protraction headgear may be necessary to maintain the maxillary position and settle the occlusion.

Unsuccessful primary surgery

Inexpert primary surgery can present a number of challenges to the orthodontist. Traumatic surgery with severe residual scarring makes maxillary surgical advancement inevitable and orthodontics is limited to arch alignment. Pre-bone graft incisor alignment and transverse expansion will take longer to achieve and be subject to relapse well into adulthood (Figure 19.15). Arch expansion, merely to achieve bilateral crossbite, may be the only realistic option.

Eruption of the posterior teeth is impeded when there is no interincisal contact or when maxillary constriction causes the tongue to spread laterally. The resulting 'overclosure' exaggerates the anteroposterior discrepancy and may make the retention of brackets on the upper teeth difficult. It may be necessary to provide a removable lower anterior bite plane for a short time to allow bracket placement and to encourage posterior tooth eruption.

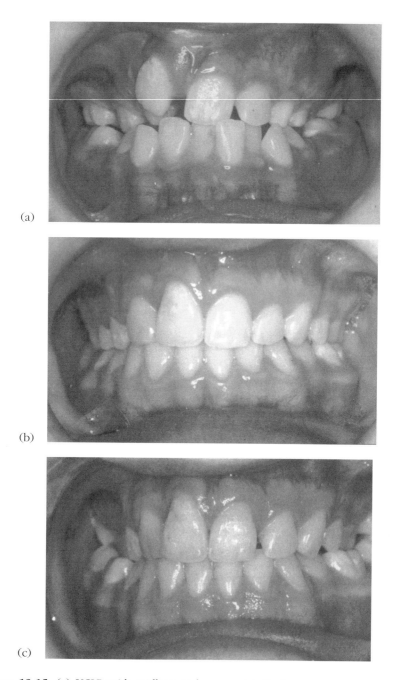

(a)

(b)

(c)

Figure 19.15. (a) UCLP with midline and segmental displacement pre-treatment. (b) Archform achieved by orthodontics. (c) Transverse relapse despite the use of a bonded retainer.

When specialized primary cleft surgery is not available, inexpert technique may produce large palatal fistulae. In BCLP the worst of these may extend through the alveolus and make successful bone grafting impossible. In these circumstances, some levelling of the occlusal plane may be necessary so that an overdenture is not required. Figure 19.16 shows a removable anterior bite plane incorporating buccal springs for extrusion of the buccal teeth.

Other cleft types

Incomplete CLP (I-CLP)

Patients with an incomplete cleft lip and palate can usually be treated according to non-cleft principles even though both the anterior and posterior of the maxilla are involved. This cleft subgroup is fairly small and has not received much attention in the literature. However, from clinical experience, facial growth in this cleft subtype seems to be more similar to non-cleft development. The same considerations as for patients with cleft lip/alveolus (see below) concerning the lateral incisor, bone grafting and the need for any lip/nose revisions are relevant for this group.

Cleft lip and alveolus (CLA)

Since patients with CLA have normal maxillary growth (Dahl, 1970), they can be treated according to orthodontic principles for non-clefts. But even though the alveolar arch at birth seems little affected by the cleft, in most instances irregularities of the number, size, shape and form of the lateral incisor on the cleft side will be found. Where two lateral incisors are present, the one with the poorest form should be removed to allow the best possible chance for development and eruption of the remaining lateral incisor. In many cases the cleft side lateral incisor will have a diminutive shape and will therefore need a composite build-up. The orthodontist should provide appropriate space so that the restored tooth can assume the same size and form as the non-cleft lateral incisor.

Some patients with CLA have an alveolar bony defect large enough to restrict orthodontic closure of the space in the cleft region, and in these cases alveolar bone grafting may be required.

Cleft palate only (CPO)

In patients with CPO both the maxilla and the mandible are smaller and more retrusive than in non-clefts (Dahl, 1970; Bishara and Iversen, 1974; Jonsson and Thilander, 1979; Viteporn et al., 1991). However, in most instances the degree of retrusion is similar in both jaws and therefore the relationship

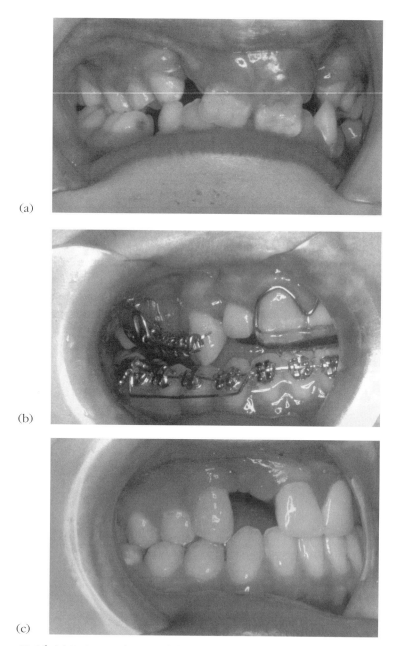

(a)

(b)

(c)

Figure 19.16. (a) Patient with vertical displacement of the premaxilla. As the patient had a large palatal fistula, alveolar bone grafting was ruled out. (b) The permanent buccal teeth were extruded by buccal arms attached to an acrylic base plate and anterior bite plane. (c) Occlusal levelling permitted the placement of small bone grafts to stabilize the premaxilla and facilitate the provision of a partial denture (obturator).

between the jaws is usually satisfactory. The mandibular plane is usually steep and the gonial angle obtuse. The incisors in both jaws are often retroclined. Patients with CPO also have a higher frequency of missing teeth than their non-cleft counterparts. The dental arches are slightly narrower and shorter (Athanasiou et al., 1987; Friede et al., 1993), and therefore dental crowding is a common feature. However, conventional orthodontics, often including extraction of teeth in both jaws, usually achieves an acceptable occlusion.

The orthodontist treating patients with CPO should, however, be aware of their vertical growth pattern and the greater tendency towards relapse because of the palatal scar tissue.

References

Åbyholm F, Bergland O, Semb G (1981) Secondary bone grafting of alveolar clefts. Scandinavian Journal of Plastic and Reconstructive Surgery 15: 127–140.

Andreasen JO (1992) Atlas of Replantation and Transplantation of Teeth. Fribourg: Mediglobe.

Athanasiou AE, Mazaheri M, Zarrinnia K (1987) Longitudinal study of the dental arch dimensions in hard and soft palate clefts. Journal of Pedodontics 12: 35–47.

Bergland O, Sidhu SS (1974) Occlusal changes from the deciduous to the early mixed dentition in unilateral complete clefts. Cleft Palate Journal 11: 317–326.

Bergland O, Semb G, Åbyholm F (1986) Elimination of the residual alveolar cleft by secondary bone grafting and subsequent orthodontic treatment. Cleft Palate Journal 23: 175–205.

Bishara SE, Iversen WW (1974) Cephalometric comparisons on the cranial base and face in individuals with isolated clefts of the palate. Cleft Palate Journal 11: 162–175.

Bjerklin K, Kurol J, Paulin G (1993) Ectopic eruption of the maxillary first permanent molars in children with cleft lip and/or palate. European Journal of Orthodontics 15: 535–540.

Bøhn A (1963) Dental anomalies in harelip and cleft palate. Acta Odontologica Scandinavica 21(suppl. 38): 1–109.

Bokhout B, Hofman FX, van Limbeek J, Kramer GJ, Prahl-Anderson B (1996) Increased caries prevalence 2, 5-year-old children with cleft lip and/or palate. Eur J Oral Sci 104: 518–522.

Boyne PJ, Sands NR (1972) Secondary bone grafting of residual alveolar and palatal defects. Journal of Oral and Maxillofacial Surgery 30: 87–92.

Boyne PJ, Sands NR(1976) Combined orthodontic-surgical management of residual palato-alveolar cleft defect. American Journal of Orthodontics 70: 20–37.

Dahl E (1970) Craniofacial morphology in congenital clefts of the lip and palate. An x-ray cephalometric study of young males. Dissertation. Acta Odontologica Scandinavica 28, suppl. 57.

Enemark H (1993) Orthodontic considerations in cleft orthognathic surgery patient. Abstract 336. 7th International Congress on Cleft Palate and Related Craniofacial Anomalies. Brisbane, Australia.

Enemark H, Sindet-Pedersen S, Bundgaard M (1987) Long-term results after secondary bone grafting of alveolar clefts. Journal of Oral and Maxillofacial Surgery 45: 913–918.

Enemark H, Bolund S, Jørgensen I (1990) Evaluation of unilateral cleft lip and palate treatment: Long-term results. Cleft Palate Journal 27: 354–361.

Fishman LS (1970) Factors related to tooth number, eruption time, and tooth position in cleft palate individuals. ASDC Journal of Dentistry for Children 37: 303–306.

Foster TD, Lavelle CLB (1971) The size of the dentition in complete cleft lip and palate. Cleft Palate Journal 8: 307–313.

Friede H, Persson EC, Lilja J, Elander A, Lohmander-Agerskov A, Søderpalm E (1993) Maxillary dental arch and occlusion in patients with repaired clefts of the secondary palate. Influence of push back palatal surgery. Scandinavian Journal of Plastic and Reconstructive Surgery and Hand Surgery 27: 297–305.

Haas R, Mensdorff-Poilly N, Mailath G, Watzek G (1996) Survival of 1,920 IMZ implants followed up to 100 months. International Journal of Oral and Maxillofacial Implants 11: 581–588.

Harvold E (1947) Observations on the development of the upper jaw in harelip and cleft palate. Odontologisk Tidsskrift 55(3): 289–305.

Jonsson G, Thilander B (1979) Occlusion, arch dimensions and craniofacial morphology after palatal surgery in a group of children with clefts in the secondary palate. American Journal of Orthodontics 76: 243–255.

Kramer G (1994) Early dento-maxillary development in children with cleft lip and/or palate. Dissertation. Academic Centre for Dentistry, Amsterdam.

McCance AM, Roberts-Harry D, Sherriff M, Mars M, Houston WJB (1990) A study model analysis of adult unoperated Sri Lankans with unilateral cleft lip and palate. Cleft Palate Journal 27: 146–154.

Nordquist GG, McNeill RW (1975) Orthodontic vs. restorative treatment of the congenitally absent lateral incisor. Long term periodontal and occlusal evaluation. Journal of Periodontology 46: 139–143.

Paulin G, Thilander B (1991) Dentofacial relations in young adults with unilateral cleft lip and palate. A follow-up study. Scandinavian Journal of Plastic and Reconstructive Surgery and Hand Surgery 25: 63–72.

Paulin G, Åstrand P, Rosenquist JB, Bartholdson L (1988) Intermediate bone grafting of alveolar clefts. Journal of Cranio-Maxillo-Facial Surgery 16: 2–7.

Pöyry M (1987) Dental development in 0–3-year-old children with cleft lip and palate. Dissertation. University of Helsinki.

Proffit WR (1993) Contemporary Orthodontics. St Louis: Mosby-Year Book.

Pruzansky S, Aduss H (1967) Arch form in the deciduous occlusion in complete unilateral cleft lip and palate. European Orthodontic Society Transactions 43: 365–382.

Ramstad T, Semb G (1997) The effect of alveolar bone grafting on the prosthodontic/reconstructive treatment of patients with unilateral complete cleft lip and palate. International Journal of Prosthodontics 10: 156–163.

Ramstad T (1998) Fixed prosthodontics in cleft palate. In: McKinstry RE, ed. Cleft Palate Dentistry. Arlington: ABI Professional Publications. Chapter 9, pp 236–262.

Ranta R (1972) The development of the permanent teeth in children with complete cleft lip and palate. Proceedings of the Finnish Dental Society 68, suppl. 3.

Ranta R (1983) Developmental course of 27 late-developing second premolars. Proceedings of the Finnish Dental Society 79: 9–12.

Ranta R (1986) A review of tooth formation in children with cleft lip/palate. American Journal of Orthodontics 90: 11–18.

Ranta R (1990) Orthodontic treatment alternatives for unilateral cleft lip and palate patients. In: Bardach J, Morris HL (eds) Multidisciplinary Management of Cleft Lip and Palate. Philadelphia: WB Saunders, Ch. 77, pp. 637–641.

Ross RB (1970) The clinical implications of facial growth in cleft lip and palate. Cleft Palate Journal 7: 37–47.

Ross RB (1987) Treatment variables affecting facial growth in complete unilateral cleft lip and palate. Part I: Treatment affecting growth. Cleft Palate Journal 24: 5–23.

Ross RB, Johnston MC (1972) Cleft Lip and Palate. Baltimore: Williams & Wilkins.

Schwartz O (1992) Cryopreservation of teeth before replantation or transplantation. In: Andreasen JO (ed.) Atlas of Replantation and Transplantation of Teeth. Fribourg: Mediglobe, pp. 241–256.

Semb G (1991a) A study of facial growth in patients with unilateral cleft lip and palate treated by the Oslo CLP Team. Cleft Palate–Craniofacial Journal 28: 1–21.

Semb G (1991b) A study of facial growth in patients with bilateral cleft lip and palate treated by the Oslo CLP Team. Cleft Palate–Craniofacial Journal 28: 22–39.

Semb G, Schwartz O (1997) The impacted tooth in patients with alveolar clefts. In: Andreasen JO, Petersen JK, Laskin DM (eds) Textbook and Color Atlas of Tooth Impaction. Copenhagen: Munksgaard, pp. 331–348.

Semb G, Shaw WC (1996) Facial growth in orofacial clefting disorders. In: Turvey TA, Vig KWL, Fonseca RJ (eds). Facial Clefts and Craniosynostosis. Principles and Management. Philadelphia: WB Saunders, Ch. 2, pp. 28–56.

Sindet-Pedersen S, Enemark H (1993) Management of impacted teeth in congenital clefts. In: Alling CC, Helfrick JF, Alling RD (eds) Impacted Teeth. Philadelphia: WB Saunders, pp. 344–352.

Stenvik A, Semb G, Bergland O, Åbyholm FE, Beyer-Olsen EMS, Gerner NW, Haanæs HR (1989) Experimental transplantation of teeth to simulated maxillary clefts. Scandinavian Journal of Plastic and Reconstructive Surgery 23: 105–108.

Suzuki A, Watanabe C, Nakano M, Takakama Y (1992) Maxillary lateral incisors of subjects with cleft lip and/or palate. Part 2. Cleft Palate–Craniofacial Journal 29: 380–384.

Turvey TA, Vig KWL, Fonseca RJ (eds) (1996) Midface advancement and contouring in the presence of cleft lip and palate. In: Facial Clefts and Craniosynostosis. Principles and Management. Philadelphia: WB Saunders, Ch. 20, pp. 441–503.

Vargervik K (1978) New bone formation secured by oriented stress in maxillary clefts. Cleft Palate Journal 15: 132–140.

Vargervik K (1990) Orthodontic treatment of cleft patients: Characteristics of growth and development/treatment principles. In: Bardach J, Morris HL (eds) Multidisciplinary Management of Cleft Lip and Palate. Philadelphia: WB Saunders, Ch. 78, pp. 642–649.

Viteporn S, Enemark H, Melsen B (1991) Postnatal craniofacial skeleton development following a pushback operation of patients with cleft palate. Cleft Palate–Craniofacial Journal 28: 392–396.

CHAPTER 20

Alveolar Bone Grafting

M. Mars

Introduction

Alveolar bone grafting (ABG) in the mixed dentition, before eruption of the permanent canine, is now established as the treatment for the residual alveolar defect in patients with cleft lip and palate. It was introduced into the UK in the early 1980s and many centres now have ten years' experience of this procedure. Medullary bone from a distant site (most commonly, the iliac crest but sometimes the tibia, mandibular symphysis or cranium) is placed in the alveolar defect. Within three months of successful surgery, grafts appear to be indistinguishable radiologically and behave clinically as normal alveolar bone.

The benefits of alveolar bone grafting in clefting deformities are well recognized, and are outlined below (Witsenburg, 1985; Bergland et al., 1986; Amanat and Langdon, 1991; Andlin-Sobocki et al., 1995). Many different grafting materials have been applied (Freihofer et al., 1993). Autogenous cancellous bone from the anterior iliac crest is used and advocated most frequently (Witsenburg, 1985). Secondary alveolar bone grafting is considered to be the appropriate strategy (Boyne and Sands, 1972, 1976; Åbyholm et al., 1981; Enemark et al., 1985; Bergland et al., 1986; Amanat and Langdon, 1991). Better results are achieved when the secondary alveolar bone grafting is performed before the eruption of the cleft canine (Bergland et al., 1986; Freihofer et al., 1993).

At the time of primary lip and palate repair the bony defect in the alveolar process is not repaired. The cleft segments abut one another but are not in bony union. Frequently, and often deliberately, a small buccal and sometimes palatal fistula remains. Attempts to bone graft the alveolar process at the time of lip repair using rib struts (so called primary bone grafting) were common practice. Inconsistent results and the suggestion that maxillary growth might have been impaired have led to the abandonment of this procedure (Johanson and Ohlsson, 1961; Johanson et al., 1974). One centre alone continues to advocate primary bone grafting, though the technique is very different from that originally proposed, using 'minced' rib rather than struts (Rosenstein et al., 1982).

Aims of alveolar bone grafting

The objective of alveolar bone grafting is the elimination of the bony alveolar defect, to provide the following benefits:

1. To permit eruption of the permanent canine in the cleft site into sound bone.
2. To provide bony support for teeth on either side of the cleft site.
3. To improve stability of the cleft segments, especially the mobile premaxilla in bilateral cleft lip and palate cases.
4. To facilitate fistula closure.
5. To obviate or minimize the need for prosthetic replacement of teeth in the cleft site.
6. To improve the contour of the alar base.

Timing

It is generally agreed that the optimum timing for alveolar bone grafting is before eruption of the permanent canine relating to the cleft site (Boyne and Sands, 1972; Hall and Posnick, 1983; Sindet-Pedersen and Enemark, 1985; Bergland et al., 1986; Paulin et al., 1988; Kortebein et al., 1991; Freihofer et al., 1993).

Some authorities state that bone grafting should take place when one-half to two-thirds of the canine root is formed. There is no precise recommended chronological age but a range of between eight and a half and ten and a half years is normal. Later bone grafting, after eruption of the canine adjacent to the cleft site, still offers many advantages but the success rate is reduced, particularly in bilateral cleft lip and palate cases (Åbyholm et al., 1981; Hall and Posnick, 1983; Jia et al. 1998).

The lateral incisor in cleft lip and palate patients is frequently absent. In a small number of cases the presence of a diminutive lateral incisor, which may, however, be useful, is an indication for earlier bone grafting at around seven to eight years of age.

A short period of orthodontic treatment, usually not more than six months, prior to bone grafting is often required. Incisors in crossbite should be proclined and lateral segments which are collapsed should be expanded.

The quad-helix appliance (Figure 20.1) with additional buccal fixed appliances is most often used. Simple removable appliances may also be beneficial though fixed appliances are used more commonly. The aim of such treatment is to create the best possible access for the surgeon to place the graft and to reveal the true extent of any fistulae. A wide view of the nasal floor and its repair is facilitated by orthodontic expansion. There is no need for orthodontic treatment where good surgical access already exists.

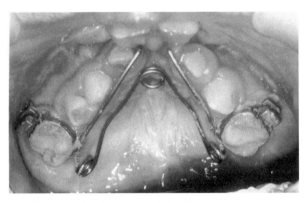

Figure 20.1. A modified quad-helix (a tri-helix) where the narrowness anteriorly before expansion provides insufficient room for two helices.

In bilateral cleft lip and palate cases, proclination of incisor teeth which are sometimes severely retroclined (Figure 20.2) is essential preoperatively, if proper vision and access to the palatal fistula is to be achieved. The mobile premaxilla must be stabilized by fixed appliances; this is achieved by a heavy buccal archwire which is removed during surgery and replaced in the operating theatre immediately after surgery. This appliance is retained for three to four months after surgery.

A very thin bony covering of the central incisor next to the cleft site is a common feature before bone grafting. Often, there is just a lamina dura with no cancellous bone. In such cases the incisor should not be bodily uprighted because of the possibility of bone loss and fenestration of the thin cortical lamina. Bodily movement is best deferred until after successful alveolar bone grafting as part of definitive orthodontic treatment. Some three to four weeks before surgery, it is often advisable that any erupted supplemental teeth and the deciduous canine should be extracted. This permits healing of the mucosa, so that at surgery an intact mucoperiosteal flap, which must be of attached gingivae, can be advanced over the surgical site without 'holes'. A common error is the use of flaps of reflected mucosa. These do not have a periosteal sub-lining and hence do not provide support for underlying bone or the eruption of teeth.

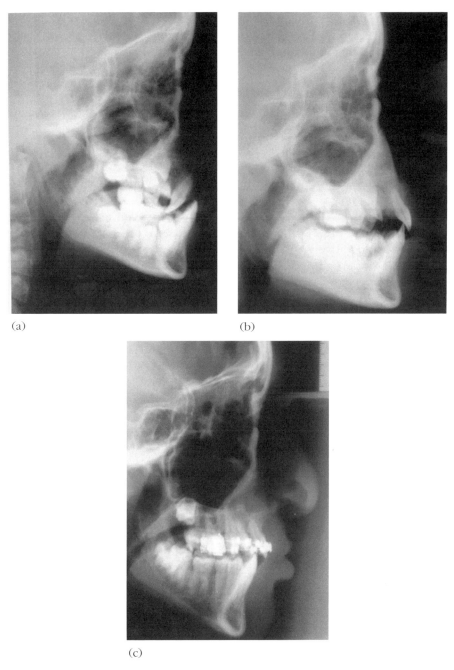

(a)   (b)

(c)

Figure 20.2. Lateral skull X-rays: (a) before proclination of the severely retroclined incisors, (b) after proclination and before bone grafting, and (c) after bone grafting during definitive orthodontic treatment.

Grafting is a combined orthodontic and surgical procedure and decisions regarding timing, orthodontic treatment and the need to extract teeth in the cleft site should be jointly discussed.

Records, audit and review

High quality records comprising dental study models, intra- and extraoral photographs and especially good quality intraoral radiographs are required for clinical and audit purposes. Upper occlusal X-rays should present a detailed picture of the whole cleft site and related teeth. If taken at high angles (70° to the horizontal) magnification is eliminated. Patients are reviewed on a joint clinic one week, three weeks, six weeks, 12 weeks, 26 weeks and 52 weeks after surgery. They are then seen annually until the time for definitive orthodontic treatment. X-rays are taken at 12 weeks, and one year postoperatively and annually thereafter. The eruption of the canine through the bone graft occurs spontaneously in most cases, but this may take over two years. Canines which present with an aberrant eruption pattern, or which are bodily displaced, may need to be uncovered and orthodontic brackets with trailing wires or chains attached, so that they can be aligned properly.

The principal aim of alveolar bone grafting is to permit eruption of the canine into the cleft site. The canine must, when erupted, be supported by bone of as near normal height and contour as possible. A simple system of analysis (Bergland et al., 1986) has been described in which four groups of bony height can be readily determined:

Group 1, where there is normal interdental bony height.
Group 2, where there is more than three-quarters normal interdental bony height.
Group 3, where there is less than three-quarters interdental bony height.
Group 4, where there is no bony bridge at all.

For clinical purposes Bergland considers groups 1 and 2 as successful, and groups 3 and 4 as unsuccessful. Most reports demonstrate between 85% and 95% success rate, e.g. (Bergland et al., 1986; Amanat and Langdon, 1991; Collins et al., 1998). Such reports usually relate to mixed unilateral and bilateral cleft lip and palate groups. In contrast, one study reports a significantly worse outcome for late operated bilateral cleft lip and palate cases with a 67% success rate (Jia et al., 1998).

All assessments claiming a high success rate have been undertaken by those centres performing the surgery, i.e. internal assessment. It is salutary to note that in the recent Clinical Standards Advisory Group (CSAG) Report on Cleft Lip and Palate (1998) two independent external assessors were employed to review results from units around the UK. They under-took allocation to Bergland's four groups in a blind manner, thereby elimi-nating bias. Of 183 films assessed, 26 were considered to be unreadable due to poor film quality or tooth position. Of the remaining 157 films examined, 58% showed a successful outcome whilst 42% were seriously deficient or total failures. Therefore, it would seem that independent assessment performed blindly, has shown poorer outcome than previ-ously reported.

Complications

Complications of alveolar bone grafting, apart from inadequate alveolar interdental bony height, have been discussed in previous reports. (Bergland et al., 1986; Sindet-Pederesen and Enemark, 1988; Amanat and Langdon, 1991). Proliferation of granulation tissue intraorally, infection of donor and/or recipient site, and occasional paraesthesia of skin around the hip incision, are rare problems. A few cases of internal or external resorption of the canine have been reported. These are thought to be due to surgical instrumentation of the root surface at the time of grafting, resulting in loss of the protective layer of cementum overlying the root dentine.

Clinical examples

The following cases demonstrate features of alveolar bone grafting.

Figure 20.3(a) is an oblique upper occlusal X-ray which displays the extent of the alveolar bony defect. Figure 20.3(b) shows the same site three months after successful bone grafting, in which the bony trabecular pattern is indistinguishable from the rest of the maxillary bone.

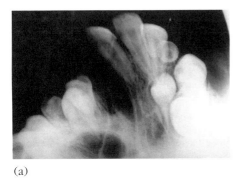 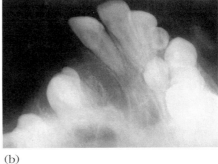

(a)   (b)

Figure 20.3. (a) An upper occlusal X-ray showing the extent of the bony defect. (b) The same site three months after bone grafting.

Figures 20.4(a, b and c) are upper oblique occlusal X-rays: (a) before expansion, with supernumerary teeth present in the cleft; (b) one month after bone grafting – the supernumerary teeth have been removed and expansion has previously been undertaken; (c) one year after alveolar bone grafting. Figures 20.4(d and e) show the occlusion four years after bone grafting and definitive orthodontic treatment. The malformed lateral incisor has been built up with composite dental material and a permanent palatal retainer is in place.

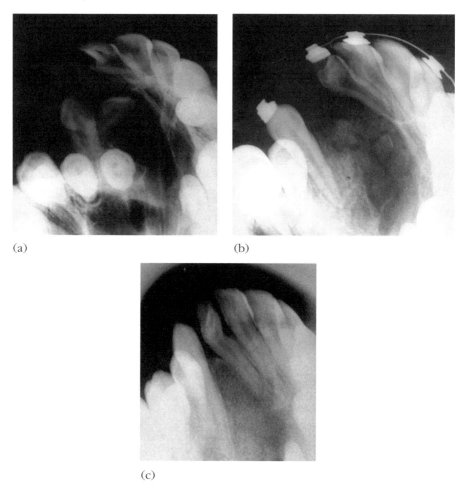

(a)   (b)

(c)

Figure 20.4. (a) An upper occlusal X-ray, before expansion, with supernumerary teeth present. (b) One month after bone grafting; expansion has previously been undertaken, and supernumerary teeth have been removed at operation. (c) Normal trabecular bone one year after alveolar bone grafting.

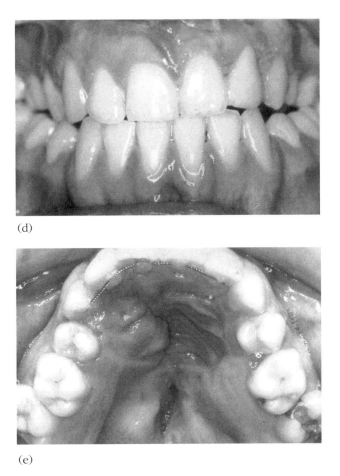

(d)

(e)

Figure 20.4. (contd) (d) Occlusion four years after bone grafting. (e) A permanent palatal retainer in place.

Figures 20.5(a, b and c) show the benefit of alveolar bone grafting even after the ideal time when the canine tooth has already erupted. Note that the canine takes the position of the absent lateral incisor next to the central incisor.

The patient in Figures 20.6(a, b, c, d, e and f) demonstrates preliminary proclination of incisors and extraction of deciduous teeth before alveolar bone grafting (Figures 20.6a and b). Figures 20.6(c, d and e) show views at surgery where buccal and palatal mucoperiosteal flaps are elevated: the unerupted permanent canine is visible and after repair of the nasal floor the cleft is packed with cancellous bone; the buccal flaps are advanced over the cleft and sutured. Figure 20.6(f) shows the incisions for the buccal flaps.

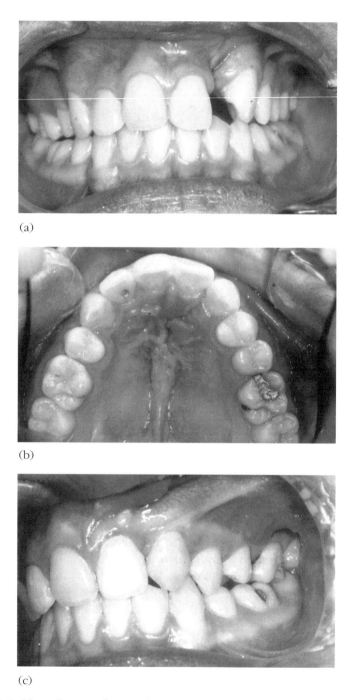

(a)

(b)

(c)

Figure 20.5. (a) Pre bone grafting occlusion. (b and c) Occlusion after grafting and after orthodontic treatment.

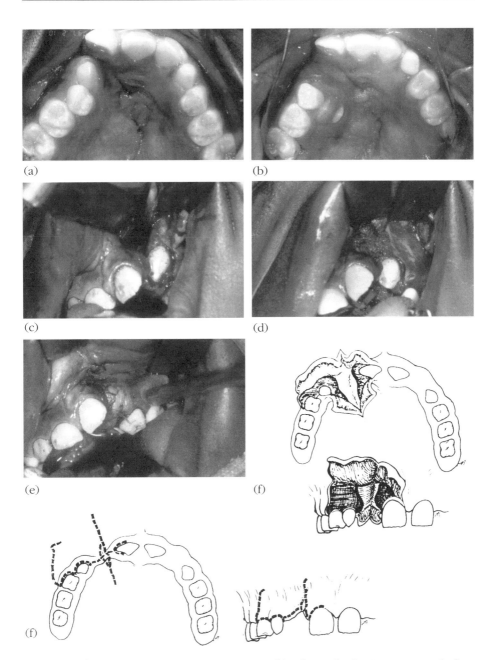

Figure 20.6. (a) Before orthodontic treatment. (b) After orthodontic treatment, before bone grafting. (c) At surgery, the permanent canine is exposed and the defect is visible. (d) The defect is filled with cancellous bone. (e) The mucoperiosteal flaps are sutured over the bone. (f) Incisions and flap design for alveolar bone grafting (drawings courtesy of F. Åbyholm).

Summary

Alveolar bone grafting has been a major advance in cleft lip and palate treatment. In particular, it has enabled an orthodontic programme combined with a surgical procedure to eliminate or minimize the need for prosthodontic rehabilitation. Alveolar bone graft surgery, though not major, is precise, requiring strict attention to detail; in particular, the nasal floor must be repaired with a 'water-tight' seal. The advanced buccal flap must be of attached mucoperiostium (gingivae) not of reflected mucosa. Patients must have a high standard of oral hygiene pre- and postoperatively. Successful alveolar bone grafting necessitates a joint orthodontic and surgical involvement pre-, peri- and postoperatively.

Audit of results should ideally be undertaken by independent assessors, working 'blind', based on a consecutive series of cases.

References

Åbyholm F, Bergland O, Semb G (1981) Secondary bone grafting of alveolar clefts. Scandinavian Journal of Plastic Reconstructive Surgery 15: 127–140.

Amanant N, Langdon JD (1991) Secondary alveolar bone grafting in clefts of the lip and palate. Journal of Cranio-Maxillo-Facial Surgery 19: 7–14.

Andlin-Sobocki A, Eliasson LA, Paulin G (1995) Periodontal evaluation of teeth in bone grafted regions in patients with unilateral cleft lip and cleft palate. American Journal of Orthodontics and Dentofacial Orthopedics 107: 144–152.

Bergland O, Semb G, Åbyholm F (1986) Elimination of the residual alveolar clefts by secondary bone grafting and subsequent orthodontic treatment. Cleft Palate Journal 23: 175–205.

Boyne PJ, Sands NR (1972) Secondary bone grafting of residual alveolar and palatal clefts. Journal of Oral Surgery 30: 87–92.

Boyne PJ, Sands NR (1976) Combined orthodontic-surgical management of residual palato-alveolar cleft defects. American Journal of Orthodontics 70: 20–37.

Clinical Standards Advisory Group (CSAG) (1998) Cleft Lip and Palate. Report of a CSAG Committee. London: HMSO.

Collins M, James DR, Mars M (1998) Eight years experience of alveolar bone grafting: a review of 115 patients. European Journal of Orthodontics, 20: 115–120.

Enemark H, Simonsen EK, Schramm JE (1985) Secondary bone grafting in unilateral cleft lip and palate patients: indications and treatment procedure. International Journal of Oral Surgery 14: 2–10.

Freihofer HPM, Borstlap WA, Kuijpers-Jagtman AM, Voorsmit RACA, Damme PAV, Heidbuchel KLWM, Borstlap-Engels VMF (1993) Timing and transplant materials for closure of alveolar clefts, a clinical comparison of 296 cases. Journal of Cranio-Maxillo-Facial Surgery 21: 143–148.

Hall DH, Posnick JC (1983) Early results of secondary bone grafts in 106 alveolar clefts. Journal of Oral and Maxillofacial Surgery 41: 289–294.

Jia Y, James DR, Mars M (1998) Bilateral alveolar bone grafting – a report of 55 consecutive cases. European Journal of Orthodontics 20: 299–307.

Johanson B, Ohlsson A (1961) Bone grafting and dental orthopaedics in primary and secondary cases of cleft lip and palate. Act Chirurgica Scandinavica 122: 112–124.

Johanson B, Ohlsson A, Friede H, Ahlgren S (1974) A follow-up study of cleft lip and palate patients treated with orthodontics, secondary bone grafting and prosthetic rehabilitation. Scandinavian Journal of Plastic and Reconstructive Surgery 8: 121-135.

Kortebein MJ, Nelson CL, Sadove AM (1991) Retrospective analysis of 135 secondary alveolar cleft grafts using iliac or calvarial bone. Journal of Oral and Maxillo Facial Surgery 49: 493–498.

Paulin G, Astrand P, Rosenquist JB, Bartholdson L (1988) Intermediate bone grafting of alveolar clefts. Journal of Cranio Maxillo-Facial Surgery 16: 2–7.

Rosenstein SW, Monroe CW, Kernahan DA, Jacobson BN, Griffith BH, Bauer BS (1982) The case for early bone grafting in cleft lip and palate. Journal of Plastic and Reconstructive Surgery 70: 297–309.

Sindet-Pedersen S, Enemark H (1985) Comparative study of secondary and late secondary bone-grafting in patients with residual cleft defects. Short term evaluation. International Journal of Oral Surgery 14: 389–398.

Witsenburg B (1985) The reconstruction of anterior residual bone defects in patients with cleft lip, alveolus and palate. A review. Journal of Maxillofacial Surgery 13: 197–208.

CHAPTER 21

Orthognathic Surgery

G.E. LELLO

Introduction

A number of children who have had repair of a cleft lip and palate develop an increasing deformity as they grow, particularly as they pass through adolescence. This is due to under-development of the maxilla and relatively greater growth of the mandible which leads to a concave facial profile and disproportion between the height of the middle and lower thirds of the face. This deformity can be corrected by dividing and repositioning the bones, a technique known as orthognathic surgery. Usually this involves a maxillary osteotomy at Le Fort I level; less often osteotomy at a higher level may be needed, or mandibular or genial osteotomies (Figures 21.1, 21.2 and 21.3).

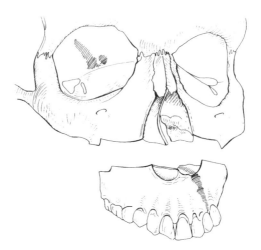

Figure 21.1. Le Fort I maxillary osteotomy with step.

338

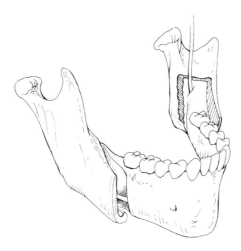

Figure 21.2. Sagittal split mandibular osteotomy.

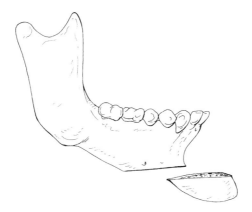

Figure 21.3. Genial osteotomy.

The retromaxillism and micromaxillism can give rise to increasing psychosocial problems (see Bradbury, Chapter 23), difficulties in mastication, pain and speech abnormalities, all of which would make early surgical correction desirable. Unfortunately, extensive surgery to the maxilla at an early age may cause damage to unerupted teeth, contribute to retardation of future maxillary growth, or create an ideal occlusion which is later disrupted by disproportionate maxillary and mandibular growth. For these reasons orthognathic surgery is usually delayed until facial growth is complete. The duration and nature of orthodontic management is an important and complicating factor. In a complete alveolar cleft, bone grafting will normally have been completed prior to the patient's pubertal growth spurt. Any associated orthodontic management at this stage, to position erupting teeth within or through the alveolar graft and align the dental arches, may leave the orthodontist faced with the difficulty of having to maintain the arch forms and tooth inclinations in compensated positions relative to surrounding active muscle forces until growth ceases and orthognathic surgery is undertaken. This prolonged period of retention may compromise the health of the teeth and surrounding structures and embarrass the patient during important psychosocial formative years.

If psychosocial pressures are great, it is possible to proceed with surgery early on, on the understanding that a repetition of the surgery may be necessary at a later date.

Sometimes an adult patient presents for orthognathic surgery who has been lost to review and has had no surgical procedures during adolescence. In such a patient, the problems of facial aesthetics, malocclusion, oronasal fistulae and alveolar bone grafting can be addressed simultaneously, but better and more stable results, with fewer complications, are more likely to be achieved when alveolar grafting and orthodontic management have been completed prior to the maxillary osteotomy.

The preparations for orthognathic surgery can be prolonged and the surgery is complex. It should never be undertaken unless the patient understands what is involved and is prepared to cooperate fully.

Orthodontic preparation

Before orthognathic surgery is carried out, orthodontic management is necessary to provide a stable dental base upon which to perform the surgery and to prevent relapse.

Retromaxillism is often accompanied by a degree of micromaxillism, and this smaller than normal bony base should contain no more teeth than can be accommodated. Tooth angulation and inclination to the bone base should be optimal, and the arches should be aligned, coordinated and levelled (in segments, when segmental surgery has been planned). Presurgical orthodontics often unavoidably makes worse the apparent jaw and tooth discrepancy (overjet and overbite) and holds the teeth in a decompensated position, awaiting surgery. The attached mucosa must be healthy preoperatively, with no marginal gingivitis present and oral hygiene should be meticulous.

Close cooperation between surgeon and orthodontist is essential to ensure that orthodontic appliances which may impede surgery are removable and that arch wires will not prevent differential maxillary segmental movement when necessary but will also contribute to stabilization of the relocated maxillary segments.

Initial orthodontic preparation may have been undertaken for the alveolar bone grafting procedure (see Mars, Chapter 20). Thereafter, once healing is complete (usually within three months of grafting), further preparation of teeth and occlusion for the surgical relocation of the maxilla by conventional osteotomy procedures or distraction osteogenesis techniques is undertaken.

Adolescents

Le Fort I downfracture osteotomy

General principles and considerations

The goal of orthodontic and surgical intervention is to establish a good occlusion and improve facial aesthetics from a concave to a convex profile without deleteriously affecting other features and functions such as the appearance of the nose and speech (Obwegeser et al., 1985). This requires adequate mobilization of the maxilla, despite soft tissue scarring, to enable a tension-free advancement of the maxilla while maintaining adequate blood supply to the tissues.

Three factors need to be taken into account when planning, and contribute significantly to relapse:

- the degree of surgical advancement of the maxilla;
- the nature and extent of soft tissue scarring;
- the blood supply to the mobilized maxilla.

The temptation to retrude surgically an already small mandible in the cleft patient to decrease the negative overjet should be resisted. Patient, careful mobilization of the maxilla enables most negative overjets of up to approximately 15 mm to be corrected. If scarring, diminished blood supply or the degree of maxillary retrusion precludes adequate maxillary advancement using the standard Le Fort I technique, the Converse and Shapiro (1952) technique may be considered, although it is not without undesirable complications. This entails advancing the maxilla by means of a transverse palatal osteotomy at the juncture of the palatine and maxillary bones, and it has been suggested that it reduces the incidence of postoperative velopharyngeal dysfunction (James and Brook, 1985; Sell et al., 1993).

In these circumstances, distraction osteogenesis may prove to be a feasible alternative. Elongation, hypertrophy and hyperplasia of muscle, soft tissue and overlying skin has been shown by Yagui et al. (1991) and Molina and Ortiz-Monasterio (1995) in response to bone distraction. Extrapolation of these findings to the distraction of the cleft maxilla may imply the possibility for the soft palate to adapt to the gradual advancement of the maxilla, with a reduced deleterious effect on velopharyngeal dysfunction.

Poor blood supply to the maxilla may necessitate an osteotomy being planned at a higher level than Le Fort I (e.g. Le Fort III), which may also be called for in terms of facial aesthetics and to avoid damage to unerupted permanent teeth. Many modifications to the Le Fort osteotomies exist to achieve the best appearance for an individual patient, including moving the maxilla in segments.

In planning the maxillary advancement, consideration must be given to likely changes in facial features. These may include elevation of the nasal tip and broadening of the nasal alae (rhinoplasty being deferred until after the osteotomy), decreasing the nasolabial angle, altering the maxillary tooth and upper lip relationship in both vertical and anteroposterior aspects, changing the facial profile and possibly causing the chin to appear small (which would require an advancement genioplasty).

Planning considerations for movement of the maxillary segments should include alveolar bone grafting if it has not already been done, the possibility of the placement of osseo-integrated implants and the onlaying of lyophilized, autogenous or allogeneic material to the zygomatic eminences (Sailer, 1983).

If oronasal fistulae are present they can be closed simultaneously.

Preparation and planning

Orthognathic surgery involves a comprehensive assessment of the patient's facial features in the context of stature, body build, head shape, sex, race, and opinion of what changes the patient would wish to see following surgery.

Clinical evaluation is the most important aspect of planning, and conclusions are supported by standard radiographs including cephalometric analyses and prediction tracings (manual or computerized – Figure 21.4) and photographs. Plaster cast study models of the dentition are used to simulate surgical movement of the jaws, to measure approximate jaw movement in three dimensions, and to ascertain that an acceptable occlusion is attainable. The models may be articulated in a simple hinge articulator, or in functional articulators of varying degrees of complexity and sophistication mimicking the position and function of the masticatory apparatus and dentition. The production of stereolithographic models, computer three-dimensional and virtual-reality simulations of the surgery offer scope for improved prediction of surgical moves and changes, but the weak link remains the accurate transfer of planned surgical procedures from the simulation to the patient during surgery.

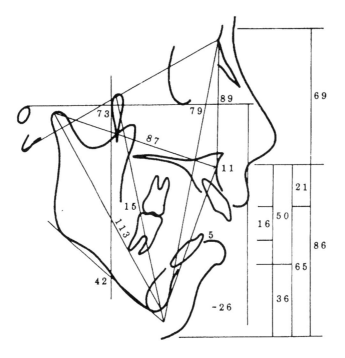

Figure 21.4. Example of prediction tracings from lateral cephalometric radiograph (measurements in millimetres).

Maxillary advancement can cause borderline velopharyngeal closure to become incompetent. The assessment and evaluation of speech and velopharyngeal function by a speech and language therapist, nasendoscopy and videofluoroscopy (see Sell and Grunwell, Chapter 16 and Mercer and Pigott, Chapter 17; Wakamuto et al., 1996), acoustic and aerodynamic methods such as nasometry (Dalston et al., 1991) should be undertaken both pre- and postoperatively to determine the likely effect of the operation on the patient's speech (Witzel and Vallino, 1992).

Following the surgical attainment of the planned intermaxillary relationship by means of a maxillary (and possibly mandibular) osteotomy, closure of any oronasal fistulae, alveolar bone grafting and genioplasty, the orthodontic refinement of the occlusion is completed and endosseous implants may then be placed in the alveolus if required.

Technique

In the non-cleft patient (Epker and Wolford, 1980) nasoendotracheal intubation under general anaesthesia allows for a buccal maxillary vestibular incision extending from one first molar across the midline to the opposite first molar, to expose the lower extent of the piriform rim, the infra-orbital nerve and cortex of the lateral wall of the maxillary sinus posteriorly as far as the pterygoid plates. A horizontal osteotomy (Figure 21.1) through this cortex bilaterally, together with separation of the caudal end of the vomer and cartilaginous septum of the nose from the maxilla, a horizontal osteotomy of the lateral nasal wall beneath the inferior turbinate and the chiselling of the maxillary tuberosities free from the pterygoid plates, allow downward pressure on the anterior maxilla to fracture the posterior wall of the maxillary sinus and to mobilize the maxilla. Pedicled on the soft palate and buccal mucosa distal to the first molars, the maxilla may be relocated anteriorly, superiorly or inferiorly. Prefabricated acrylic occlusal wafer splints from the plaster cast dental model simulation allow for relatively accurate location of the maxilla, which is fixed in position by osteosynthesis plates and screws (metal or, less frequently, resorbable material).

Postoperatively the jaws may be placed into intermaxillary fixation (inter-arch wires or elastics) for periods ranging from one to three weeks. The acrylic inter-occlusal splint may be secured to the maxillary teeth during this period to facilitate interdigitation of the opposing teeth during the initial phase of healing prior to resumption of orthodontic treatment. Presurgical orthodontic preparation includes the placement of tooth brackets and dental arch wires, which in turn facilitate intermaxillary fixation during and, if necessary, after surgery.

Specific modifications for cleft lip and palate

When previous alveolar bone grafting has been undertaken (Turvey and Tejera, 1996) the maxilla is moved as a single unit unless specific segmental orthodontics and surgery have been planned. While the object of the surgical intervention is to achieve the same goals as for the non-cleft patient, the potential for surgical relapse due to inelastic scar tissue is greater in the cleft patient. For this reason, modifications to the above procedure are generally considered important to increase the stability of the end result.

The grafted cleft alveolus

When the alveolus has been successfully grafted, the maxillary osteotomy at the Le Fort I level is essentially similar to that described for a non-cleft maxillary procedure. However, if extensive scarring is thought to jeopardize maxillary vascularity, the bone may be approached through bilateral small vertical incisions over the zygomatic buttress, with vertical or short horizontal incisions in the anterior sulcus to maintain vascular pedicles.

The osteotomy (Figure 21.1) of the lateral maxillary sinus wall should incorporate a vertical step down for approximately 1 cm in the region of the first molar tooth. This so-called L-step osteotomy allows a corticomedullary pelvic bone graft to be wedged into the vertical gap once the maxilla has been advanced, to resist posterior or superior relapse, and to facilitate bony union across the osteotomy gap.

The nasal mucosa should be elevated carefully from the lateral nasal wall and nasal septum/nasal floor junction, on either side of the cleft nasal floor and hard palate. This allows for the cutting of the nasal mucosa free from the palatal mucosa along the previous line of repair of the palatal cleft, prior to downfracturing the maxilla. This horizontal cut should be placed through the nasal mucosa rather than through the palatal mucosa, so that, following the downfracturing of the maxilla, only repair of the nasal mucosa may be necessary. Repair of the palatal mucosa can be very difficult once the maxilla has been mobilized, and may result in an oronasal fistula.

An acrylic occlusal wafer splint with deep insets for the maxillary teeth is utilized to ensure that the mobilized maxilla is placed without any undue tugging into a good occlusion with the mandible, while the osteotomy gap is bone grafted and osteosynthesis plates are placed. The occlusal splint is wired to the maxillary teeth or orthodontic appliances to support the tooth arch configuration and prevent medial collapse of the maxillary segments. The splint may also serve to stabilize a relatively poor inter-occlusal inter-digitation prior to final orthodontic treatment, and may allow for the mandibular teeth to lock into their indentations within the splint, thereby supporting and stabilizing the relocated maxilla.

It is unusual to have to apply intermaxillary fixation postoperatively, but inter-arch elastics are frequently necessary to retain the relocated maxilla during the weeks following surgery to prevent scar contraction-induced relapse. Intermaxillary fixation for a prolonged period will not prevent relapse of a maxilla that has not been adequately mobilized or supported by appropriate bone grafting and plate fixation following a significant move, but may only serve to extrude teeth and prolong the patient's period of discomfort.

The non-grafted cleft alveolus

When the maxillary osteotomy is undertaken simultaneously with the grafting of the alveolus, differential segment movement may be used to establish the occlusion and close the alveolar gap. The immediate place-ment of a new complete dental arch wire or provision of support across the break in the arch wire by splinting, using the occlusal wafer or other methods of linking the adjacent teeth, may suffice to retain the arch form. Equally, careful consideration must be given to the design of soft tissue flaps to cover the alveolar bone graft and to close the oronasal fistula, as the blood supply of the soft tissue is likely to be jeopardized by scarring from previous surgery and by the degree of mobilization and advancement of the maxilla necessary to obtain the desired occlusion.

Le Fort I distraction osteogenesis osteotomy

General principles

When a bone is fractured or cut it heals by callus formation. Gradual distraction of callus to provide new bone and stabilize relocated bone was popularized by Ilizarov (Ilizarov et al., 1980). It has for many years been employed to relocate virtually every major bone in the craniofacial complex (McCormick, 1995), including the maxilla (McCarthy et al., 1992, Rachmiel et al., 1995, 1999; Cohen et al., 1997).

Distraction osteogenesis of the maxilla is undertaken once preparatory orthodontic management, alveolar bone grafting with subsequent eruption of the canine through the graft, and orthodontic alignment of the dental arches is complete.

Preparation and planning

Planning is similar to that for a standard osteotomy, involving a clinical evaluation of the patient, analysis of a lateral cephalogram and plaster cast dental model operation. An occlusal acrylic wafer is constructed for the predicted final occlusion in order to stabilize and support the relocated maxilla.

Technique

A short vertical maxillary sulcus mucosal incision is placed over each zygomatic buttress, and a short horizontal incision in the anterior sulcus is completed. Subperiosteal tunnelling allows osteotomies to be carried out as described for the cleft maxilla. The maxilla is downfractured and mobilized, taking care to preserve the soft tissue pedicles, and gentle stretching of the soft tissues is undertaken by attempting to mobilize and advance the maxilla to its final planned occlusion, or as near as possible without tearing tissue. The maxilla is then seated back into the pre-osteotomy position and occlusion, without any form of fixation, and the wounds are sutured. No other procedures are undertaken, and the patient is discharged one day after surgery, with a clinically loose maxilla. A soft diet is prescribed, and the patient is asked to note the mobility of the maxilla each day and to inform the surgeon or orthodontist when the mobility becomes noticeably less, usually five to seven days after surgery. Regular clinical checks to confirm the loss of maxillary mobility are necessary. Light analgesia during this period may be necessary. Antibiotics are administered as a bolus on general anaesthesia induction only.

As soon as the maxilla is no longer mobile to gentle finger pressure or light occlusion, it is gradually distracted at 1 to 2 mm a day by means of a reverse face frame or appropriate intraoral device. When the desired position of the maxilla is achieved, retention of the established occlusion with inter-arch elastics is necessary for about three to six months.

Orthognathic surgery in adult cleft lip and palate patients

Dentulous patients

In most instances the adult patient with a dentulous maxilla is managed similarly to the older child and adolescent. Prediction of the final relationship between the maxilla and mandible is more accurate, as further facial growth will not occur to disrupt the achieved occlusion. Unerupted or developing teeth are less likely to interfere with the placement of the osteotomies, but perioperative dental management may still be necessary to achieve an acceptable and stable occlusion. Surgery may involve immediate and full relocation of the maxilla, often accompanied by simultaneous grafting of the cleft alveolus and closure of an oronasal fistula, or a distraction osteogenesis technique may be acceptable to the patient.

Precautions including bone grafts, resilient arch wires, osteosynthesis plates and frequently inter-arch elastics to prevent relapse are essential. The effect of maxillary movement on speech must be taken into account and monitored.

Edentulous patients

The greatest difficulty in the management of the edentulous maxilla occurs as a result of teeth not being available to assist in planning accurately the degree and direction of relocation of the maxilla, to facilitate intermaxillary fixation during surgery while bone plates and grafts are being secured, and to serve as an early-warning guide to postoperative relapse.

The cleft alveolus should always be bone grafted successfully prior to the undertaking of a definitive osteotomy. Following the integration of an alveolar bone graft, an L-step maxillary osteotomy should be attempted, using acrylic dentures or splints secured to the maxilla to assist in the desired placement of the maxilla during operation. Reliance is placed solely upon corticomedullary interpositional bone grafts and metal osteosynthesis plates to maintain the maxilla's position, obviating the need for postoperative intermaxillary fixation.

If the bone is very atrophic (Obwegeser et al., 1985), additional measures may include further bone grafting to stabilize the repositioned maxilla and simultaneously increase the alveolar height and improve the nature of the buccal vestibular mucosa for denture retention.

Other considerations

Le Fort I modifications, Le Fort II and Le Fort III osteotomies

Sometimes, for aesthetic reasons or if there are doubts about the blood supply of the osteotomized maxilla at the Le Fort I level, it may be necessary to modify the maxillary osteotomy at a Le Fort I, II or III level (Obwegeser et al., 1985; Bell et al., 1992; Keller, 1992).

Mandible

There are occasions when a simultaneous osteotomy of the mandible and maxilla may be planned. A mandibular body or ramus osteotomy, such as a bilateral ramus sagittal split to retrude the mandible, may be required to help achieve an acceptable dental occlusion, especially when excessive maxillary advancement is necessary. However, this compromise almost invariably gives less than satisfactory aesthetic results, as the mandible is usually already smaller than normal. It would be better to attempt a distraction osteogenesis procedure. This would stretch the limiting scar tissue gradually and allow for adaptation of the vascular supply until the desired advancement of the maxilla has been achieved or, failing that, until the maxillary advancement is such that any subsequent mandibular osteotomy retrusion will be minimized.

Chin

If the chin is retruded, a pedicled, horizontal sliding genioplasty to bring it forward (Figure 21.3) is preferable to the onlaying of synthetic materials or free grafting of autogenous material, as the end result is more predictable and stable and there are fewer complications.

Rhinoplasty

Altering the position of the maxilla will alter the support of the nose and the configuration and projection of the nasal tip, bridge and nares. Advancement of the maxilla tends to spread the alae laterally, close the nasolabial angle and lift the nasal tip, particularly if the nasal spine is not removed. While some nasal changes may be favourable after a maxillary osteotomy, others will be unfavourable. It is therefore advisable to defer definitive nasal correction until after the completion of maxillary osteotomies (see Watson, Chapter 17).

Implants

Osseo-integrated dental implants simulate tooth roots and allow for the construction of a dental superstructure. They may be used (Chiapasco et al., 1996) with teeth attached to complete a deficient dental arch, to retain dentures, or to facilitate orthodontic anchorage.

Fine tuning of facial aesthetics may require the onlaying of material, preferably autogenous bone or cartilage, to areas such as the nasal bridge, zygomatic eminences, paranasal or piriform rim region (Figure 21.5).

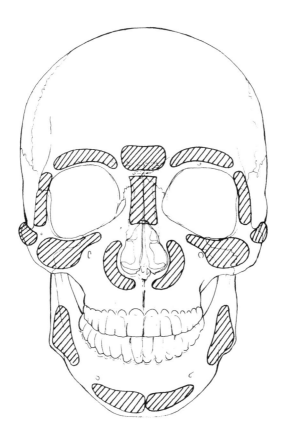

Figure 21.5. Sites for onlays on craniofacial skeleton.

References

Bell WH, Darab D, You Z (1992) Maxillary and midface deformity. In: Bell WH (ed.) Modern Practice in Orthognathic and Reconstructive Surgery. Philadelphia: WB Saunders, p. 2210.

Chiapasco M, Ronchi P, Frattini D (1996) Endosseous implants in bone grafted alveolar clefts. Journal of Craniomaxillofacial Surgery 24 (Suppl. 1): 28.

Cohen SR, Burstein FD, Stewart MB, Rathburn MA (1997) Maxillary–midface distraction in children with cleft lip and palate: a preliminary report. Plastic and Reconstructive Surgery 99(5): 1421–1428.

Converse JM, Shapiro HH (1952) Treatment of developmental malformations of the jaws. Plastic and Reconstructive Surgery 10: 473.

Dalston RM, Warren DW, Dalston ET (1991) Use of nasometry as a diagnostic tool for identifying patients with velopharyngeal impairment. Cleft Palate–Craniofacial Journal 28: 184.

Epker BD, Wolford LM (1980) Dentofacial Deformities, Surgical-Orthodontic Correction. St Louis: Mosby.

Ilizarov GA, Devyatov AA, Karnerim UV (1980) Plastic reconstruction of longitudinal bone defects by means of compression and subsequent distraction. Acta Chirurgiae Plasticae 22: 32.

James DR, Brook K (1985) Maxillary hypoplasia in patients with cleft lip and palate deformity – the alternative surgical approach. European Journal of Orthodontics 7: 231–247.

Keller EE (1992) Quadrangular Le Fort I and II Osteotomies. In: Bell WH (ed.) Modern Practice in Orthogathic and Reconstructive Surgery. Philadelphia: WB Saunders, p. 1797.

McCarthy JG, Schreiber J, Karp N (1992) Lengthening of mandible by gradual distraction. Plastic and Reconstructive Surgery 89: 1.

McCormick SU (1995) Osteodistraction: Selected Readings in Oral and Maxillofacial Surgery, Vol. 4, No. 7. University of Texas, South Western Medical Center, pp. 1–24.

Molina F, Ortiz-Monasterio F (1995) Mandibular elongation and remodelling by distraction: A farewell to major osteotomies. Plastic and Reconstructive Surgery 96: 825.

Obwegeser HL, Lello GE, Farmand M (1985) Correction of secondary cleft deformities. In: Bell WH (ed.) Surgical Correction of Dentofacial Deformities. Philadelphia: WB Saunders, p. 592.

Rachmiel A, Levy M, Laufer D (1995) Lengthening of the mandible by distraction osteo-genesis. Journal of Oral and Maxillofacial Surgery 53: 838.

Rachmiel A, Aizenbud D, Ardekian L, Peled M, Laufer D (1999) Surgically-assisted ortho-pedic protraction of the maxilla in cleft lip and palate patients. International Journal of Oral Maxillofacial Surgery 28: 9–14.

Sailer HF (1983) Transplantation of Lyophilised Cartilage in Maxillo-Facial Surgery: Experimental Foundations and Clinical Success. New York: Karger.

Sell D, Ma L, James DR, Mars M, Sheriff M (1993) A pilot study to investigate the effects of transpalatal Le Fort 1 maxillary osteotomy on velopharyngeal function in cleft palate patients. Paper presented at Seventh International Congress on Cleft Palate and Related Craniofacial Anomalies, Broadbeach, Australia.

Turvey TA, Tejera TJ (1996) Cleft maxillary advancement: previously bone grafted vs simultaneously bone grafted repaired patients. Journal of Craniomaxillofacial Surgery 24 (Suppl. 1): 118.

Wakamuto M, Isaacson K, Friel S, Gibbon F, Suzuki N, Nixon F, Hardcastle W, Michi K (1996) Articulatory reorganisation of fricative consonants following osteotomy. Folia Phoniatrica Logopedica 48: 275–289.

Witzel MA, Vallino LD (1992) Speech problems in patients with dentofacial or craniofacial deformities. In: Bell WH (ed.) Modern Practice in Orthognathic and Reconstructive Surgery, Vol. 2. Philadelphia: WB Saunders, p. 1721.

Yagui N, Kojimoto H, Shimoizu H, Shimomura Y (1991) The effect of distraction upon bone muscle and periosteum. Orthopedic Clinics of North America 22: 563.

CHAPTER 22

Restorative Dental Treatment

B. GRIFFITHS

Introduction

Treatment for patients with cleft lip and palate is best provided in a specialist centre by a multidisciplinary team (Shaw et al., 1992; CSAG, 1998). The role of the restorative dentist within the cleft team is to provide advice and treatment, most particularly for patients between the ages of 11 and 20 years, but also for adult patients. The role also includes liaison with the patient's own general dental practitioner with regard to primary dental care.

The aim of specialist restorative dental care is to restore appearance and function of the dentition, especially where orthodontic and surgical options are unable to provide an optimum outcome. The techniques range from periodontal therapy, to fixed and removable prosthodontics involved in the restoration of teeth and the replacement of missing teeth. Additionally, the provision of prostheses to improve arch form, obturate palatal fistulae, provide a speech bulb or orthodontic retention may be required.

The outcome of treatment should be evaluated not only in terms of clinical appearance and function, but also from the patient's perspective. Sound treatment planning involves the whole of the team (Shaw et al., 1996). Involvement of restorative dentists at the planning stage of orthodontic and secondary surgical treatment helps to avoid unnecessary and/or prolonged treatment.

Special anatomical considerations

The term cleft lip and palate embraces patients with a variety of cleft anatomy and dental anomalies, self-motivation, and expectations of treatment. These factors will influence the type of treatment chosen. In favourable circumstances definitive treatment may be provided by surgical and orthodontic treatment with little intervention by the restorative dentist, whereas other patients will require extensive restorative reconstruction after orthodontic and surgical treatment to meet their aesthetic and functional needs (Figures 22.1 and 22.2).

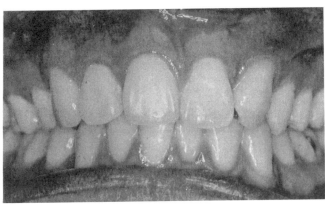

Figure 22.1. Post-surgical and orthodontic result for a unilateral cleft patient with good oral hygiene, no caries experience and a missing upper left lateral incisor in the line of the cleft. The lateral space has been closed. Re-contouring of the upper left canine can be aided by acid-etch composite restorations.

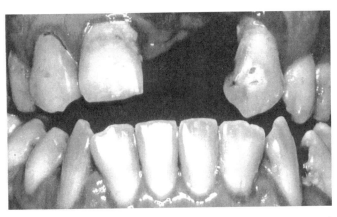

Figure 22.2. Poorly motivated teenager with unilateral cleft lip and palate. A large alveolar defect and missing teeth (congenitally absent and extracted). Poor oral hygiene and dentition with a poor prognosis.

A number of anatomical features, arising either as a result of the cleft, or as a result of surgical treatment, deserve special consideration when planning restorative dental treatment as they are unique to cleft patients.

• Tissue defect

Soft tissue – scarred lip and labial sulcus

The lip repair may result in an upper lip which is relatively immobile. This does have the advantage of helping to conceal any alveolar defects and irregularities in gingival contour. However, the scarring may present difficulties in the toleration of local anaesthetic administration, access for oral hygiene measures and adequate extension of denture flanges. Due to underlying dental and skeletal abnormalities the lip may also appear to lack support and require improved support with a prosthesis. Revision of the lip scar is often performed during late adolescence and the timing of this surgery needs to be coordinated with definitive restoration of the upper anterior teeth.

Hard tissue

The severity of the tooth and bony defects may limit orthodontic and surgical treatment. In turn this will influence the requirement for and design of restorative treatment. The range of residual defects in the line of the cleft includes hypoplastic teeth, hypodontia (most commonly affecting the lateral incisor), deficiency of alveolar bone, and palatal or buccal fistulae.

• Arch discrepancies

Development of the maxillary arch may be compromised. A class III relationship and profile may remain if untreated with surgical and orthodontic procedures.

• Mobility of the maxillary segments and teeth

The independent movement of maxillary segments across the line of the cleft, even after cleft closure and alveolar bone grafting is unique to cleft patients. Teeth adjacent to the cleft commonly have reduced bone support and associated mobility, especially in the absence of a successful alveolar bone graft (see Mars, Chapter 20).

• Stability of the orthodontic result

With the advances in both surgical and orthodontic techniques, the stability of the final tooth position at the end of these stages of treatment is now much improved. However, the long-term stability needs to be considered as part of the restorative treatment.

Prevention of caries and periodontal diseases

Prevention of caries and periodontal diseases in this group of patients is extremely important because of the anatomical difficulties in providing prosthetic replacements for the maxillary teeth. However, establishing good oral hygiene and maintaining dental care in children and adolescents is particularly difficult. This reflects the demands on the patient and family by surgical and medical interventions necessitated by the cleft and any associated syndromes. It may also relate to the focus on the mouth demanded by oral hygiene procedures and local anatomical difficulties which may make access for cleaning more demanding.

Local anatomical factors as a result of the cleft and corrective surgery, in addition to extensive dental treatment, contribute to the difficulties in maintaining plaque control. Even at the ages of five and six years, children with clefts have an increased incidence of gingival inflammation and caries compared to non-cleft children (Dahllof et al., 1989), and despite a coordinated team approach to treatment, Bragger et al. (1992) reported that cleft patients aged 18–20 had poorer oral hygiene and more periodontal disease (documented as clinical loss of periodontal attachment and radiographic loss of alveolar bone height) than non-cleft patients. However, with increasing age into adulthood, there was no evidence that this trend continued (Ramstad, 1989; Bragger et al., 1992).

Comparing sites adjacent to and distant from the cleft, teeth adjacent to the cleft had a poorer periodontal condition as a result of the prosthodontic treatment (Ramstad, 1989) and had reduced bone support (Bragger et al., 1992). In addition, root length of the upper anterior teeth may be compromised by extensive orthodontic tooth movement.

Prosthodontic treatment options

Fixed or removal prostheses may be used to replace missing teeth and restore the maxillary arch. Communication between surgeon, orthodontist and restorative dentist is imperative so that the definitive restoration can be planned. Appearance, function, long-term outcome and patient expectations are the key features in the planning. Primary dental disease and anatomy related to the cleft need to be considered alongside the tooth position, the size and position of residual spacing and occlusion.

Many patients opt for surgery, orthodontic treatment and a fixed restorative solution. This option offers complex treatment and involves the patient in many out- and inpatient episodes over many years. Other patients prefer a less extensive approach with limited orthodontic and surgical treatment and a removable prosthesis to produce a functional and aesthetic result. However, even after extensive orthodontic treatment and surgery, the final restorative treatment options may be limited by anatomical factors, medical conditions or by the patient's ability to cooperate.

A simple fixed prosthesis is considered to be the treatment of choice, especially as palatal inflammation is common when a removable prosthesis is worn. This option may be excluded by the extent and site of tooth loss, the need to restore an alveolar bone defect or palatal fistula or the need to disguise an arch discrepancy. In addition, removable prostheses may be used as a provisional solution whilst awaiting completion of growth and/or treatment in other disciplines.

There has been much debate about orthodontic retention for this group of patients. With current orthodontic and surgical techniques, it would appear that premolar and molar collapse is not a major problem, even when bridgework with a minimum of abutments is provided (Bragger et al., 1991).

Fixed prosthodontics

Conventional crown and bridgework

Historically extensive fixed bridgework involving several teeth on either side of the cleft was advocated (Kantorowicz, 1975). Such complex restorations were aimed at providing stability of the maxillary segments and tooth position after rapid maxillary expansion. Other authors have reported less extensive crown and bridgework with one or two abutments on either side of the cleft (Ramstad, 1973; Johanson et al., 1974). Before alveolar bone grafting became a routine part of treatment, residual defects in alveolar bone were common. These were obturated with removable (acrylic) or fixed (pink porcelain) extensions of the bridgework and today these techniques may still be used in older patients with alveolar defects which have not been restored by alveolar bone grafts.

Currently conventional principles of bridgework design are employed, with avoidance of fixed restorations across the cleft where possible. The extensive preparation of teeth required for conventional bridgework is a disadvantage, especially in young patients. Bennington et al. (1979) emphasized the importance of resisting pressures from the patient and family to provide elaborate fixed restorations in the young patient.

Adhesive dentistry

Advances in adhesive restorative materials, a general reduction in the incidence of caries, together with more stable orthodontic and surgical results have transformed the restorative treatment options available, especially for younger cleft patients.

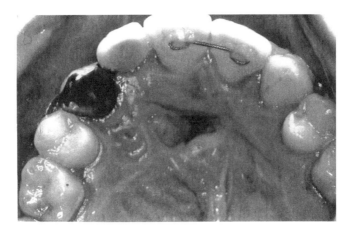

Figure 22.3. Unilateral cleft with residual fistula (left without obturation), cantilever resin-bonded bridge to replace upper left lateral incisor and multi-strand wire retention of the central incisors.

Adhesive techniques including resin composite restorations and porcelain veneers may be used to improve the appearance of teeth which need re-contouring; for example peg shaped lateral incisor teeth or canines in the position of lateral incisor teeth (Figure 22.1).

The development of resin-bonded bridges has been important, especially in the treatment of young adult cleft patients (Figure 22.3). The major advantage is the minimal preparation of the teeth. The essential elements of design are as for non-cleft patients, using a cantilever design where possible. A variety of hybrid designs have been described (Kelleher, 1984), and the resin-bonded bridge may be combined with composite build-up of the abutment teeth where tooth position and size need improving. A success rate of 94% has been reported for cantilever resin-bonded bridges for non-cleft patients (Hussey and Linden, 1996). Despite earlier concerns of increased failure in cleft patients, the techniques have improved to make this an ideal option for the restoration of the anterior sextant in many cleft patients.

Adhesive techniques may also be used for anterior orthodontic retention by the use of multi-strand wire on the palatal surfaces of the anterior teeth (Figure 22.3).

Removable prosthodontics

The design and construction of dentures in patients with clefts may be complicated by short clinical crowns, crown angulation and a flat palate. In addition, the palatal gingivae and mucosa are commonly inflamed and hyperplastic, especially where the patient is committed to wearing a prosthesis full-time (Figures 22.5 and 22.6). A variety of techniques have

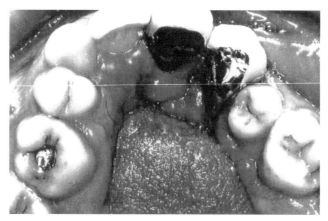

Figure 22.4. Palatal tongue flap to close palatal fistula. Conventional crowns to correct arch form and disguise tooth form. The loss of palatal gingivae, upper right premolar, and the presence of the tongue flap have made oral hygiene procedures more difficult for the patient.

been used to improve retention of removable prostheses. These include recontouring the teeth with composite restorations, construction of cast gold copings or crowns, with or without precision attachments (Bennington et al., 1979; Patterson, 1987), and the use of dental implants (Figures 22.5–22.8).

Removable prostheses may need to be designed to obturate palatal defects, disguise arch discrepancies or provide orthodontic retention, in addition to replacing missing teeth.

Palatal defects

Although in most cases closure of palatal clefts is possible, some patients are left with residual fistulae. Small defects which do not interfere with speech, drinking or eating do not require obturation (Figure 22.3).

The closure of residual fistulae with tongue flaps (Coghlan et al., 1989) (Figure 22.4) gives high patient satisfaction but such flaps may complicate restorative dentistry; the grafts provide a poor base where a denture is required and may interfere with oral hygiene measures.

Palatal fistulae may be closed by an obturator, constructed as an integral part of a conventional denture. The aim of the obturator is to form a seal between the nose and the mouth, to prevent the escape of food, drink or air during eating and speaking. The part of the obturator forming the seal is fabricated in acrylic so that it can be easily adjusted in function if required (Figures 22.7 and 22.8).

Speech bulbs which extend into the velopharynx may be required where there is an unrepaired cleft of the hard and soft palate or velopharyngeal

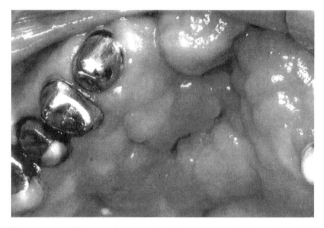

Figure 22.5. Illustration of hyperplastic palatal tissues and short clinical crowns. In this case the crowns have been modified with gold copings.

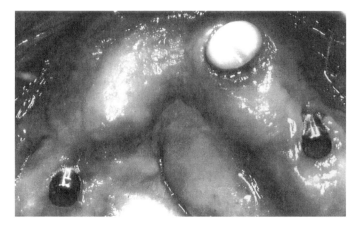

Figure 22.6. Flat palate in a patient with one remaining tooth and two implants in the posterior maxilla with magnets to aid denture retention.

dysfunction. Once the conventional denture construction is complete, functional impressions allow the speech bulb to be formed *in situ* during speech (Bennington et al., 1979). Nasopharyngoscopy may be used to aid the assessment and fitting of the speech bulb (see Sell and Grunwell, Chapter 16).

Arch discrepancies

In some instances correction of the contracted maxillary arch form by orthodontic and surgical treatment may not be possible or desired by the patient (Figures 22.9 and 22.10). The class III occlusion with reverse overjet and buccal crossbite is often accompanied by an anterior open bite with failure

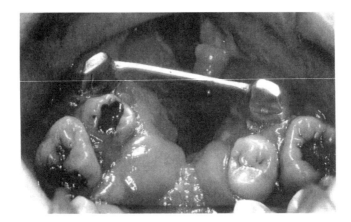

Figure 22.7. Bilateral cleft, with premaxilla removed, residual fistula and very contracted arch. Designs made with fixed elements across the line of the cleft are prone to failure. In the long term, this design with milled bar and copings failed due to movement across the line of the cleft. An obturator of similar design, without the milled bar, was worn successfully.

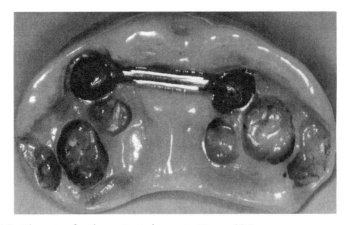

Figure 22.8. Obturator for the patient shown in Figure 22.7.

of the lesser segment to reach the occlusal plane. Thus there is a failure to develop in both the horizontal and vertical planes. Such arch discrepancies may be disguised for appearance and function by the use of an overdenture which covers the teeth (Figures 22.11 and 22.12). This type of denture allows the prosthetic teeth to be placed in a position to improve the appearance of the dentition, lip support and profile. The maintenance therapy for these patients is particularly important as the risk of caries is increased by covering the teeth with a denture.

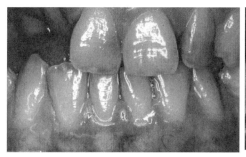
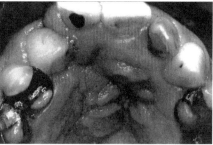

Figures 22.9, 22.10. A contracted arch in a repaired unilateral cleft; the greater segment is of normal contour, and the lesser segment closer to the midline.

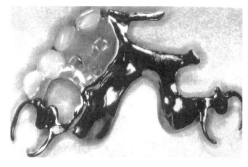
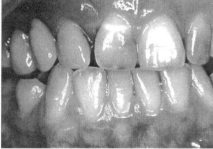

Figures 22.11, 22.12. Overdenture: removable prosthesis with overlay for the patient shown in Figures 22.9 and 22.10. The design avoids coverage of the gingivae where possible and has additional bracing components for orthodontic retention.

Orthodontic retention

If retention is needed around the arch, a fixed solution may not be appropriate for the reasons outlined above. The disadvantage of providing orthodontic retention with a denture is that the prosthesis needs to be worn day and night and the risk of caries, periodontal disease and inflammation of the palatal mucosa is increased. However, to minimize these risks, a denture with minimal gingival coverage (Figure 22.12) is preferable to an orthodontic type retainer.

The edentulous patient and complete dentures

The architecture of the repaired cleft palate after the loss of the teeth is never ideal from the point of view of providing a retentive complete maxillary denture. The palate is often flat and the buccal sulcus reduced by scarring. The residual edentulous alveolar ridge is small, especially in the anterior region. In addition, the palatal mucosa may be hyperplastic and may not provide a firm base for the denture. This underlines the great importance of maintaining the teeth, even as roots for overdenture abutments.

There is a relatively small group of older edentulous UK residents with unoperated cleft palates who present for prosthetic treatment. These patients are of interest in demonstrating the maxillary arch development and form without the influence of surgery and scar tissue. They are generally extremely adept at coping with a complete denture with obturator and speech bulb, both in retaining the denture and having developed adaptive speech patterns (Figures 22.13 and 22.14). This type of obturator with speech bulb is constructed in two parts, as described earlier.

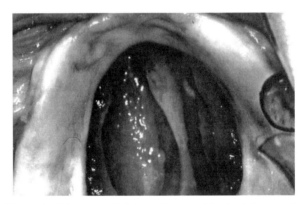

Figure 22.13. Unrepaired bilateral cleft in a 90-year-old edentulous patient.

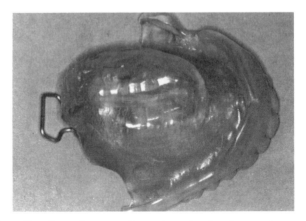

Figure 22.14. Hollow box obturator. Posterior wire for the attachment of the speech bulb, which will be made by a functional impression in gutta percha and then constructed in acrylic resin.

Dental implants may provide additional help for edentulous cleft patients where denture retention is a problem.

Dental implants

Treatment with dental implants is considered separately as this treatment is relatively new, especially in patients with cleft palates. Patients with clefts are one of the priority groups for receiving implants funded under the NHS (National Clinical Guidelines – Faculty of Dental Surgery, 1997). The potential benefits are to provide single tooth replacements for congenitally missing teeth and to provide retention and support for prostheses where several teeth are missing and the provision of a conventional prosthesis is difficult. The major limitation to implant treatment in cleft patients is finding adequate bone of good quality, particularly in the line of the cleft. Figure 22.6 demonstrates the use of dental implants and magnets to stabilize a complete denture in a patient with a repaired cleft palate. Development of bone grafting and guided tissue generation to produce bone in selected sites increases the possibilities for successful treatment.

There is a lack of longitudinal data to assess implant treatment for patients with clefts, but several case reports have appeared in the literature (Verdi et al., 1991; Matsui et al., 1993). Guidelines for implant treatment are beginning to be published both with regard to the appropriate age for implants and the use of implants in the line of the cleft (Kearns et al., 1997).

Conclusions

The degree of clefting, corrective surgery and orthodontics, together with patient motivation, influence the requirements, design and the success of restorative dental treatment. The importance of prevention of caries and periodontal diseases, treatment planning and maintenance cannot be underestimated.

References

Bennington IC, Watson IB, Jenkins WMM, Allan GRJ (1979) Restorative treatment of the cleft patient. British Dental Journal 146: 14–17, 47–50, 79–82, 115–118, 144–148, 183–186.

Bragger U, Burger S, Ingevall B (1991) Long term stability of treatment results in cleft lip and palate patients. Special print (translated to English) from: Schweizer Monatsschrift Zahmedizin 101: 1542–1548.

Bragger U, Schurch JRE, Salvi G, Von Wyttenbach T, Lang NP (1992) Periodontal conditions in adult patients with cleft lip, alveolus and palate. Cleft Palate–Craniofacial Journal 29: 17–185.

Clinical Standards Advisory Group (CSAG) (1998) Cleft Lip and/or Palate. London: The Stationery Office.

Coghlan K, O'Regan B, Carter J (1989) Tongue flap repair of oro-nasal fistulae in cleft palate patients. Journal of Cranio-Maxillo-Facial Surgery 17: 255–259.

Dalhoff G, Ussisoo-Joandi R, Ideberg M, Modeer T (1989) Caries, gingivitis, and dental abnormalities in pre school children with cleft lip and/or palate. Cleft Palate Journal 26: 233–237.

Faculty of Dental Surgery (1997) National Clinical Guidelines (ed. TA Gregg). The Faculty of Dental Surgery of the Royal College of Surgeons of England.

Hussey DL, Linden GJ (1996) The clinical performance of cantilevered resin-bonded bridgework. Journal of Dentistry 24: 251–256.

Johanson B, Ohisson A, Frede H, Ahegren J (1974) A follow up study of cleft lip and palate patients treated with orthodontics, secondary bone grafting and prosthetic rehabilitation. Scandinavian Journal of Prosthetic and Reconstructive Surgery 8: 121–135.

Kantorowicz CF (1975) Bridge prostheses for cleft palate patients. British Dental Journal 139: 91–97.

Kearns G, Perrott DH, Sharma A, Kaban LB, Vargervik K (1997) Placement of endosseous implants in grafted alveolar clefts. Cleft Palate–Craniofacial Journal 34: 520–525.

Kelleher MGD (1984) A movable joint composite attached bridge for a cleft palate patient. Restorative Dentistry 27–31.

Matsui Y, Ohno K, Ichi K, Yamagata K (1993) Application of hydroxyapatite coated implants as support for palatal lift prostheses in edentulous patients with cleft palate: a clinical report. International Journal of Oral Maxillofacial Implants 8: 316–322.

Patterson N (1987) Prosthetic treatment of Cleft Palate Patients. Dental Update 352–361.

Ramstad T (1973) Post orthodontic retention and post prosthodontic occlusion in adult complete unilateral and bilateral cleft subjects. Cleft Palate Journal 10: 34–50.

Ramstad T (1989) Periodontal condition in adult patients with unilateral complete cleft lip and palate. Cleft Palate Journal 26: 14–20.

Shaw WC, Asher-McDade C, Dahl E, Mars M, Brattstrom V, McWilliam J, et al. (1992) A six centre international study of treatment outcome in patients with clefts of the lip and palate. Cleft Palate–Craniofacial Journal 29: 413–418.

Shaw WC, Sandy JR, Williams AC, Devlin HB (1996) Minimum standards for the management of cleft lip and palate: efforts to close the audit loop. Annals of the Royal College of Surgeons of England 78: 110–114.

Verdi FJ, Lanzi GL, Cohen SR, Powell R (1991) Use of the Branemark Implant in the cleft palate patient. Cleft Palate–Craniofacial Journal 28: 301–304.

CHAPTER 23

Growing up with a Cleft: the Impact on the Child

E. Bradbury

Introduction

As children grow up with a cleft, they have to learn ways of coping with the knowledge that their appearance and their speech may be different from those of other children, in a society where appearance is an important determinant of social acceptability. Some children adapt well to this task and grow up to lead normal social lives. However, other children are burdened by a sense of inferiority and difference which leaves them with low self-esteem, poor social skills and a pervasive lack of confidence.

For many decades, the literature on the psychology of clefts was focused on psychopathology, that is a search for clinically significant levels of anxiety and depression in these children. The findings were conflicting, but it is clear from the literature that there is no inevitable relationship between a cleft and psychological problems. (See, for example, Clifford, 1983.)

However, psychologists and other clinicians working in the field have recognized that many of these children were unhappy and that some children were struggling to cope with social relationships and feelings of low self-esteem (Lansdown, 1990). There have certainly been consistent findings of dissatisfaction with appearance. Richman (1976) demonstrated that a significant number of adolescent subjects expressed dissatisfaction with appearance whilst being otherwise well adjusted. There is an association between this dissatisfaction and low self-esteem (Kapp, 1979).

The work of Macgregor (1982), Kreuckeberg et al. (1993), Speltz et al. (1993) and others have found there are unifying themes in the psychology of children with clefts. The characteristic profile to emerge was that of a child who was anxious, passive, socially withdrawn and family-dependent (Pillemer and Kaye, 1989). In our own research, we have found that children with clefts scored lower than their normal peers for levels of disturbed and difficult behaviour, but higher than the matched child psychiatry population for levels of anxiety (Bradbury, 1995).

Children are a moving target – they are growing and moving through different stages of development in which they have different needs, abilities and aspirations. This discussion about children with a cleft will take the developmental perspective into account. Just as there are differences in responses at different ages, so there are differences between children. Not every child responds in the same way and it is important to recognize both common stressors and factors which influence individual differences. Some children have a resilient temperament which enables them to overcome difficulties. These children may find that they are successful in other areas of their lives. They can gain self-esteem by striving to excel in activities such as sport or music. A further factor which influences individual responses is the ability of the family to support and sustain the child (Fonagy et al., 1994). Thus any discussion about the psychological impact of a cleft must take into account both common stressors and individual differences within a developmental framework.

Common stressors and individual differences: resilience and vulnerability

The physical consequences of a cleft

Physical factors relating to a cleft lip and/or palate are described elsewhere in this book. They may include impaired speech and hearing and altered physical appearance. These factors are potential stressors because of the burden of coping they place on children and because the children have to go through treatment to improve their physical state.

The impact of physical difference

The child with a cleft often has problems with hearing and speech. Undetected hearing loss can cut children off from the world and make them less socially responsive. However, having had grommets inserted, the child cannot take part in some normal activities such as swimming underwater. Speech problems can also be isolating; especially if children are self-conscious about their speech and therefore less likely to speak out in class or talk to others. The use of the telephone to contact friends becomes stressful. The regurgitation of food down the nostril can make a child embarrassed to eat in public, particularly those foods that are runny, such as ice cream and chocolate. A school trip in summer to an outdoor swimming area can be fraught with potential problems for a child with a cleft.

There is also the effect of facial appearance. Children vary in their concerns about the details of their face. For some it is the asymmetrical nose, for others the vermilion border of the lip, or scarring to the alar base. For younger children, any feature that is difficult to explain may be the source of teasing. In some ways, scarring is easier to explain and some children talk more freely about scarring as the result of an accident than about congenital anomalies. They feel more entitled to elicit sympathy following an accident, whereas they may feel confused and uncertain about physical anomalies which are less easy to explain. This difficulty becomes particularly acute if parents who are distressed about the cleft have not discussed the condition with their child in a clear and straightforward way.

Body image issues become intense at adolescence, when the body is going through a period of change and instability and when appearance is of vital importance for self-esteem. Increased self-consciousness is part of normal adolescent development. Adolescents often consider how their appearance would seem to an imaginary audience (Elkind, 1967) and become enmeshed in an egocentric view of the world in which they feel that they are being constantly watched by others. The added issue of physical difference intensifies this perception and makes it more acute. This is a time when sexual identity becomes highly significant. The adolescent girl with a class III malocclusion can feel less feminine. The quiet and withdrawn boy may feel he is not sufficiently assertive and competitive to fit a male stereotype.

The impact of treatment

Treatment imposes a very real cost on the child and the family. The children miss time at school, which has implications for their social relationships as well as for their education. For the anxious child who may suffer from needle phobia or from a gagging response, treatment can be a source of great stress. Families have to organize for other children to be cared for, take time off work, travel to clinics for regular appointments and they also experience the trauma of seeing their child through surgery.

Occasionally, children who are having difficulties at school welcome time spent at the hospital or speech and language therapy clinic, as this is an escape from their peers into the world of friendly adults. The child who is eager to attend for treatment may be having very real problems which are hidden from the adults to whom he or she relates so well.

The impact of treatment changes as the child grows. Infants generally cope better with surgery than their parents, but a child between the ages of 18 months and three years can be very distressed by any restraint and become resistant to hospitalization. Children aged 7–12, when orthodontics and bone-grafting may happen, are often able to cope well and are well-motivated to have treatment. Adolescence brings its own problems, and young adolescents are often very anxious about treatment which involves appearance, such as wearing fixed appliances. They may also develop fears about surgery which involves anaesthetic and loss of control. In addition, at a time of physical transition, they often find it hard to cope with further changes to their body image. However, when treatment such as osteotomy goes well and the result is successful for the adolescent, the rewards can be very great. The young person often describes the feeling of having lost the stigma of the 'cleft appearance' and can now relate to others with more social confidence. There is also a sense of relief that the final treatment hurdle has been overcome.

Parental adjustment

The parents of a baby with a cleft go through a process of adjustment in which they have to let go of their hopes for an anticipated perfect baby and adjust to the baby with a cleft (Solnit and Stark, 1962). Some parents find it easy to adjust to their new baby. For others, it can be a troubled and prolonged process (Bradbury and Hewison, 1994). At its extreme, parents become fixed in a chronic mourning process and show continuing signs of denial or ongoing grief.

Children are connected to their parents by invisible wires. They are intensely aware of their parents' responses. Babies as young as ten weeks old will scan their mother's face for emotional reactions, and will behave more anxiously if the mother seems angry or distressed (Haviland and Lelwicka, 1987). Older children can become protective of their parents and not mention any problems in case the parents become upset. If the parents have never come to terms with the cleft, the child may internalize feelings of shame and guilt. Thus for some children with a cleft, coping with their parents' feelings, can be a stressor. When parents give unconditional love the child is more able to face the world.

The social world of the child

There are real social pressures for children with clefts. Richardson and Royce (1968) identified stigmatizing responses to visible difference in children. This work has been corroborated by Sigelman et al. (1986), who described early stigmatizing reactions to disfigurement by other children and suggested that there is a process of social learning – the older children in the study were more negative about disfigurement than the younger children. This was particularly true for girls, who were more negative about cosmetic defects than boys. However, boys are confronted with a more competitive social world, and are less likely to build the type of close confiding relationship that can help a girl to cope.

Children with clefts will commonly describe being teased because of their appearance or their speech. Teasing and bullying is not uncommon in schools. In a survey of 1000 primary school children, Stephenson and Smith (1987) found that 23% reported being bullied, and the incidence of occasional teasing is likely to be much higher. Although physical appearance plays a role in being the victim of bullying, its importance is often over-estimated (Lane, 1992). Bullies will pick on any characteristic, including personality or behavioural ones.

Olweus (1993) described the characteristics of *passive victims* in this context as being anxious and insecure, cautious, sensitive and quiet. They suffer low self-esteem, feel isolated from their peers and are family-dependent. It is interesting that he says that they also commonly feel unattractive. This profile fits the characteristic psychological picture of a child with a cleft, and thus the bullying that happens may not just be a consequence of the cleft, but of the way in which the child's personality has developed. Olweus (1993) also talks about the *provocative victims*, who are characterized by both anxious and aggressive reaction patterns and whose behaviour can provoke bullying. It is useful to identify patterns of interaction in order to understand the extent to which the child is making bullying more likely.

Friendship is an important part of a child's development and sense of self-worth. Good friends can mitigate the impact of teasing. Children with clefts whose appearance or speech provokes unease in other children may be isolated, whilst the aggressive child is more likely to be rejected. Thus children who react to teasing with aggression may find themselves quickly rejected if there is already an element of avoidance and unease. Amongst the factors affecting popularity are appearance (Langlois and Stephan, 1981) and social skills. A child with a cleft who is socially withdrawn and lacking the confidence to interact with others may have poorly-developed social skills. Rejection or avoidance on the basis of appearance or speech difference will also reduce the child's popularity and limit friendships. Longitudinal studies have shown that unpopularity in children is often enduring and affects their ability to form relationships in adulthood. This is particularly true for the rejected child (Rutter, 1988).

Friendship needs follow a developmental pattern (Sullivan, 1965). Children between the ages of four and nine years tend to prefer a group of friends rather than particular individuals. In the pre-adolescent period onwards, friendships become closer and more enduring, with greater intimacy. Friendship at this stage becomes crucial for the growth of self-esteem and as a buffer against adversity. If early friendship patterns do not occur, then the adolescent is less likely to have developed the social and empathic skills needed to build closer friendships (Rutter and Rutter, 1992).

Thus the social world of the child is a complex environment. Children with clefts may have social problems, but these need to be understood within the framework of their social development and within the context of their particular needs.

The internal world of the child: the development and regulation of self-esteem

Self-esteem is the term used to describe the evaluation we make about ourselves in relation to others. Studies have shown apparently conflicting results when self-esteem for those with clefts has been measured. Some studies describe heightened self-esteem (Brantley and Clifford, 1979) as there is a sense of having overcome adversity. Others found lowered self-esteem resulting from a sense of difference, which was associated with dissatisfaction with appearance (Kapp, 1979). It is possible that both these processes can be found in individual children and that self-esteem is a fluctuating construct in childhood but becomes more fixed in later adolescence and adulthood (Rutter and Rutter, 1992).

The development of self-esteem and self-awareness comes from early relationships with parents and close family, interactions with other children and also from the internal beliefs and emotions of the child. Children thus learn a sense of self which comes from external and internal representations of reality. Those born with a congenital anomaly have known no other self and grow up feeling normal until they start to compare themselves with their parents, their siblings and their peers. This process of comparison begins at an early age, but its impact on the child takes longer to develop (Bradbury, 1993).

From the age of about three or four, children with clefts will begin to notice that there are differences about their facial appearance and may comment on this. If the child has not internalized any maternal distress, then the comment may be both inquisitive and wishful: 'Why is my lip like this? I want to look like ...' At this age, there is still a belief in magic and the child may believe that any imperfections will disappear. If they recognize real hurt, shame and distress in their parents, they will wish to look and sound normal in order to eradicate that which upsets their parents. They want to get rid of the cleft so that their parents will truly love them.

> Children can learn to live with a disability. But they cannot live well without the conviction that their parents find them utterly loveable ... If the parents, knowing his defect, love him now, he can believe that others will love him in the future. With this conviction he can live well now and have faith in the years to come. (Bettelheim, 1972)

As they reach the age of about six or seven years, they come to recognize that there is a limit to any improvement. This can be a traumatic time. The forming of friendship groups at this age leads to teasing and bullying as some children are inevitably excluded from the group. The child has limited ability to handle teasing at this age, yet has a great need for affiliation. This sense of rejection interacts with the sense of loss of hope and often provokes a crisis for the child. It is a crisis characterized by uncertainty, sadness and lowered self-esteem. It can be recognized by altered behaviour in the child, who may be more tearful and irritable at home and less communicative. If this is not acknowledged, then the child may never resolve this crisis and may go through childhood feeling unaccepted and unacceptable. However, if the child is given the opportunity to talk about this, then he or she can be strengthened and develop a greater sense of self-esteem (Bradbury, 1996).

The next significant stage in terms of children's emotional development comes as they reach adolescence (Richman et al., 1985). This is a time of change and altered body image which affects all young people. If they enter adolescence already feeling unaccepted by their parents and rejected by their peers, then they will be anxious and uncertain with low self-esteem and a lack of confidence in their ability to cope. On the other hand, adolescents who feel secure in their attachments, popular with their friends and confident in their coping skills will generally be able to deal with adversity. They need all the confidence they can get, because they are entering a world obsessed with appearance and dating, where judgements about worth are based on the appearance of the person being dated. At this age, adolescents with clefts whose appearance and/or speech are different have to find ways of succeeding and retaining their self-esteem. They may do this by becoming very defensive and denying any problems, making it difficult to help them if there are real problems. In addition, some issues are very sensitive and difficult to discuss; for example, the adolescent who is self-conscious about the lip may be very reluctant to kiss or get physically close to anyone.

Development does not end with adolescence, but goes on into adulthood. Psychological outcome can be assessed by considering whether the adult with a cleft is leading the life he or she would want, for example, to gain and keep a job, form a long-term intimate relationship, have children. One study suggests that adults with clefts are less likely to marry (Ramstead et al., 1995) and adults who feel that they do not want children because they do not want their child to have to repeat their experience are expressing a deep sense of unhappiness about having grown up with a cleft. Lowered vocational aspirations are another sign that self-esteem is not high (Goldberg, 1974).

Decision-making about treatment and surgery

Parental decision-making

Primary repair of the lip and the palate is essential for the well-being of the baby and there are no decisions that the parent has to make about whether or not there should be surgery. However, they may be asked to decide on their preferred timing of surgery – whether the repair should be carried out immediately after birth or a few months later. There is a tendency on the part of surgeons to believe that their own regime is the best for the psychological well-being of the parents. This is a natural consequence of observing the gratitude expressed by the parents. However, clinical experience has taught that not every parent wants a neonatal repair and may feel the need to take the baby home and spend time with their child before any surgery (see Watson, Chapter 12). Similarly, not every parent wants to wait for surgery and may be much happier and more able to bond with the child once the early repair is out of the way. The surgeon should take time to understand the needs of the individual parents if a choice of timing is possible (Bradbury and Hewison, 1994).

Decision-making by the families starts to be an issue as the child grows and secondary surgery is being considered. A child who is being teased may ask for surgery to improve the nose, although this may not be the optimum time to carry out this procedure. The child would benefit from help in dealing with the teasing. An immediate response which alters appearance without improving coping strategies can confirm in the child's mind the sense that only external means of help are possible and thus encourage external thinking, which relies on others, rather than internal thinking, which comes from within and enables the child to feel competent and able to cope.

The competence of the child

How can you judge the competence of the child to be involved in the decision-making process? Children as young as four or five can be actively involved in that process if they are told about things in a language they can understand (Bradbury et al., 1994). Involving children in decisions about their treatment helps them to feel more involved in the process and reduces their anxiety about loss of control (Alderson, 1993).

Some very anxious children will have problems tolerating procedures such as nasopharyngoscopies, and may resist surgery to improve function, such as a pharyngoplasty, because of fears about surgery, hospitals or needles. Such a child should be helped to deal with these fears. If these are disregarded, then they confirm for the child that they have a real reason to be afraid, making further treatment more traumatic. Early intervention can desensitize children by encouraging them to communicate their fears and by gradually increasing their exposure to the feared situation in a supportive and protected way. This will enable them to feel they have some control and raise their self-esteem with the knowledge that they have faced the problem and dealt with it. It will also prepare them for future treatment.

Decision-making in adolescence

Decision-making about treatment and surgery in adolescence can be fraught. This is likely to be the first time the young person is required to make his or her own decision. Until then, parents have been the primary decision-makers. If the adolescent is rather shy and family-dependent, it is too easy for all concerned to have the dialogue with the parents, with the adolescent nodding assent. All adolescents contemplating surgery to improve their appearance, including osteotomy and rhinoplasty, should have the opportunity to talk alone away from the group in clinic and away from their parents (see Lello, Chapter 21). This should be with a counsellor or psychologist who is able to identify the issues, facilitate communication and allow the adolescent to reach a considered decision. This process is particularly important as aesthetic surgery at this time can provoke a crisis for adolescents. They may have struggled to come to terms with how they look and have reached a point where their body image has been stabilized. The offer to alter their appearance may threaten that stability and provoke feelings of anger and distress. A counsellor will be able to help the adolescent work through this and reach a decision which is disentangled from all the other issues. Adolescents often go through a period akin to grieving – they feel that it is unfair that they have had to go through all this treatment which disrupts their life and reminds them that they are different. They feel a sense of loss for the person they would have been without the cleft. With skilled help, they can learn to integrate this into their own self-concept (Lansdown et al., 1997).

When is it enough?

It is often easier for all those concerned to continue with surgery than it is to say no to it. Some people may be offered surgery they do not want. However, this can be very hard to express in clinic. They may feel that they are letting down their relatives and friends who want the best for them, they may feel that they are letting down the surgeon who has cared for them over the years and above all, they know that this means that they now have to accept how they look. There are no more hopes of improvement, no more magic. It can take considerable courage to reach this point of self-acceptance. Enabling the young person to do this is as important for the team as it is to offer further treatment.

The organization of the clinic

The care of the child with a cleft is multidisciplinary, involving many different professionals. Families have to travel to outpatient appointments and it seems logical that they should be seen by different professionals together in the same room. Thus the multidisciplinary outpatient clinic has developed. It can reach quite awesome proportions, with a room crowded with surgeons, orthodontists, speech and language therapists, audiologists, health visitors, etc., plus students, observers and trainees. Some will wear white coats, some will be familiar to the family, others will be strangers who may never be introduced. It can be overwhelming to both parents and their children. There is the 'goldfish bowl' effect, in which the family feels that they are on centre stage.

For the parent who is feeling tearful, for the shy child, for the adolescent who wants to talk about decision-making, this scenario can be very traumatic. It certainly makes it difficult for a true two-way discussion. The families may find it hard to say all that they want to say and the clinician may find that some of what is said has not been taken in or understood.

In a recent study (Shaw et al., 1996), parents identified a need to be seen by individual clinicians who are relevant to their child's care at that time. They preferred a one-to-one consultation with each clinician, but on the same day in order to reduce the time spent travelling and to minimize absence from school for the child. This may not be possible if the rooms are not available, but it is possible to set some guidelines in terms of the psychological needs of the families when they come to clinic:

1. New families should be given information about the organization of the clinic and likely waiting times, parking places, etc.
2. They should be introduced to the people in the room they do not know, whose role in the clinic should be clear.
3. The room should be arranged so that there is space for them, toys for the children and the opportunity to talk face-to-face with the relevant clinician.
4. They should be included in any conversation: there should be no casual discussions between the people in the room.
5. If sensitive issues are being discussed, such as whether a child is being teased, then this should be done away from the main room in a quiet and private place.

6. Adolescents facing decision-making about treatment should always have the opportunity to talk to someone who is responsible for the psychological care of the patients.

Ways of helping

Helping parents

Parents can be given general advice to help them cope with their own concerns and anxieties about their children. It is important for parents to understand that comments made by the young child do not necessarily mean that the child is disturbed about the cleft. Coming from a child before the age of about five or six, these comments are often based on curiosity and the need for reassurance. Parents can be encouraged to answer these questions in a straightforward and reassuring way, such as by saying 'the reason your lip is like that is because you were born with a cleft [showing photos of how the child had looked before the repair]. The doctors mended it when you were little and it has left you with this mark. We love you and we think you look lovely now, it's nothing to worry about, everything is fine'. In this way, the parent tells the truth, illustrates the situation to explain to the child, and reassures that they love and accept the child and that all is well. If the parents find this too difficult and become too upset, then they need help to talk through their feelings and work through their sadness. The ability of the parent to provide clear and reassuring explanations is the most important early intervention that can be made.

When the children start school, they may report teasing and bullying. If they have already built up a dialogue with the parents about the cleft, then it is easier for them to talk about this. Parents can be helped to help their children by the knowledge that the physical appearance or speech of their child is not likely to be as important as the way their child behaves and responds. Comments or taunts about difference can become bullying if the child responds by displaying victim behaviour – passivity, tearfulness, anxiety. Bullying can also develop if the child becomes provocative and aggressive in response (see section of teasing and bullying above).

The best way to help the child is a combination of encouragement and support at home and the involvement of the school. Discussing the situation with the teacher can be very helpful. The organization Changing Faces (1/2 Junction Mews, London W2 1PN) has produced a pack for schools containing videos and suggested intervention by the school.

The next stage in a child's development when particular help may be needed is in adolescence. Adolescents with clefts may be very dependent on their parents and the parents may feel very protective and find it difficult to expose them to the world of adolescence. At this stage, the adolescent needs to gain more independence, take more chances, move from their primary affiliation being the family to being with their peers. In clinic, adolescents need to be encouraged to talk for themselves. They should be given the opportunity to discuss treatment on their own on a one-to-one basis.

This general advice can be helpful and encourages parents to develop a sense of competence in their own parenting skills. However, if the child or adolescent is showing signs of behavioural disturbance such as withdrawn and anxious behaviour, regression, sleep disturbance, tearfulness, then the parents need further advice from the psychologist or specialist counsellor in the cleft team (Bradbury, 1996; Lansdown et al., 1997; Royal College of Surgeons, 1995).

Working with children and adolescents

The most important principle in working with children and adolescents is to form a relationship based on mutual regard, respect and empathy. Children should never be 'talked down to'. They pick up a patronizing or dismissive attitude very quickly and will not feel safe to communicate. This principle applies to children of any age, but most acutely in adolescence.

Ways of helping children and adolescents include giving them the opportunity to talk away from the clinic in privacy, encouraging them to express their feelings about the ongoing treatment to ensure that they are fully part of the process, and preparing them for treatment.

Conclusions

There is no direct relationship between the severity of the cleft and psychological distress. Psychological processes are more subtle and affected by a variety of factors including parental reactions and the temperament of the child. All those with a cleft have to find ways of coping with it and some are more successful than others. In order to offer good psychological care, it is important to have a psychologist or specialist counsellor within the cleft team to assess the child, to advise those treating the families and to offer psychological intervention when necessary. By learning to cope with any problems that arise, children become more resilient and develop a sense of self-worth which will sustain them in the face of future adversity.

References

Alderson P (1993) Childrents Consent to Surgery. Buckingham: Open University Press.
Bettelheim B (1972) How do you help a child who has a physical handicap? Ladies Home Journal 9: 34.

Bradbury ET (1993) Psychological approaches to children and adolescents with disfigurement. ACPP Review and Newsletter 15 (1): 1–6.

Bradbury ET (1995) The psychosocial impact of visible congenital deformity. Unpublished PhD thesis. University of Leeds.

Bradbury ET (1996) Counselling People with Disfigurement. Leicester: British Psychological Society.

Bradbury ET, Hewison J (1994) Early parental responses to visible congenital disfigurement. Child: Care, Health and Development 20: 251–266.

Bradbury ET, Kay SPJ, Tighe CT, Hewison J (1994) Decision-making by parents and children in paediatric hand surgery. British Journal of Plastic Surgery 47: 324–330.

Brantley HT, Clifford B (1979) Cognitive, self-concept and body image measurements of normal, cleft palate and obese adolescents. Cleft Palate Journal 16(2): 177–182.

Clifford B (1983) Why are they so normal? Cleft Palate Journal 20(1): 83–84.

Elkind D (1967) Egocentrism in adolescence. Child Development 38: 1025–1034.

Fonagy P, Steele M, Steele H, Higgin A, Target M (1994) The Emmanuel Miller Memorial Lecture 1992. The theory and practice of resilience. Journal of Child Psychiatry and Psychology 35(2): 231–257.

Goldberg RT (1974) Adjustment of children with invisible and visible handicaps – congenital heart disease and facial burns. Journal of Counselling Psychology 21(5): 428–432.

Haviland JM, Lelwicka M (1987) The induced affect response: 10-week-old infants' responses to three emotional expressions. Developmental Psychology 23: 844–849.

Kapp K (1979) Self-concept of the cleft lip and/or palate child. Cleft Palate Journal 16(2): 171–176.

Kreuckeberg SM, Kapp-Simon KA, Ribordy SC (1993) Social skills of pre-schoolers with and without craniofacial anomalies. Cleft Palate–Craniofacial Journal 30(5): 475–481.

Lane DA (1992) Bullying. In: Lane DA, Miller A. (eds) Child and Adolescent Therapy: a Handbook. Buckingham: Open University Press, pp. 138–156.

Langlois JH, Stephan CW (1981) Beauty and the beast: the role of physical attractiveness in the development of peer relations and social behavior. In: Brehm SS, Kassin SM, Gibbons FX (eds) Developmental Social Psychology: Theory and Research. New York: Oxford University Press.

Lansdown R (1990) Psychological problems of patients with cleft lip and palate: discussion paper. Journal of the Royal Society of Medicine 83: 448–450.

Lansdown R, Rumsey N, Bradbury ET, Carr A, Partridge J (eds) (1997) Visibly Different. Oxford: Butterworth-Heinemann.

Macgregor FC (1982) Social and psychological studies of plastic surgery. Clinics in Plastic Surgery 9(3): 283–288.

Olweus D (1993) Bullying at School. Oxford: Blackwell.

Pillemer FG, Kaye VC (1989) The psychosocial adjustment of pediatric craniofacial patients. Cleft Palate Journal 26(3): 201–208.

Ramstead T, Ottem F, Shaw WC (1995) Psychological adjustment in Norwegian adults who had undergone standardised treatment for complete cleft lip and palate. 1: Education, employment and marriage. Scandinavian Journal of Plastic and Reconstructive and Hand Surgery 29: 251–257.

Richardson SA, Royce J (1968) Race and physical handicap in children's preference for other children. Child Development 39: 467–480.

Richman LC (1976) Behavior and achievement of cleft palate children. Cleft Palate Journal 13: 4–10.

Richman LC, Holme CS, Ehason MJ (1985) Adolescents with cleft lip and palate: self-perceptions of appearance and behaviour related to personality adjustment. Cleft Palate Journal 22(2): 93–96.

Royal College of Surgeons of England (1995) The Treatment of Cleft Lip and Palate: a Parents' Guide. London: RCS.

Rutter M (1988) Continuities and discontinuities from infancy. In: Osofsky JD (ed.) Handbook of Infant Development. New York: Wiley.

Rutter M, Rutter M (1992) Developing Minds: Challenge and Continuity across the Life Span. London: Penguin.

Shaw WC, Williams AC, Sandy JR, Devlin HB (1996) The minimum standards for the management of cleft lip and palate: efforts to close the audit loop. Annals of the Royal College of Surgeons of England 78: 110–114.

Sigelman CK, Miller TE, Whitworth LA (1986) The early development of stigmatising reactions to physical differences. Journal of Applied Developmental Psychology 7: 17–32.

Solnit A, Stark MH (1962) Mourning and the birth of a defective child. Psychoanalytic Study of the Child 16: 9–24.

Speltz ML, Morton K, Goodell EW, Ciarren SK (1993) Psychological functioning of children with craniofacial anomalies and their mothers: follow-up from late infancy to school entry. Cleft Palate–Craniofacial Journal 30(5): 482–489.

Stephenson P, Smith P (1987) Bullying in the junior school. In: Tattum DP, Lane DA (eds) Bullying in Schools. Stoke-on-Trent: Trentham Books.

Sullivan HS (1965) Personal Psychopathology. Norton: New York.

CHAPTER 24

The Role of Parent Support Groups

G. Davies

The need for parents' groups

While health professionals can provide appropriate and effective clinical treatment for cleft lip and palate, there is another dimension to care. This is the dimension of feeling able to cope, being confident, and, above all feeling reassured. Those directly affected by cleft lip and palate are perhaps uniquely placed to provide this care. Health professionals may sympathize but rarely can they empathize.

Even the best approach around breaking the news, even the most approachable surgeon, even the most informed cleft nurse, cannot fully alleviate the feelings of distress and loneliness which are sometimes felt by parents immediately after the birth of a child with a cleft. Yet such feelings can be greatly reduced by meeting another family with an older cleft child; a family who has been through it all before and come out the other end – usually smiling. Such encounters can provide the type of reassurance for the future that no health professional could really hope to emulate, unless they themselves had had personal experience of clefts.

Not just self-help

The role of parent support groups can be far broader than self-help and experience-sharing. A partnership between health professionals and parents can bring about a comprehensive package of care extending to information provision, awareness raising, funding equipment and research.

This overall care package might include the following elements:

• Empathy

New parents gain from meeting those who have experience of cleft surgery, who can answer many of the practical questions surfacing in the early days that require not medical advice, but merely the support of someone who has been through it all themselves. A local network of parents should be on hand to be called on to make hospital and home visits and provide this support.

• Information provision

Information sheets and booklets on various aspects of cleft lip and palate can be produced with some support from the cleft team. As well as general notes on treatment these should include 'before' and 'after' pictures, ideally of different types of cleft so they can be selected according to the individual circumstances.

• Education/teaching

Education is best done in a low-key way through organizing local talks and seminars, not only for the benefit of parents but also for those health professionals who routinely care for children but who are unconnected with the cleft team (nurses, midwives, health visitors). Specific topics might include a presentation on the establishment of feeding and range of equipment available, or a talk on any of the areas of concern in the care of cleft children.

• Awareness raising

Awareness of cleft lip and palate amongst the population at large might be increased through talks to schools and higher education establishments, dissemination of leaflets in health centres, hospitals, dental surgeries, maternity units, health education departments, libraries, citizens advice bureaux, social services and nurseries. General fundraising events may additionally generate local press interest.

• Lobbying/pressure group activity

People can be made aware of good practice in cleft management and the guidelines on minimum standards set out following the Clinical Standards Advisory Group Report on cleft care (CSAG, 1998). Parents should be encouraged to ask questions about the care they are receiving and if there are concerns the support group may wish to lobby health care purchasers, as well as providers, for better service provision.

• Fundraising

Fundraising for local hospital equipment and national research is usually central to a group's dynamics and will often be a focus of group activities. Effective fundraising will often have knock-on effects in terms of local publicity – especially if shops and companies become involved.

• **Social activities**

Social activities are central to the support provided by parents' groups. Whilst not directly addressing any specific issues such activities provide an opportunity for people who may not necessarily be seeking support to benefit from meeting others who have experienced similar situations. Above all, social activities can be fun. Media coverage of such events can raise awareness of cleft lip and palate.

Role of the cleft team

The type of support offered by parents' groups is unique but can only be effective if there is regular liaison with the cleft team. The team and the support group should work in partnership. The cleft team is in essence the support group's PR department. Only via the cleft team can new parents hear about the group and be encouraged to participate in local activity.

The cleft team should:

- Support and encourage the development of a local parents' group.
- Inform new parents of the existence of a local group, giving up-to-date contact details, preferably with a phone number.
- Appoint a named individual on the team to be responsible for maintaining contact with the local group, ensuring the team is informed of services offered and activities planned by the group. Equally it is that individual's responsibility to provide the group with up-to-date information on the cleft team.
- Assist in, and approve the production, of all medical or medically related information on cleft lip and palate.

Problems and precautions

Parent support groups provide the opportunity for members to explore their own issues and responses to having a child born with a cleft. Part of this exploration involves recognition of any issues that may affect the support they offer to new parents. People need to recognize that it is not appropriate for them to offer advice and support on issues that they themselves have not yet resolved. There can be dangers of parents off-loading their own problems on to new parents who may in fact be coping very well. It may be appropriate to facilitate active recognition of any such issues by arranging training opportunities in basic listening skills and/or befriending training – especially for those routinely involved in making the initial contact with new parents.

Antenatal diagnosis

More and more people are becoming aware that conditions such as cleft lip and palate can be diagnosed antenatally (see Chitty and Griffin, Chapter 7). Such diagnosis raises issues similar to those associated with postnatal diagnosis but can also raise questions around the continuation of pregnancy, particularly since this is sometimes an option raised by the medical staff involved in the diagnosis.

The support offered to parents expecting a baby with a cleft must ensure that they are given the opportunity of making informed decisions about the future. Parents of babies born with clefts should be aware that they may not be in a position to give impartial advice and support in this situation and should recognize that this is an area perhaps best dealt with by trained health professionals.

About CLAPA – the Cleft Lip and Palate Association

History and development

CLAPA was set up in 1979 as a partnership between parents and health professionals. Two consultant orthodontists at Great Ormond Street Hospital (Dr M. Mars and Mr D.A. Plint) recognized the need for support for new parents over and above what the health service could realistically provide. An initial meeting was organized to explore the viability of establishing a parent support group and any doubts about whether there was indeed a need were dispelled by the fact that numbers attending the meeting far exceeded all expectations. With the involvement of a core of enthusiastic parents (Jill and Barry White deserve special mention), the Cleft Lip and Palate Association was formally constituted in May 1979 and awarded charitable status.

During the 1980s CLAPA developed rapidly as a national charity with local branches emerging around many of the main cleft centres. A specialist mail order feeding equipment service was developed by CLAPA Essex and run single-handedly by Jan Robertson from her home. It was perhaps this excellent service that put CLAPA firmly on the map – not only amongst parents but also amongst health professionals and hospital departments. Throughout this period the charity's first point of contact for all enquirers was Cy Thirlaway, who was appointed as national secretary in 1981. Working from her home in Newcastle, Cy ran a national telephone advice line and saw the 10 letters per month grow to a hundred letters and a hundred phone calls a month. Always putting first the emotional welfare of cleft patients and their families, Cy became a familiar name at conferences and seminars. In a memorable presentation to the Craniofacial Society in

1994 she and Monica Turner offered a blueprint of good practice in cleft care.

There are now more than forty CLAPA groups around the UK (all staffed by volunteers) and many other regional contacts in the UK, each committed to providing the support needed by families affected with cleft lip and palate. Groups are run by people who have benefited from CLAPA, often working in partnership with local health professionals.

In 1995 CLAPA moved into a new phase of its development following a successful application for funding from the Department of Health to appoint a chief executive. This enabled the charity to set up and staff a national office, which has led to a greater public profile, increased range of services and better coordination of activities throughout the country. In 1996 a survey was undertaken examining parents' experiences of their child's cleft care and the results of this formed the basis for prioritizing service development. As a direct result of this, the charity was awarded a substantial grant from the Kings Fund to develop information and training for midwives, health visitors and nurses, who are normally the first point of contact for parents of a cleft baby. More recently, CLAPA has been turning its attention to the needs of young people and teenagers with clefts. In 1999, it launched a new magazine, Left Clip, aimed at teenagers and established an internet clubsite of the same name. Both new services are receiving excellent feedback.

A measure of the respected force that CLAPA has now become is the fact that CLAPA was invited on to and played a key role in the Clinical Standards Advisory Group committee on cleft lip and palate, which examined the future of cleft care in the UK in 1996–1997 (CSAG, 1998). It continues to be involved with the CSAG process and has been instrumental in advising health authorities on practical aspects of implementing some of the CSAG recommendations.

Whilst the taking on of paid professionals to develop services is leading to a more business-like approach in running and developing the charity, it is important not to lose sight of the organization's core values. CLAPA's strengths are the thousands of individuals around the country who, with a wisdom that can only be gained through personal experience, have given up their time to support others.

Quote from a parent helped by CLAPA:

> We are absolutely clear in our belief that the most important feature of CLAPA's work lies in the network of parent contacts. There is no substitute for hearing how other families have dealt with the experiences the family of a cleft child will experience, and for the reassurance these contacts provide. We also think there is a great value in CLAPA's ability as a recognized body to organize meetings and lectures with medical professionals to explore the many aspects of the treatment of clefts and research its causes. Individuals alone would not be able to arrange such meetings with professionals.

CLAPA

Aims

CLAPA is the only national voluntary organization specifically helping those with, or affected by, cleft lip and palate. It is unique. CLAPA seeks to ameliorate the distress often experienced by parents in bringing up a child with a cleft and to improve the quality of life for those with clefts

Activities

- Organizing local parent-to-parent support through its nationwide network of branches
- Running a specialist service for parents and health professionals seeking help with feeding babies with clefts
- Developing and supporting training for children and adolescents affected by clefts at school and in social settings
- Encouraging and supporting research into the causes and treatment of cleft lip and palate
- Representing the interests of patients and parents, influencing policy on future treatment of cleft lip and palate
- Conducting educational seminars for health professionals and the general public
- Raising funds in the community for specific treatment and equipment
- Publishing and distributing a range of information leaflets, increasing public awareness of the condition

Addresses

CLAPA
Cleft Lip and Palate Association
3rd Floor
235–237 Finchley Road
London NW3 6LD
website: www.clapa.com
email: info@clapa.com

Other support organizations

Changing Faces
1 and 2 Junction Mews
London W2 1PN
Tel: 020 7706 4232
website: www.changingfaces.co.uk

Pierre Robin Support Group UK
PO Box 27913
London SE7 7WL
Tel: 020 8858 6274
website: www.pierrerobinuk.org

Wide Smiles
PO Box 5153
Stockton
CA 95205
USA
Tel: 001 (209) 942 2812
website: www.widesmiles.org

References

CSAG (1998) Clinical Standards Advisory Group Report. London: HMSO.

CHAPTER 25

Choosing the Best Treatment for the Child with a Cleft

W.C. SHAW AND G. SEMB

For cleft lip and palate care providers there are some challenges ahead. The present scientific basis of the discipline is weak since virtually no elements of treatment have been subjected to the rigours of contemporary clinical trial design (Roberts et al., 1991). Thus highly complex and varied protocols of care are practised by different teams. Generally speaking, choices in surgical technique, timing and sequencing, and choices in ancillary procedures such as orthopaedics, orthodontics and speech therapy are arrived at following disappointment in the results of former practices rather than firm evidence that the new protocol has succeeded elsewhere. As a consequence the unsubstantiated testimony of enthusiasts for a particular treatment (often advocated with near religious zeal) has done much to shape current practices. Typically, enthusiastic claims are made for a new type of therapy; the procedure is widely adopted; a flow of favourable clinical reports ensues; little or no positive evidence develops to support the desirability of the procedure; there is a sharp drop in the number of clinical reports, again without evidence to support the change (Spriestersbach et al., 1973).

In choosing the best treatment for the child with a cleft consideration of therapeutic effectiveness, financial cost, and the burden imposed upon the patient and family by the treatment process is necessary.

Judging evidence of effectiveness

The general rules of 'health technology assessment' are well established and the quality of treatment comparisons conforms to a widely accepted hierarchy, from anecdotal reports to randomised trials (Byar, 1980). Even greater strength of evidence may be derived from systematic reviews of groups of trials (Chalmers and Altman, 1995).

Anecdotal case reports

Though case reports may signal important new developments in surgical practice, the evidence they contain for a widespread change in practice remains generally unconvincing in the absence of subsequent confirmatory series. A positive example is secondary bone grafting, which was first reported on a small scale (Boyne and Sands, 1972, 1976), adopted elsewhere and eventually the subject of published reports of large series of cases. (e.g. Bergland et al., 1986).

Case series

Reports of a series of cases treated by the same method provide more substantial evidence of the merits of a particular technique or programme of treatment, and provide the professional community with a general impression of relative efficacy. They are of particular value in demonstrating that new procedures can be reliably performed and have a low risk of serious morbidity. Rather commonly, however, outcome is measured in the short term and the enthusiasm of the reporters may impair true objectivity. Thus primary bone grafting, first heralded as an important breakthrough in case series reports, was later shown by randomized control trials to be harmful to facial growth (Rehrmann et al., 1970; Jolleys and Robertson, 1972). On the other hand, case series of secondary bone grafting using cancellous iliac crest grafts revealed persuasive evidence that one aspect of outcome, the patient's dentition, could be reliably restored beyond levels previously attainable (Bergland et al., 1986). The immediacy of these benefits ruled against the need for a randomized trial though potential growth disturbances still deserved consideration (Semb, 1988). Future trials of bone grafting may, however, still be necessary to examine individual aspects of surgical technique or timing, or to test the suitability of alternative graft materials.

Case series rarely provide evidence of the superiority of one technique over others where a choice of broadly similar methods exists and in which any improvement may be incremental rather than dramatic. This is a major problem in the evaluation of primary surgical repair since this may be achieved with apparently similar success by methods that differ in technique, timing and sequence. Meaningful comparison of reports of case series in the literature is often prohibited by methodological inconsistencies in assessment, and by the absence of strict and well-defined entry criteria such as consecutive cases with an equivalent prognosis (Semb and Shaw, 1998).

Case series reports may include equivalent data for the non-cleft population, the implication being that the closer the cleft lip and palate (CLP) data conform to normal, the better treatment has been. However, such benchmarks do little to enhance comparability with other techniques and if samples are small, real differences between the cleft and non-cleft patient may not be detected statistically.

Retrospective comparative studies

Opportunities for non-experimental comparisons of therapies or programmes of care can arise in several ways: through coexisting therapies at the same centre, through the replacement of one therapy with a second, or by the comparison of treatment centres using different therapies. However, any lack of equivalence between the cases prior to treatment or lack of equivalence in the competence of the clinicians will undermine the conclusions.

(a) Comparison of coexisting therapies

In using retrospective material such as case notes or clinical databases, checks can be made on the equivalence of the groups, commonly in terms of gender, age or cleft subtype. Preferably, they can be matched pairwise on these characteristics. Alternatively, adjustments can be made in the analysis by stratification or the use of multivariate statistical methods. In either case doubt may remain that important prognostic factors have been masked, for if two or more therapies were being used concurrently within a single centre, selective allocation to treatment must be suspected.

Factors that may have influenced clinical decision-making could be unrecorded or unreliably recorded. For example, decisions as to when (at what age) to perform primary surgery may be influenced by unrecorded aspects of the morphology of the cleft, the availability of personnel, the health of the child or parental attitudes towards the cleft. Should these factors influence outcome, confounding would occur in any study of the effect of age on surgical outcome.

The possibility of confounding in this way is especially likely when treatment has been provided 5 or 10 years previously and different staff were involved. Retrospective ascertainment of details of primary surgery or cleft subtype is difficult and descriptive terminology may have changed in subtle ways. It may be possible to match or adjust data to remove bias due to gender, age or cleft subtype but this gives no guarantee that some other prognostic factor that may affect outcome is not associated with choice of treatment. A critical factor in surgical outcome would appear to be the competence of the surgeon, high volume operators being apparently more likely to achieve good results (Shaw et al., 1992a; CSAG, 1998). Thus, if treatment A is 5% better than treatment B but surgeon X is 10% better than surgeon Y, and X does B and Y does A, the difficulty in judging the relative effectiveness of the two treatments is obvious.

(b) Comparison with historical controls

These studies may arise as natural experiments by changes in therapy within a treatment centre. Such research is particularly valuable when durable records (radiographs, study casts, speech recordings, photographs etc.) are obtained in a standardized way for both those subjects treated by a previous method (the historical controls), and those subjects treated by the new method, allowing simultaneous unbiased evaluation. Data may already exist on two well-documented treatments that have been used in different time periods.

An alternative circumstance in which such studies arise is where data for a group of patients receiving a standard treatment already exists and can be gathered in a similar way when a new treatment is introduced. This design requires only half the number of patients to be gathered prospectively as a randomized clinical trial and is clearly attractive where recruitment of cases is slow. Furthermore, it has been argued that in circumstances of poor outcome it may be unethical to withhold new treatment in order to create a control group (Gehan, 1984). There are nevertheless several biases and possibilities for confounding that generally tend to favour the newly introduced procedure.

In practice, changes in technique at a treatment centre often come about as a result of changes in personnel who may have performed differently in respect of the previous method. This leads to bias due to differences in skill of personnel associated with either treatment method. For example a new method of treatment is often tested by an experienced and innovative surgeon who may be expected to achieve better results than the average surgeon. This clearly introduces the confounding effect of operator skill with treatment. Even where there is stability of staff, bias reflecting gradual changes of ability and technique are highly likely and definition or ascertainment of prognosis may change. New methods may be initially applied with some selectivity to 'suitable' cases as experience is gained. Other aspects of clinical management may have been altered with the intention of improving outcome, creating additional possibilities for bias in favour of the innovative procedure. Multivariate methods have been suggested as a way to adjust for these biases, but serial changes in treatment are likely to take place in parallel, resulting in a strong association between treatment variables. This is one reason why historical control design is generally unsuited to evaluating primary surgery since other changes in the total programme of care are likely to have occurred during the extensive recruitment period.

The bias favouring the innovative procedure is a major cause for concern with historical control studies as they may either fail to resolve a controversy or alternatively create ethical concerns that preclude further more rigorous comparisons. Favourable outcomes suggested for a new procedure by historical control studies have been disputed by subsequent randomized controlled trials (Pinsky, 1984; Pollock, 1986). Thus the danger exists that historical control studies could set in motion an unwarranted cycle of change with no benefit to the patient and consequently delay the process of development.

The reduction in recruitment time for a historical control study in which data are gathered prospectively on a new method is also less important when evaluating primary surgery due to the extended follow-up required of each case. If, for example, the proposed follow-up of a trial of two methods of primary surgery is 10 years and the recruitment time of patients sufficient for a randomized trial is 4 years, the total duration would be 14 years. The potential saving of time in a partially prospective historical control study would only be 2 years (14%).

Inter-centre audit

In even the busiest CLP treatment centres the generation of adequate samples within specific cleft subtypes treated by contrasting treatment modalities is extremely difficult. Consequently, the multicentre approach offers distinct advantages. Prospectively planned recall of cases at participating centres allows data on outcome to be collected in a standardized way, and rigorous planning and execution across the centres can ensure consecutive case recruitment and unbiased evaluation (Shaw et al., 1992b).

Provided procedures for entry into the study are equivalent in all participating centres, this strategy is extremely valuable in assessing the outcome of primary surgery together with other major components of the treatment programme at respective centres. However, it is difficult, if not impossible, to establish the key beneficial or harmful features of a specific treatment as a general scientific conclusion, due to the invariably complex and arbitrary mix of surgical technique, timing, and sequence, ancillary procedures, and surgical personnel (Shaw et al., 1992a). For example, if two centres differ in the use of presurgical orthopaedics and types of primary lip and palate surgery, there is no way to determine which of these procedures might be responsible for any difference in outcome between centres, nor would a null result allow the conclusion that individual aspects of the treatment programme are equivalent. The method is therefore better suited to comparative clinical audit and quality assurance than definitive clinical research. Nevertheless, the existence of significant disparities in outcome of the overall treatment process provides a basis for speculating as to the possible cause and inter-centre studies should therefore be highly motivating towards the generation of specific hypotheses for subsequent more detailed testing.

An ambitious audit of this kind was conducted in the UK to determine the standards of cleft care in the country as a whole and included a comparison with centres in other European countries (Sandy et al., 1998; Bearn et al., 2000). Prospectively planned recall of all five-year-olds and 12-year-olds with unilateral cleft lip and palate and standardized recording of a range of outcomes allowed a series of subgroup comparisons as well as comparison with standards elsewhere. The conclusions of this study formed the basis for government recommendations to reconfigure cleft services (CSAG, 1998).

Randomized controlled trials

For the comparison of therapies there is little doubt that the randomized control trial is generally the method of choice scientifically and ethically (Shaw, 1995). Randomization avoids conscious or unconscious bias in treatment allocation. Prognostic factors, whether known or unknown to the investigator, tend to be balanced between treatment groups. Since patients are followed up prospectively according to a clearly defined protocol, missing data are less likely as the potential loss to follow-up is reduced. If loss does occur it may be possible to quantify any induced bias, in contrast with retrospective studies where the researcher may be unaware of patients lost to follow-up and hence the scale of bias this may have introduced into the results.

Almost thirty years ago, Spriestersbach et al. (1973) identified the need for prospective research to resolve central problems of cleft management, but remarkably few randomized trials have been performed in CLP surgery, despite being the surest means of advancing the discipline in the face of overwhelming uncertainty about the relative efficacy of countless different programmes of care around the world. In 25 years of the Cleft Palate Journal only five controlled clinical trials were identified with only one involving a follow-up of surgery for more than four years (Roberts et al., 1991). However, at the end of the 1990s a series of randomized trials on different topics is underway or completed in Europe, the USA and Latin America (e.g. Jigjinni et al., 1993; Brine et al., 1994; Sloan et al., 1996; Prahl et al., 1996; Semb and Shaw, 1998; Williams et al., 1998; Ysunza et al., 1998; Lee, 1999; Shaw et al., 1999).

Measuring treatment outcome

The ultimate goal of cleft care is restoration of the patient to a 'normal' life, unhindered by handicap or disability. However, the measurement of 'normalcy' is a highly complex proposition and there is certainly no index at present that would allow sufficiently sensitive comparison between alternative treatment protocols. Clinical research will focus more on 'proximate' outcomes. These will mainly represent different aspects of anatomical form and function in the parts affected by the clefting process, often reflecting the particular interests of individual disciplines and provider groups. In essence, most measures will be an indication of the degree of handicap that persists despite (or as a result of) treatment, such as shortcomings in speech, hearing and dentofacial development.

Outcome measures

Outcome measures must satisfy several criteria. The easiest to meet is that the measurement should be *reproducible* between and within examiners.

The most suitable statistic for comparing the reproducibility of different measurement scales is the intra-class correlation coefficient (ICC) also referred to as the reliability coefficient. In a research setting a measurement may be broken up into two components, firstly the 'true' or 'error-free' measurement of each case, and secondly the measurement error or 'noise' in the measurement that one would wish to minimize. The intra-class correlation coefficient is a ratio of the variation of the error-free measurement to the total variation including measurement error. As a ratio it is dimensionless and hence independent of the units of measurement whether they be distances, angles or scale points in a rating scale. Consequently, it allows cross-comparison of reproducibility between different methods of measurement.

In the unlikely circumstance that a measurement scale is applied without any measurement error the variation of error-free measurement will equal the total variation, so the ICC is 1. On the other hand, a scale containing substantial error will have a much smaller ICC. In the worst case, where the measurement error is so great that the scale is unable to distinguish between cases, the ICC is equal to zero. At the design stage of a study, poor reproducibility of an outcome measure may be offset by an increase in sample size. The sample size required is increased (relative to that for an entirely reliable scale) by a factor $1/R$ where R is the ICC. It is generally estimated using analysis of variance. If the scale used is categorical, the weighted kappa statistic may be used (Cohen, 1968). This is equivalent to the ICC if squared weights are used (Fleiss and Cohen, 1973).

Another strategy to improve the reproducibility of a measure, is to use the total or mean of a set of measurements from a panel of observers working independently. This also reduces any bias that may related to the idiosyncratic perceptions of a particular observer. It is possible to estimate the reliability of such a pooled value by using the Spearman Brown formula (Fleiss, 1986). If R is the ICC for a single observer, then the ICC for a measurement obtained by totalling the scores of m observers is given by the result:

$$Rm = \frac{mR}{(1 + (m - 1)R)}$$

More difficult is the requirement of *validity*, that the measure truly represents what it is supposed to. For example, do the results of a nasopharyngoscopy examination reflect how well the patient sounds to others? Or does a series of cephalometric measurements actually reflect how well the patient looks to others? External facial appearance is a crucial outcome for the patients, since this after all, is what they and society around them actually see. Cephalometric analysis, with its central place in the thinking of ortho-dontists, is assumed to be an important outcome in its own right, if only as a 'surrogate' measure (Herson, 1989). It is, however, an invalid measure of many aspects of external facial appearance.

A particular problem in the study of a congenital condition such as CLP arises when outcomes are assessed in childhood though eventual form and function will not be known until adulthood. This is especially so for aspects of facial growth such as maxillary prominence, since this feature deterio-rates steadily while growth is occurring (Semb, 1991). A useful way to identify potential outcome measures that are valid and predictive is to examine longitudinal archives. The relative prominence of the maxilla in patients with complete clefts is an important outcome for evaluating the success of primary surgery. One common method for doing this is to measure angle ANB, the relationship of the anterior outlines of the maxilla and mandible to the frontonasal suture. However, identification of point A on the maxillary outline is difficult in early childhood because of the position of the unerupted permanent incisors. In the Eurocleft study (Mølsted et al., 1992), soft tissue analysis at age 10 for unilateral cleft lip and palate (UCLP) was broadly consistent with that derived from hard tissues (Figure 25.1) and if soft tissue ANB angle could be shown to be adequately predictive, it would be a good alternative. Indeed, it has the further advan-

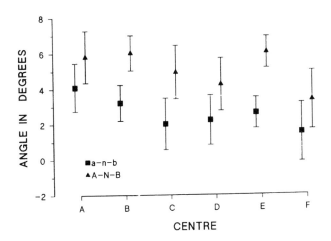

Figure 25.1. Comparison of maxillo-mandibular profile measurements for UCLP: hard tissue (anb), soft tissue (ANB). Derived from data collected in the Eurocleft study.

tages of being measurable on photographs, obviating the need for irradiation, and reflecting the actual facial outline observable in everyday life.

Data from the Oslo Archive (Semb, 1991) were examined at a number of age points to assess how well early measurement of ANB angle would predict the situation in adulthood. To assess the strength of any linear predictive relationship r^2 was calculated between soft tissue ANB at age 6 ± 1 year and measurements at a later stage (Table 25.1). Small groups of 20 to 30 UCLP patients from Manchester and Oslo have been compared in a number of studies at different ages. In Figure 25.2, average soft tissue ANB angle for each centre at ages 6, 9 and 12 years are shown. Though the levels of significance for the differences fall just below the 5% level, the differences between each centre at different ages are of similar magnitude, reinforcing the predictive worth of soft tissue ANB angle at age 6 ± 1 year.

Table 25.1. Correlation between measurement of maxillo-mandibular profile at age six and subsequently in the same cases. Data from the Oslo Archive.

	Strength of linear relationship with ANB at age 6 years ($\pm$ 1) measured by r^2 ($n = 56$)		
	12 years	15 years	18 years
anb	0.67	0.45	0.27
ANB	0.74	0.57	0.46

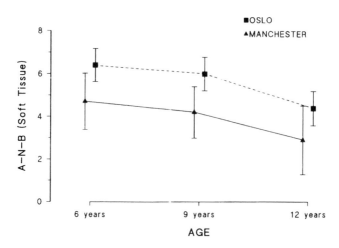

Figure 25.2. Comparison of Oslo and Manchester samples with UCLP for different age groups. Group means with 95% confidence limits.

Measurement scales

The development of measurement scales that are both reproducible and valid for cleft outcomes is still at an early stage. Preliminary experience derives from attempts to compare dentofacial form and relationships in the Eurocleft study using cephalometric analysis for skeletal form (Mølsted et al., 1992), dental arch relationships (Mars et al., 1992), and nasolabial appearance (Asher-McDade et al., 1991, 1992).

Cephalometric measurements though reproducible suffer a lack of *content validity*, since they measure three-dimensional structures in a two-dimensional way. None-the-less, cephalometric relationships can tell a great deal about potential growth inhibition for structures undoubtedly affected by surgical procedures (Semb and Shaw, 1996), and they successfully discriminated between different centres (Mølsted et al., 1992).

To compare dental arch relationships the Goslon Yardstick (Mars et al., 1987), an index designed to systematize subjective perception, was used. Originally a large sample of study casts was graded by a panel of orthodontists and a series of five groups containing representative cases ranging from the best (group 1) to the worst (group 5) dental arch relationships. These reference groups were subsequently used to assist in grading new cases.

In the Eurocleft study five observers assessed a sample of 149 study casts using the yardstick, and a good level of reliability with an intra-class correlation coefficient of 0.80 was obtained (Table 25.2). The mean of the five measurements was then used as a summary score. Application of the Spearman Brown formula suggests that the reliability of this average score is excellent. From the formula above, the estimated value for the mean of five assessments was 0.95. The mean of the five examiners' scores was found to be sensitive to differences between treatment centre (Mars et al., 1992).

In a subsequent study (Morris et al., 1994), an attempt was made to discover whether certain measurements could be made directly without the need to assemble a panel of orthodontists. In order to relate the subjective assessment of the Goslon Yardstick to objective measurement, overjet, overbite, incisor angulation, and various arch form and crossbite relationships were measured on the same series of study casts using a reflex metrograph. These objective measurements were then used as predictors of the mean Goslon score in a multiple regression analysis. Overjet of the incisor on the unaffected side (all cases were UCLP) explained a substantial proportion of the variance (r^2 equal to 0.87). The other measures explained only an additional 3% of variance.

In an attempt to compare the nasolabial appearance of the patients in the Eurocleft study using photographs, several difficulties were confronted. Technical issues such as film quality, lighting, sharpness of image, the patients' facial expression and the background general facial appearance

Table 25.2. Evaluation of reproducibility for study cast (Goslon) and features of nasolabial appearance. Derived from data from the Eurocleft study.

	Goslon	Nasal	Symmetry	Vermilion	Profile	Total
Intra-class correlation coefficient	0.80	0.47	0.36	0.47	0.48	0.49
Lower 95% confidence limit	0.76	0.41	0.30	0.40	0.42	0.43
Sample size	149	115	115	115	115	115
Number of examiners (N)	Spearman Brown estimates of reliability of total of independent scores by N examiners					
3	0.92	0.73	0.62	0.72	0.74	0.75
5	0.95	0.82	0.73	0.81	0.82	0.83
6	0.96	0.84	0.77	0.84	0.85	0.85

All based on six observers except Goslon, involving 5.

were all factors that could influence an observer's opinion. To assess the influence of background appearance such as hair, eyes and complexion, a panel of observers was asked to examine independently three frontal views: the nasolabial area in isolation, the full face, and the surrounding features without the nasolabial part (Asher-McDade et al., 1991). Each view was scored in terms of attractiveness using a visual analogue scale. There was found to be a strong correlation between the full face and surrounding area ($r = 0.53$, $p < 0.001$), indicating that indeed the full face is likely to be influenced by surrounding features.

Consequently, a more valid measure would be based on restricting the areas under consideration to those directly affected by the anomaly and its repair. Thus the Eurocleft examiners were asked to make assessments of a standardized view of the frontal and lateral view of the nasolabial area. We considered it important to break down the task into four components: (i) nasal form (frontal view); (ii) deviation of the nose from the midline; (iii) shape of the vermilion border; and (iv) profile including the upper lip. Each observer was asked to score each of the components with a five-point subjective scale with scale points from very good appearance to very poor appearance. A total score was also computed by aggregation of the scores of the four components. The reliability of each component and the total score were ranged from 0.47 for nasal form and vermilion border to 0.36 for symmetry (Table 25.2).

We found reproducibility poor compared to that obtained for dental arch relationships and the reliability of the total score was little better than that for the component scores. In this case the strategy of splitting the assessment into components appeared to have a limited ability to improve the quality of measurement. Detailed analysis of the data suggested that if one observer scored higher than another observer for one of the four components the observer was likely to do so for the other three.

For future work we will test whether the reproducibility is improved by reducing the subjective element by providing reference examples or 'benchmarks', as with the Goslon Yardstick, or by the enumeration of specific features for rating. Elsewhere we have found this to improve reproducibility. For example, rating of dental aesthetics is assisted by providing an illustrated ten-point scale, and orthodontic treatment need on dental health grounds is reproducibly rated when clear diagnostic categories are used (Brook and Shaw, 1989).

The provision of benchmarks must be done with some caution, however, as the choice of categories for each scale and the subject of each subscale determine the content validity of the total measurement. Thus there is a danger of imposing the researchers' perceptions of what is important.

An alternative strategy for rating appearance is to rank subjects pairwise against each other. All possible pairs of subjects are compared (Tobiasen, 1989). For each pair a score of one is allocated to the preferred photograph. The score for each case is then its total after comparison with all other cases. One practical difficulty, however, is that the number of comparisons escalates with sample size. The number of possible pairs is equal to $N(N-1)/2$ for a sample of N cases. So for a sample of 10 subjects 45 comparisons are needed; with 50 subjects the number rises to 1225. However, the pairwise technique might be modified by comparing each case against a random or systematic sample of other subjects. For example, the photographs for the complete sample might be arranged in a random sequence and then a score for each case obtained by comparing against the next k subjects. The larger choices for k would improve the reliability of the score for each case but increase the total time to perform the task. A more fundamental limitation is that the scale is only meaningful as the relationship between subjects within the same sample since the comparison is not transferable from one study to another.

The static nature of a still photograph is a major weakness in respect of validity since the lip in function cannot be judged. Consequently, the use of video recording has been explored (Morrant and Shaw, 1996). An edited sequence for a series of 30 subjects using a number of standardized views of the nasolabial area at rest and function was prepared. A panel of judges then rated the cases using a scoring chart with nine responses for the lip and ten for the nose.

Assessment was made of the nose and the lip separately, with eight components and an overall score for lip and nine components and an overall score for the nasal area. For the nasal area the ICC for individual components ranged from 0.40 to 0.27, with 0.52 for the overall score and 0.49 for the sum of the components. For the lip the ICC ranged from 0.39 to 0.10, with 0.28 for the overall score and 0.34 for the sum of components.

Whilst such a dynamic view may be more valid, the inter-examiner agreement was generally worse than that achieved from a static image. This may reflect the significantly higher content of information contained in the video format; by further discussion of the items to be rated and possible provisions of improved descriptive categories or illustrated examples, an appearance scale of high validity seems feasible.

Treatment costs

In most developed countries the high medical costs of rehabilitating the child with a cleft are borne or at least supported in part by the state. Economic pressures around the world now force a re-examination of the true financial costs of treatment and with reducing budgets, clinicians must either be involved in cost controls or have arbitrary choices imposed upon them. Surgical operations are invariably expensive treatment episodes and successful primary operations that minimize the need for multiple secondary revisions are highly desirable. Furthermore, successful primary repairs are likely to reduce the duration and complexity of ancillary procedures such as speech therapy, orthodontics and maxillary osteotomy (Shaw, 1997).

In economic terms the cheapest care will certainly be that which is provided with a high degree of planning and coordination. Common examples might be combining the placement of drainage tubes with another operation, timing alveolar bone grafting so that natural space closure is facilitated and the duration of subsequent orthodontics is minimized, and recognizing a later need for maxillary osteotomy so that inappropriate early orthodontics is avoided.

The burden of care

Since the consequences of an orofacial cleft are apparent through every phase of childhood and adolescence, there is seldom a time when the disciplines involved in care could not recommend some or other intervention. The powerful desire of patients and parents to reach the point where the stigma of clefting will be completely eradicated makes it likely that they will accept most proposals. Most patients and parents will willingly comply with protocols of care recommended by all members of their team, no matter how demanding they may be. They have little choice.

So far, 'burden of care' has received little attention in cleft care, yet the combined total of operations, other treatment episodes, and review appointments for the first twenty years of life, including all the disciplines that may be involved, can easily exceed one hundred. Apart from pain and suffering and the disruption of family life and school attendance, the dependent role that this places the patient in may have an adverse effect on the patient's sense of self-determination, or locus of control.

Balancing outcome, cost and burden

Decision analysis (utility theory) is the science of relative utilities or preferences, and can be employed to formulate global outcome measures that are more relevant to patients than the short-sighted proximate outcomes that absorb clinicians. Clearly it behoves the providers of cleft care to seek optimal balance in the development of protocols of care spanning the years from birth till late adolescence.

Undoubtedly, there are intriguing discussions ahead. Take the use of early orthopaedics and delayed palatal closure. Patients receiving this treatment have to be brought on many additional visits to the treatment centre during infancy and childhood, and endure the minor risk of impression taking together with the greater risk of some discomfort associated with the appliances. For the years until the hard palate is closed they will have to tolerate a residual cleft or an obturator, all the while having a rather clear sense of being an orthodontic *patient*. How much benefit does this additional treatment have to produce over treatment without early orthopaedics to justify its inclusion in care? An average increase in angle SNA (maxillary prominence) of 1°, a 10% reduction in osteotomy rate in the teens or a better cosmetic repair of the lip? (if differences do exist, how would they be measured?) Similar questions arise about other elements of care. How often should lip or nasal revision be attempted? When does the law of diminishing returns start to apply? Surgical management of velopharyngeal incompetence is not without some risk, so how bad does the problem have to be to justify the average gain from pharyngoplasty or flap? How much orthodontics should be performed in childhood if the duration and outcome of definitive treatment in the permanent dentition will not be radically altered?

These are issues about which patients and parents deserve honest information and the opportunity to have their preferences taken into account.

Conclusion

Regrettably, the choice of best treatment for the child with a cleft cannot be made reliably at present. However, there is clear evidence that simple treatment protocols that minimize the burden on the child can produce equivalent or better results than complex ones (Shaw et al., 1992a, Shaw, 1997), and no evidence that the opposite is true. Furthermore, centralization of treatment, with therapy provided by high volume operators, provides the best setting for good and comprehensive care and at least allows quality assessment within a reasonable period (Shaw et al., 1996).

It has been said that doctors make choices about treatment in three ways – seduction, induction or deduction. In the seductive method the clinician simply adopts what he or she has been taught or encouraged to do by teachers or colleagues, i.e. treatment based on faith. The inductive method includes choices based on clinical experience – what seems to work, or on theories of what ought to work – e.g. 'Do extensive muscle repositioning during primary lip repair because this will encourage growth' or 'do minimal tissue mobilization and disturbance during surgery because more surgery means more scar induced growth disturbance'. Or – 'Don't touch the vomer during lip repair because it is a growth centre' or 'do use a vomerine flap because there is no evidence for growth disturbance and it permits good arch development, minimizes fistulae, and providing a good nasal floor for later bone grafting'.

Finally, there is the deductive or hypothetico-deductive method – decisions made on the unbiased evidence of randomized trials. Initiating the multicentred collaborations and protocols for these trials is the challenge that has to be grasped by today's clinicians who do wish to choose the best treatment for the children they care for. In time, randomized trials will be aggregated in systematic reviews (Chalmers and Altman, 1995), providing as never before a sound evidence base for provision of cleft care.

Following a recent survey of European cleft centres, the register of 201 teams revealed the use of 194 protocols for one cleft subtype (Shaw et al., 2000). The end of the millennium would seem to be a timely point for concerted action to leave this morass of clinical uncertainty behind. The unfortunate consumers of cleft care certainly deserve better.

References

Asher-McDade C, Roberts CT, Shaw WC, Gallagher C (1991) The development of a method for rating nasolabial appearance in patients with clefts of the lip and palate. Cleft Palate–Craniofacial Journal 28: 385–391.

Asher-McDade C, Brattström V, Dahl E, McWilliam J, Mølsted K, Plint DA, Prahl-Andersen B, Semb G, Shaw WC, The RPS (1992) A six-centre international study of treatment outcome in patients with clefts of the lip and palate: Part 4. Assessment of nasolabial appearance. Cleft Palate–Craniofacial Journal 29: 409–412.

Bearn D, Mildinhall S, Murphy T, Murray J, Sandy JR, Sell D, Shaw WC, Williams AC (2000) Cleft lip and palate care in the United Kingdom – The Clinical Standards Advisory Group (CSAG) Study: Part 4 – Outcome comparisons, training and conclusions. Cleft Palate – Craniofacial Journal, in press.

Bergland O, Semb G, Åbyholm FE (1986) Elimination of the residual alveolar cleft by secondary bone grafting and subsequent orthodontic treatment. Cleft Palate Journal 23: 175–205.

Boyne PJ, Sands NR (1972) Secondary bone grafting of residual alveolar and palatal clefts. Journal of Oral Surgery 30: 87–92.

Boyne PJ, Sands NR (1976) Combined orthodontic surgical management of residual alveolar clefts defects. Journal of Oral Surgery 70: 20–37.

Brine EA, Rickard KA, Brady MS, Liechty EA, Manatunga A, Sadove M, Bull MJ (1994) Effectiveness of two feeding methods in improving energy intake and growth of infants with cleft palate: a randomized study. Journal of the American Dietetic Association 94: 732–738.

Brook PH, Shaw WC (1989) The development of an index of orthodontic treatment priority. European Journal of Orthodontics 11:309–320.

Byar DP (1980) Why databases should not replace randomized clinical trials. Biometrics 31: 337–342.

Chalmers I, Altman DC (1995) Systematic Reviews. London: BMJ Publishing Group.

CSAG (1998) Clinical Standards Advisory Group Report Cleft Lip and/or Palate. London: HMSO.

Cohen J (1968) Weighted Kappa nominal scale agreement with provision for scaled disagreement or partial credit. Psychological Bulletin 70: 213–220.

Fleiss JL (1986) Design and Analysis of Clinical Experiment. New York: Wiley, p. 15.

Fleiss JL, Cohen J (1973) The equivalence of weighted Kappa and the intra-class correlation coefficient as a measure of reliability. Educational and Psychological Measurement 33: 613–619.

Gehan AE (1984) The evaluation of therapies: historical control studies. Statistics in Medicine 3: 315–324.

Herson J (1989) The use of surrogate endpoints in clinical trials (an introduction to a series of four papers). Statistics in Medicine 8: 403–404.

Jolleys A, Robertson NRE (1972) A study of the effects of early bone grafting in complete clefts of the lip and palate – five year study. British Journal of Plastic Surgery 25: 229–237.

Jigjinni V, Kangesu T, Sommerlad BC (1993) Do babies require arm splints after cleft palate repair. British Journal of Plastic Surgery 46: 681–685.

Lee TK (1999) Effect of unresticted postoperative sucking following cleft palate repair on early postoperative course. 4th Asia Pasific Cleft Lip and Palate Conference.

Mars M, Plint DA, Houston WJB, Bergland O, Semb G (1987) The Goslon Yardstick: A new system of assessing dental arch relationships in children with unilateral clefts of the lip and palate. Cleft Palate Journal 24: 314–322.

Mars M, Asher-McDade C, Brattström V, Dahl E, McWilliam J, Mølsted K, Plint DA, Prahl-Andersen B, Semb G, Shaw WC, The RPS (1992) A six-centre international study of treatment outcome in patients with clefts of the lip and palate. Part 3. Dental arch relationships. Cleft Palate–Craniofacial Journal 29: 405–408.

Morrant DG, Shaw WC (1996) Use of standardized video recordings to assess cleft surgery outcome. Cleft Palate-Craniofacial Journal 33: 134–142.

Morris TA, Roberts CT, Shaw WC (1994) Incisal overjet as an outcome measure in unilateral cleft lip and palate management. Cleft Palate–Craniofacial Journal 31: 142–145.

Mølsted K, Asher-McDade C, Brattström V, Dahl E, Mars M, McWilliam J, Plint DA, Prahl-Andersen B, Semb G, Shaw WC, The RPS (1992) A six-centre international study of treatment outcome in patients with clefts of the lip and palate. Part 2. Craniofacial form and soft tissue profile. Cleft Palate–Craniofacial Journal 29: 398–404.

Pinsky CA (1984) Experience with historical control studies in cancer immunotherapy. Statistics in Medicine 3: 325–329.

Pollock AV (1986) Historical evolution: methods, attitudes, goals. In: Troidl H, Spitzer WO, McPeak B, Mulder DS, McKneally MF (eds) Principles and Practice of Research: Strategies for Surgical Investigators. New York: Springer Verlag, pp. 7–17.

Prahl C, Kuijpers-Jagtman AM, Prahl-Andersen B (1996) In: A Study into the Effects of Presurgical Orthopaedic Treatment in Complete Unilateral Cleft Lip and Palate Patients. A Three Centre Prospective Clinical Trial in Nijmegen, Amsterdam and Rotterdam. Interim Analysis. Nijmegen: Academisch Ziekenhuis.

Rehrmann AH, Koberg WR, Koch H (1970) Long-term post-operative results of primary and secondary bone grafting in complete clefts of the lip and palate. Cleft Palate Journal 7: 206–221.

Roberts CT, Semb G, Shaw WC (1991) Strategies for the advancement of surgical methods in cleft lip and palate. Cleft Palate–Craniofacial Journal 28: 141–149.

Sandy J, Williams A, Mildinhall S, Murphy T, Bearn D, Shaw B, Sell D, Devlin B, Murray J (1998) The Clinical Standards Advisory Group (CSAG) Cleft Lip and Palate Study. British Journal of Orthodontics 25: 21–30.

Semb G (1988) Effect of alveolar bone grafting on maxillary growth in unilateral cleft lip and palate patients. Cleft Palate Journal 25: 288–295.

Semb G (1991) A study of facial growth in patients with unilateral cleft lip and palate treated by the Oslo CLP team. Cleft Palate Journal 28: 1–21.

Semb G, Shaw WC (1996) Facial growth in facial clefting disorders. In: Fonseca RJ, Vig KWL, Turvey TA (eds) Principles and Management of Facial Clefting Disorders and Craniosynostosis. Philadelphia: WB Saunders, pp. 28–56.

Semb G, Shaw WC (1998) Facial growth after different methods of surgical intervention in patients with cleft lip and palate. Acta Odontologica Scandinavica 56: 353–355.

Shaw WC, Asher-McDade C, Brattström V, Dahl E, Mars M, McWilliam J, Mølsted K, Plint DA, Prahl-Andersen B, Semb G, The RPS (1992a) A six-centre international study of treatment outcome in patients with clefts of the lip and palate. Part 5. General discussion and conclusions. Cleft Palate–Craniofacial Journal 29: 413–418.

Shaw WC (1995) Commentary to 'Ethical issues in the case of surgical repair of cleft palate' by S Berkowitz. Cleft Palate–Craniofacial Journal 32: 277–280.

Shaw WC (1997) The Eurocleft Study – Eight Year Follow Up. In: Transactions: 8th International Congress on Cleft Palate and Related Craniofacial Anomalies. Singapore: Stamford Press, p 1037.

Shaw WC, Dahl E, Asher-McDade C, Brattström V, Mars M, McWilliam J, Mølsted K, Plint DA, Prahl-Andersen B, Roberts CT, Semb G, The RPS (1992b) A six-centre international study of treatment outcome in patients with clefts of the lip and palate. Part 1. Principles and study design. Cleft Palate–Craniofacial Journal 29: 393–397.

Shaw WC, Williams AC, Sandy JR, Devlin HB (1996) Minimum standards for the management of cleft lip and palate – efforts to close the audit loop. Annals of the Royal College of Surgeons of England 78: 110–114.

Shaw WC, Bannister RP, Roberts CT (1999) Assisted feeding is more reliable for infants with clefts – A randomised trial. Cleft Palate–Craniofacial Journal 36(3):.

Shaw WC, Semb G, Nelson P, Brattström V, Mølsted K, Prahl-Andersen B (2000) The Eurocleft Project 1996–2000. Standards of care for cleft lip and palate in Europe. European commision Biochemical and Health Research. Amsterdam: IOS Press.

Sloan G, Shaw WC, Downey SE (1996) Surgical management of velopharyngeal insufficiency: pharyngeal flap and sphincter Pharyngoplasty. In: Turvey TA, Vig KWL, Fonseca RJ (eds) Principles and Management of Facial Clefting Disorders and Craniosynostosis. Philadelphia: WB Saunders, pp. 384–395.

Spriestersbach DC, Dickson DR, Fraser FC, Horowitz SL, McWilliams BJ, Paradise JL, Randall P (1973) Clinical research in cleft lip and palate: the state of the art. Cleft Palate Journal 10: 113–165.

Tobiasen JM (1989) Scaling facial impairment. Cleft Palate Journal 26: 249–254.

Williams WN, Seagle MB, Nackashi AJ et al. (1998) A methodology report of a randomized prospective clinical trial to assess velopharyngeal function for speech following palatal surgery. Controlled Clinical Trials 19: 297–312.

Ysunza A, Pamplona C, Mendoza M, García-Velasco, Paz Aguilar, Eugenia Guerrero BS (1998) Speech outcome and maxillary growth in patients with unilateral complete cleft lip/palate operated on at 6 versus 12 months of age. Plastic and Reconstructive Surgery 102: 675–679.

Index